Series editor
Daniel Horton-Szar
BSc (Hons)
United Medical and Dental
Schools of Guy's and
St Thomas's Hospitals
(UMDS),
London

Faculty advisor
Clive Page
PhD
Professor of
Pharmacology & Co-
Director of the Sackler
Institute of Pulmonary
Pharmacology,
King's College,
University of London

Pharmacology

Magali N. F. Taylor
BSc
King's College School of
Medicine and Dentistry,
London

Peter J. W. Reide
BA (Cantab)
King's College School of
Medicine and Dentistry,
London

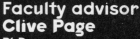

D1073707

v. Whatley
March 2002

M Mosby

London • Philadelphia
St Louis • Sydney • Tokyo

Editor	**Louise Crowe**
Development Editor	**Filipa Maia**
Project Manager	**Linda Kull**
Designer	**Greg Smith**
Layout	**Robert Curran**
Illustration Management	**Danny Pyne**
Illustrators	**Joanna Cameron**
	Deborah Gyan
	Sandie Hill
	Mike Saiz
	Annette Whalley
	Debra Woodward
Cover Design	**Greg Smith**
Production	**Gudrun Hughes**
Index	**Janine Ross**

ISBN 0 7234 3125 6

Copyright © Mosby International Ltd, 1998.

Published by Mosby, an imprint of Mosby International Ltd, Lynton House, 7–12 Tavistock Square, London WC1H 9LB, UK.

Printed in Barcelona, Spain, by Grafos S.A. Arte sobre papel, 1998.
Text set in Crash Course–VAG Light; captions in Crash Course–VAG Thin.

Cataloguing in Publication Data
Catalogue records for this book are available from the British Library and the US Library of Congress.

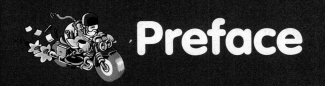

Preface

DRUGS - like them or loathe them, you have to know them!

A sound working knowledge of pharmacology is an essential part of your medical training and one which is examined on several occasions during your career as a medical student.

This book has been written by two authors who have themselves passed these exams successfully and it is designed to help you do the same. It offers a compact, yet comprehensive, knowledge of pharmacology that can be used on its own, in conjunction with your lecture course, or as a revision aid.

Good luck!

Magali N. F. Taylor
Peter J. W. Reide

This book provides a comprehensive and approachable text on pharmacology for medical students. As part of the Crash Course Series, the overall style is user friendly consisting of concise bulleted text with many informative illustrations. The content provides a comprehensive overview of the core material needed to pass the pharmacology component of the undergraduate medical curriculum. At the end of the book, there is a self-assessment section consisting of multiple-choice questions, short-answer questions and essay questions which test the reader's understanding of the topic.

In line with the new style of curricula recommended by the General Medical Council, the pharmacology is organised logically into body systems. and the clinical relevance of the pharmacology is stressed throughout.

I have no doubt that this volume will be a useful study and revision aid for students. It provides a refreshing means of bringing the medical student up to speed in pharmacology.

Clive Page
Faculty Advisor

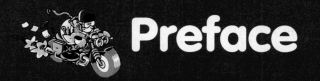

Preface

OK, no-one ever said medicine was going to be easy, but the thing is, there are very few parts of this enormous subject that are actually difficult to understand. The problem for most of us is the sheer volume of information that must be absorbed before each round of exams. It's not fun when time is getting short and you realise that: a) you really should have done a bit more work by now; and b) there are large gaps in your lecture notes that you meant to copy up but never quite got round to.

This series has been designed and written by medical students and young doctors with recent experience of basic medical science exams. We've brought together all the information you need into compact, manageable volumes that integrate basic science with clinical skills. There is a consistent structure and layout across the series, and every title is checked for accuracy by senior faculty members from medical schools across the UK.

I hope this book makes things a little easier!

Danny Horton-Szar
Series Editor (Basic Medical Sciences)

Contents

Acknowledgements

We would like to thank those who have helped us in the production of this book over the past twelve months. We owe Professor Page and King's College London a special thanks for initiating our involvement in this project, and for then acting as an invaluable source of advice and technical information.

The team at Mosby have been a constant help and liaison during the writing, editing and final publishing of the book and we are grateful to them too.

We owe thanks to our families, friends and flatmates for both their support and tolerance in putting up with us over the past year. Last, but certainly not least, we would like to thank and congratulate each other for the mutual support and work given over the past year.

Figure Credits

Figures 1.1, 1.2, 1.3, 1.10, 1.11, 1.12, 1.13, 3.1, 3.11, 4.1, 4.2, 4.3, 4.4, 4.106.1, 6.2, 6.3, 6.4, 8.1, 8.2, 8.3, 8.4, 8.5, 8.7, 8.9, 8.11, 8.16, 8.18, 9.1, 9.2, 9.3, 9.5, 9.6, 9.7, 9.8, 10.8, 10.9, 12.2, 12.3, 12.4, 12.8, 12.11, 12.12, 12.14 from *Integrated Pharmacology*, by Professor C Page, Dr M Curtris, Professor M Sutter, Professor M Walker, and Professor B Hoffman, Mosby International, 1997.

To my loving and ever supportive family, **MT**

To my loving Mother, and in memory of my Father, **PJWR**

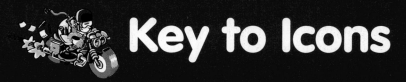

Key to Icons

Icons used throughout the book

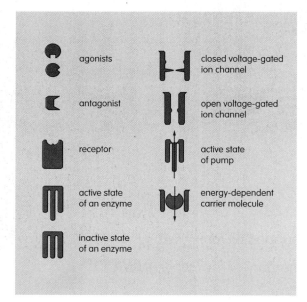

agonists	closed voltage-gated ion channel
antagonist	open voltage-gated ion channel
receptor	active state of pump
active state of an enzyme	energy-dependent carrier molecule
inactive state of an enzyme	

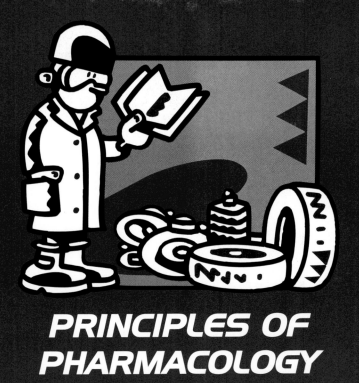

PRINCIPLES OF PHARMACOLOGY

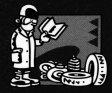

1. Introduction to Pharmacology

MOLECULAR BASIS OF PHARMACOLOGY

What is pharmacology?

The word 'pharmacology' derives from the Greek word for drug, *pharmakon*.

Pharmacology is the study of the actions, uses, mechanisms, and adverse effects of drugs.

A drug is any natural or synthetic substance that alters the physiological state of a living organism. Drugs can be divided into two groups:

- Medicinal drugs are substances used for the treatment, prevention, and diagnosis of disease.
- Non-medicinal drugs, or social drugs, are substances used for recreational purposes. Non-medicinal drugs include illegal mood-altering substances such as cannabis, heroin, and cocaine as well as everyday substances such as caffeine, nicotine, and alcohol.

Although drugs are intended to have a selective action, this is rarely achieved.

There is always a risk of adverse effects associated with the use of any drug.

Drug names and classification

A single drug can have a variety of names and belong to many classes.

Factors used for classifying drugs include their:

- Pharmacotherapeutic actions.
- Pharmacological actions.
- Molecular actions.
- Chemical nature.

The generic name of a drug is that which appears in official national pharmacopoeias. All drugs available on prescription or sold over the counter have a generic name that may vary from country to country. Newly patented drugs usually have one generic name (e.g. salbutamol) and one brand name (e.g. Ventolin). However, once the patent expires, the marketing of the drug is open to any number of manufacturers and, although the generic name is retained, the variety of brand names inevitably increases.

How do drugs work?

A drug causes a change of physiological function by interacting with the organism at the chemical level.

Certain drugs (e.g. general anaesthetics, antacids) work by means of their physicochemical properties and are said to have a non-specific mechanism of action. For this reason these drugs must be given in much higher doses (mg–g) than the more specific drugs.

Most drugs produce their effects by targeting specific cellular macromolecules. This may involve modification of DNA or RNA function, inhibition of transport systems or enzymes or, more commonly, action on receptors.

Transport systems

Ion channels

Ion channels are pores located in the cell membrane that allow selective transfer of ions in and out of the cell. Opening or closing of these channels, known as 'gating', occurs as a result of the channel proteins undergoing a change in shape. Gating is controlled either by transmitter substances or by the membrane potential (voltage-operated channels).

Some drugs modulate ion channel function directly by binding to a part of the channel protein itself, e.g. the blocking action of local anaesthetics on sodium channels. Other drugs interact with ion channels indirectly via a G-protein and other intermediates.

Carrier molecules

Transfer of ions and molecules against their concentration gradients is facilitated by carrier molecules located in the cell membrane. There are two types of carrier molecules:

- Energy-independent carriers are transporters (move one type of ion/molecule in one direction), symporters (move two or more ions/molecules), or antiporters (exchange one or more ions/molecules for one or more other ions/molecules).
- Energy-dependent carriers are termed pumps (e.g. the cardiac glycosides inhibit the Na^+/K^+ ATPase pump).

Enzymes

Enzymes are protein catalysts that increase the rate of specific chemical reactions without undergoing any net change themselves during the reaction.

All enzymes are potential targets for drugs. Drugs either act as a false substrate for the enzyme or inhibit the enzyme's activity directly by binding to other sites on the enzyme protein.

Certain drugs may require enzymatic degradation. This degradation converts a drug from its inactive form (prodrug) to its active form.

Receptors

Receptors are the means through which most drugs produce their effects.

A receptor is a specific protein molecule that is usually located in the cell membrane. Endogenous or exogenous agonist drugs bind to the receptors in the cell membrane, thereby causing activation or inactivation of the cell and a subsequent cellular response.

Synaptic transmitter substances and hormones, the body's chemical messengers, are natural ligands (i.e. molecules that bind with a molecular target) for receptors and have the following modes of action:

- Neurotransmitters are chemicals that are released from nerve terminals, diffuse across the synaptic cleft, and bind to pre- or postsynaptic receptors.
- Hormones are chemicals that, after being released into the bloodstream from specialized cells, can act at neighbouring or distant cells.

Each cell expresses only certain receptors, depending on the function of the cell.

Receptor number and responsiveness to messengers can be modulated.

In many cases there is more than one receptor for each messenger, so that the messenger often has different pharmacological specificity and different functions according to where it binds (e.g. adrenaline). This may be a result of gene splicing and other processes that led to polypeptide diversity in evolution.

Using conventional molecular biology techniques it is now possible to clone receptors and express them in cultured cells, so allowing their properties to be studied. In particular, amino acid mutations can be reproduced so that the relation between amino acid structure and function can be evaluated.

The four types of receptors for chemical messengers and growth factors are those:

- Linked directly to multimeric ion channels (ionotropic).
- Linked via G-proteins to membrane enzymes and intracellular processes (metabotropic).

- Linked directly to tyrosine kinases.
- Linked to DNA interactions (steroid receptors).

Receptors directly linked to ion channels

Receptors that are directly linked to ion channels (Fig. 1.1) are mainly involved in fast synaptic neurotransmission, where the delay between ligand binding and channel opening lasts only a matter of milliseconds. A classic example of a receptor linked directly to an ion channel is the nicotinic acetylcholine receptor (nicAChR). The nicAChR consists of five subunits—two α, one β, one γ, and one δ—each of molecular weight 40–58 kDa and of great sequence homology.

The nicAChRs possess several characteristics:

- Acetylcholine (ACh) must bind to the N-termini of both α-subunits in order to activate the receptor.
- The whole receptor oligomer incorporates 20 transmembrane segments arranged around a central aqueous channel. One of the transmembrane helices (M_2) from each of the subunits is believed to form the lining of the channel.
- The receptor shows marked similarities with the two other receptors for fast transmission, namely the γ-aminobutyric acid (GABA)$_A$ and glycine receptors.

G-protein-linked receptors

G-protein-linked receptors (Fig. 1.2) are involved in relatively rapid transduction, a response being generated in seconds. Muscarinic ACh, adrenergic, dopamine, serotonin, and opiate receptors are all examples of G-protein-linked receptors.

Molecular structure of the receptor

Most of the G-protein-linked receptors consist of a single polypeptide chain of 400–500 residues and have seven transmembrane-spanning α-helices. The third intracellular loop of the receptor is larger than the other loops and interacts with the G-protein.

The ligand-binding domain is buried within the membrane on one or more of the α-helical segments. This is unlike ion channel-coupled receptors, where the ligand binds to the extracellular N-terminal region—an area easily accessible to small hydrophobic molecules.

G-proteins

Fig. 1.3 describes the mechanism of G-protein-linked receptors:

- In the resting state the G-protein exists as an

unattached trimer consisting of α-, β-, and γ-subunits (Fig. 1.3A).

- The occupation of the receptor by an agonist produces a conformational change, causing its affinity for the trimer to increase. Subsequent association of the trimer with the receptor results in the dissociation of bound GDP from the α-subunit. GTP replaces GDP in the cleft thus activating the G-protein and causing the α-subunit to dissociate from the βγ-dimer (Fig. 1.3B).

- α GTP represents the active form of the G-protein (although this is not always the case: in the heart, potassium channels are activated by the βγ-dimer and recent research has shown that the γ-subunit alone may play a role in activation). This component diffuses in the plane of the membrane where it is free to interact with downstream effectors such as enzymes and ion channels. The βγ-dimer remains associated with the membrane owing to its hydrophobicity (Fig. 1.3C).

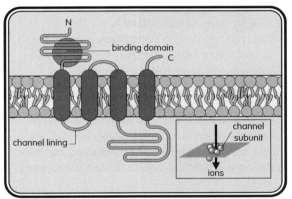

Fig. 1.1 General structure of the subunits of receptors directly linked to ion channels. (N, *N*-terminal; C, *C*-terminal.)

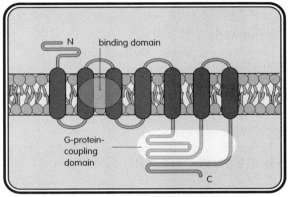

Fig. 1.2 General structure of the subunits of receptors linked to G-proteins.

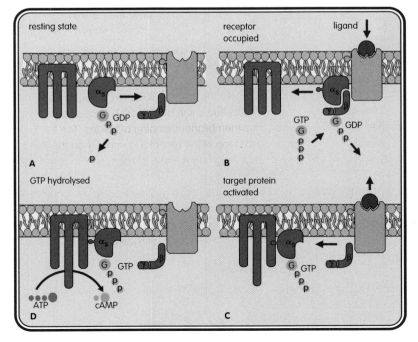

Fig. 1.3 Mechanism of G-protein-linked receptors. (α, β, γ, subunits of G-protein; cAMP, cyclic adenosine monophosphate; ATP, adenosine triphosphate; G, guanosine; GDP, GTP, guanosine di- and triphosphate; p, phosphate.)

- The cycle is completed when the α-subunit, which has enzymic activity, hydrolyses the bound GTP to GDP. The GDP-bound α-subunit dissociates from the effector and recombines with the $\beta\gamma$-dimer (Fig. 1.3D).

This whole process results in an amplification effect because the binding of an agonist to the receptor can cause the activation of numerous G-proteins which in turn can each, via their association with the effector, produce many molecules of product.

Targets for G-proteins

G-proteins interact with either ion channels or second messengers.

Ion channels

G-proteins may activate ion channels directly, e.g. muscarinic receptors in the heart are linked to potassium channels which open directly upon interaction with the G-protein, causing a slowing down of the heart rate.

Second messengers

Three second-messenger systems exist as targets of G-proteins (Fig. 1.4).

Adenylyl cyclase/cAMP system

Many types of G-protein exist. This is probably attributable to the variability of the α-subunit. G_s and G_i/G_o cause stimulation and inhibition, respectively, of the target enzyme adenylyl cyclase. This explains why muscarinic ACh receptors and β-adrenoreceptors located in the heart produce opposite effects.

The bacterial toxins cholera and pertussis can be used in order to determine which G-protein is involved in a particular situation. Each has enzymic action on a conjugation reaction with the α-subunit, such that:

- Cholera affects G_s causing continued activation of adenylyl cyclase. This explains why infection with cholera toxin results in uncontrolled fluid secretion from the gastrointestinal tract.
- Pertussis affects G_i and G_o causing continued inactivation of adenylyl cyclase. This explains why infection with *Bordatella pertussis* causes a 'whooping' cough, characteristic of this infection.

Adenylyl cyclase catalyses the conversion of ATP to cyclic cAMP within cells. The cAMP produced in turn causes activation of certain protein kinases, enzymes that phosphorylate serine and threonine residues in

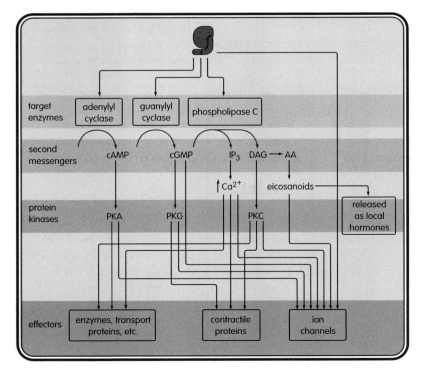

Fig. 1.4 Second-messenger targets of G-proteins and their effects. (cAMP, cyclic adenosine monophosphate; cGMP, cyclic guanosine monophosphate; DAG, diacylglycerol; IP_3, inositol (1,4,5) triphosphate; PK, protein kinase; AA, arachidonic acid.)

various proteins, thereby producing either activation or inactivation of these proteins. This can lead to:

- Increased lipolysis through activation of hormone-sensitive lipase.
- Reduced glycogen synthesis through inactivation of glycogen synthase.
- Increased glycogen breakdown through the activation of phosphorylase kinase and therefore conversion of inactive phosphorylase b to active phosphorylase a.

Activation of β_1-noradrenergic receptors found in cardiac muscle results in activation of cAMP-dependent protein kinase A, which phosphorylates and opens voltage-operated calcium channels. This increases calcium levels in the cell and results in an increased rate and force of contraction.

In contrast, activation of β_2-noradrenergic receptors found in smooth muscle causes activation of protein kinase and therefore phosphorylation, but inactivation of another enzyme—myosin light-chain kinase—needed for contraction.

Receptors linked to G_i inhibit adenylyl cyclase and reduce cAMP production. Examples of these receptors are the M_2 and M_4 muscarinic, the opioid, the 5-HT$_1$ (hydroxytryptamine) and the α_2-adrenoreceptors.

Phospholipase C/inositol phosphate system
Activation of M_1, M_3, 5-HT$_2$, peptide and α_1-adrenoreceptors, via G_q, cause activation of phospholipase C, a membrane-bound enzyme, which increases the rate of degradation of phosphatidylinositol (4,5) bisphosphate into diacylglycerol (DAG) and inositol (1,4,5) triphosphate (IP$_3$). DAG and IP$_3$ act as second messengers.

IP$_3$ binds to the membrane of the endoplasmic reticulum, opening calcium channels and increasing the concentration of calcium within the cell by 10–100-fold. Increased calcium levels may result in smooth muscle contraction, increased secretion from exocrine glands, increased hormone or transmitter release, or increased force and rate of contraction of the heart.

DAG, which remains associated with the membrane owing to its hydrophobicity, causes protein kinase C to move from the cytosol to the membrane where DAG can regulate the activity of the latter. There are at least six types of protein kinase C, with 50 or more targets including:

- Release of hormones and neurotransmitters.
- Smooth muscle contraction.
- Inflammation.
- Ion transport.
- Tumour promotion.

Guanylyl cyclase system
Guanylyl cyclase catalyses the conversion of GTP to cGMP. This cGMP goes on to cause activation of protein kinase G which in turn phosphorylates contractile proteins and ion channels.

Transmembrane guanylyl cyclase activity is exhibited by the atrial natriuretic peptide receptor upon the binding of atrial natriuretic peptide.

Cytoplasmic guanylyl cyclase activity is exhibited when bradykinin activates receptors on the membrane of endothelial cells to generate nitric oxide, which then acts as a second messenger to activate guanylyl cyclase within the cell.

Sodium nitroprusside is a nitrovasodilator that relaxes the smooth muscle of arteries and veins by increasing cGMP production. Because both central venous pressure and arterial pressure drop, there is little change in cardiac output. Sodium nitroprusside is used for angina and hypertension.

Tyrosine-kinase-linked receptors
Tyrosine-kinase-linked receptors are involved in the regulation of growth and differentiation, and responses to metabolic signals.

The response time of enzyme-initiated transduction is slow (minutes). Examples include the receptors for insulin, platelet-derived growth factor, and epidermal growth factor.

Activation of tyrosine kinase receptors results in autophosphorylation of tyrosine residues leading to the activation of pathways involving protein kinases.

DNA-linked receptors
Corticosteroids, thyroid hormone, retinoic acid, and vitamin D are all molecules with receptors that are linked so as to interact with DNA. The receptors are located intracellularly and so agonists must pass through the cell membrane in order to reach the receptor. Once in the nucleus and bound to their receptor, the complex can bind to specific DNA sequences and so alter the expression of specific genes. As a result, secondary transduction involving an increase or decrease in the synthesis of various proteins occurs. The process is very slow (hours).

The structure, mechanism, and targets of G-protein-linked receptors is a common essay question. Make sure you learn them well.

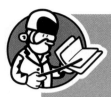

- Summarize the system of drug nomenclature and how drugs are classified.
- Distinguish between non-specific and specific drug actions.
- What are the distinguishing characteristics of the four main types of receptor?
- Describe how G-proteins function, their targets, and how each of the second-messenger systems initiates an intracellular cascade of events leading to a response.

DRUGS AND RECEPTORS

Drug–receptor interactions
Most drugs produce their effects by acting through specific protein molecules called receptors.

Receptors respond to endogenous chemicals in the body that are either synaptic transmitter substances (e.g. ACh, noradrenaline) or hormones (endocrine, e.g. insulin; local, e.g. histamine). These chemicals or drugs will do one of the following:

- Activate receptors and produce a subsequent response (agonists).
- Associate with receptors but not cause activation (antagonists). Antagonists reduce the chance of transmitters or agonists binding to the receptor and thereby oppose their action by effectively diluting or removing the receptors from the system.

Electrostatic forces initially attract a drug to a receptor. If the shape of the drug corresponds to that of the binding site of the receptor, then it will be held there

temporarily by weak bonds or, in the case of irreversible antagonists, permanently by stronger covalent bonds. The greater the number of bonds, the more complementary the fit is between drug and receptor, and so the higher the affinity of the drug for the receptor.

The affinity is defined by the dissociation constant which is given the symbol K_d. The lower the K_d, the higher the affinity. K_d values in the nanomolar range represent drugs with a high affinity for their receptor:

$$D + R \xrightarrow{K_{+1}} DR \qquad DR \xrightarrow{K_{-1}} D + R$$

The rate at which the forward reaction occurs is dependent upon the drug concentration [D] and the receptor concentration [R]:

Forward rate = K_{+1} [D][R]

The rate at which the backward reaction occurs is mainly dependent upon the interaction between the drug and the receptor [DR]:

Backward rate = K_{-1} [DR]
$K_d = K_{-1} / K_{+1}$

K_a is the association constant and is used to quantify affinity. It can be defined as the concentration of drug that produces 50% of the maximum response at equilibrium, in the absence of receptor reserve (see p. 10):

$$K_a = 1 / K_d$$

Drugs with a high affinity stay bound to their receptor for a relatively long time and are said to have a slow off-rate. This means that at any time the probability that any given receptor will be occupied by the drug is high.

The ability of a drug to combine with one type of receptor is termed specificity. Although no drug is truly specific, most exhibit relatively selective action on one type of receptor.

Agonists
Agonists bind to the receptor and the chemical energy released on binding induces a conformational change that sets off a chain of biochemical events within the cell, leading to a response. The equation for this is:

$$A + R \xrightarrow{(1)} AR \xrightarrow{(2)} AR^*$$

(1): affinity dependent
(2): efficacy dependent

Partial agonists cannot bring about the same maximum response as full agonists, even if their affinity for the receptor is the same (Figs 1.5 and 1.6).

The ability of agonists, once bound, to activate receptors is termed efficacy, such that:

- Full agonists have high efficacy and are able to produce a maximum response while occupying only a small percentage of the receptors available.
- Partial agonists have low efficacy and are unable to elicit the maximum response even if they are occupying all the available receptors.

Antagonists

Antagonists bind to receptors but do not activate them, they do not induce a conformational change and thus have no efficacy. However, because antagonists occupy the receptor, they prevent agonists from binding and therefore block their action.

Two types of antagonist exist, competitive and non-competitive.

Competitive antagonists

These bind to receptors reversibly and effectively produce a dilution of the receptors, such that:

- A parallel shift is produced to the right of the agonist dose–response curve (Fig. 1.7).
- The maximum response is not depressed. This reflects the fact that the antagonist's effect can be overcome by increasing the dose of agonist, i.e. the block is surmountable. Increasing the concentration of agonist increases the probability of the agonist taking the place of an antagonist leaving the receptor.
- The size of the shift in the agonist dose–response curve produced by the antagonist reflects the affinity of the antagonist for the receptor. High-affinity antagonists stay bound to the receptor for a relatively long period of time allowing the agonist little chance to take the antagonist's place.

This concept can be quantified in terms of the dose ratio. The dose ratio is the ratio of the concentration of agonist producing a given response in the presence and absence of a certain concentration of antagonist, e.g. a dose ratio of 3 tells us that three times as much agonist was required to produce a given response in the presence of the antagonist than it did in its absence. Thus:

- Relating this to antagonist affinity involves measuring the concentration of antagonist needed to produce a

dose ratio of 2. The negative logarithm of this concentration is termed the pA_2. The pA_2 can be defined as the negative logarithm of that concentration of antagonist which requires that the concentration of agonist be doubled to achieve a given response.

- Making the assumption that the competitive antagonist is acting in a totally reversible manner,

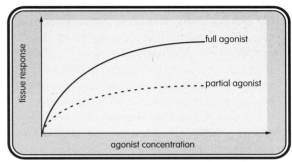

Fig. 1.5 Comparison of the dose–response curve for a partial agonist and a full agonist. (From *Medical Pharmacology at a Glance*, 2nd edition. Courtesy of Blackwell Scientific Publications.)

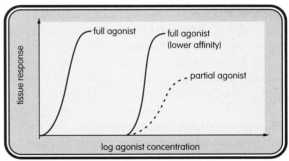

Fig. 1.6 Comparison of the log dose–response curve for a partial agonist and a full agonist. (From *Medical Pharmacology at a Glance*, 2nd edition. Courtesy of Blackwell Scientific Publications.)

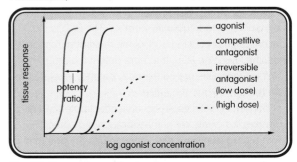

Fig. 1.7 Comparison of the log dose–response curves for competitive and non-competitive antagonists. (From *Medical Pharmacology at a Glance*, 2nd edition. Courtesy of Blackwell Scientific Publications.)

then the pA_2 is equal to the negative logarithm of the K_d for the antagonist, i.e. K_d = the concentration of antagonist required to produce a dose ratio of 2.

Non-competitive antagonists:
These are also known as irreversible antagonists. Their presence:
- Also produces a parallel shift to the right of the agonist dose–response curve (Fig. 1.7).
- Depresses the maximum response, reflecting the fact that the antagonist's effect cannot be overcome by the addition of greater doses of agonist. At low concentrations, however, a parallel shift may occur without a reduced maximum response. This tells us that not all of the receptors need be occupied in order to elicit a maximum response, since irreversible antagonists effectively remove receptors and there must be a number of spare receptors.

Receptor reserve
Although on a log scale the relationship between the concentration of agonist and the response produces a symmetrical sigmoid curve, very rarely does a 50% response correspond to a 50% receptor occupancy. This is because there are spare receptors.

This excess of receptors is known as receptor reserve and serves to sharpen the sensitivity of the cell to small changes in agonist concentration.

The low efficacy of partial agonists can be overcome in tissues with a large receptor reserve and in these circumstances partial agonists may act as full agonists.

Potency
Potency relates to the concentration of a drug needed to elicit a response.

The EC_{50}, where EC stands for effective concentration, is a number used to quantify potency. The EC_{50} is the concentration producing 50% of the maximum response. Thus, the lower the EC_{50}, the more potent the drug.

Where agonists are concerned, potency is related to both the affinity and the efficacy.

Pharmacokinetic variables also affect potency. For example, the acidic pH of the stomach may break down a drug that has been found to be very potent in a test tube but which, if given as a tablet, would have very little potency and would be ineffective.

Drugs acting on receptors are highly chemically specific, and do so at very low doses (µg, low mg levels). They are very potent and as a result overdoses may be dangerous.

- Describe the difference between the effects of agonists and antagonists.
- Outline the concept of agonist affinity in relation to the dissociation constant and the association constant.
- Describe the concept of efficacy and partial agonism.
- Describe the quantification of the concept of antagonist affinity in terms of dose ratio.
- Describe the role of receptor reserve in relation to system sensitivity.
- Outline the concept of potency in terms of EC_{50}.

PHARMACOKINETICS

Pharmacology can be divided into two disciplines. These are:
- Pharmacokinetics, which considers drug disposition and the way the body affects the drug with time, i.e. the factors that determine its absorption, distribution, metabolism, and excretion.
- Pharmacodynamics, which deals with the effect of the drug on the body.

Compliance
Compliance on the patient's behalf is very important as far as taking drugs is concerned. In order for some drugs to be effective (e.g. antibiotics), they must be taken at regular intervals and for a certain period of

time. For certain forms of treatment, patients may even need to come to hospital, in which case transport, work, and having young children may be a problem.

Compliance tends to be more of a problem in paediatric practice since it involves both parents and the child: the parent must remember to give the medication and follow directions accurately; the child must cooperate and not spit out or spill the medicine.

Practical dosage forms are important in achieving compliance. Many tablets are now sugar coated, making them easier to take, and a large number of the drugs manufactured for children are in the form of elixirs or suspensions, which may be available in a variety of different flavours, making their administration less of a problem.

The route of administration of a drug may affect compliance. Taking a drug orally, for example, is more simple than injecting it.

The dosing schedule is also an important aspect of compliance. The easier this is to follow, and the less frequently a drug needs to be taken or administered, the more likely it is that compliance will occur.

Routes of administration
Topical
Topical drugs are placed where they are needed, giving them the advantage that they do not have to cross any barriers or membranes. Examples include skin ointments; ear, nose, or eye drops; and aerosols inhaled in the treatment of asthma.

Enteral
Enteral administration means that the drug reaches its target via the gut. It is the least predictable route of administration, owing to metabolism by the liver, chemical breakdown, and the possible binding to food. Drugs must cross several barriers, which may or may not be a problem according to their physicochemical properties such as charge and size. However:

- Most drugs are administered orally unless the drug is unstable, or is rapidly inactivated in the gastrointestinal tract, or if its efficacy of absorption from the gastrointestinal tract is uncertain owing to metabolism by the liver or the intestines, vomiting, or a disease that may affect drug absorption.
- Absorption of drugs via the buccal or sublingual route avoids the portal circulation and is therefore valuable when administering drugs subject to a high degree of first-pass metabolism. It is also useful for potent drugs with a non-disagreeable taste, such as sublingual nitroglycerin given to relieve acute attacks of angina.
- Administration of drugs rectally, such as in the form of suppositories, means that there is less first-pass metabolism by the liver because the venous return from the lower gastrointestinal tract is less than that from the upper gastrointestinal tract. It has the disadvantage, however, of being inconsistent.
- Antacids have their effect in the stomach and may be considered as being topical.

Parenteral
Parenteral administration means that the drug is administered in a manner that avoids the gut. Insulin, for example, is destroyed by the acidity of the stomach and the digestive enzymes within the gut and must therefore be injected. Intravenous injection has several advantages:

- It is the most direct route of administration. The drug enters the bloodstream directly and bypasses absorption barriers.
- A drug is distributed in a large volume and acts rapidly.

For drugs that must be given continuously by infusion, or for drugs that damage tissues, this is an important method of administration.

Alternative parenteral routes of administration include subcutaneous, intramuscular, epidural, or intrathecal injections, and transdermal patches such as are used in angina.

The rate of drug absorption from the site of the injection can be decreased by binding the drug to a vehicle or co-administering a vasoconstrictor, such as adrenaline, to reduce blood flow to the site.

Drug absorption
Bioavailability takes into account both absorption and metabolism and describes the proportion of the drug that passes into the systemic circulation. This will, of course, be 100% after an intravenous injection, but following oral administration it will depend on the drug, the individual, and the circumstances under which the drug is given.

Since drugs must cross membranes in order to enter cells or to transfer between body compartments, drug absorption will be affected by both chemical and physiological factors.

Cell membranes

Cell membranes are composed of lipid bilayers and thus absorption is usually proportional to the lipid solubility of the drug. Un-ionized molecules (B) are far more soluble than those that are ionized (BH$^+$) and surrounded by a 'shell' of water.

$$B + H^+ \leftrightarrow BH^+$$

Size

Small size is another factor that favours absorption. Most drugs are small molecules (molecular weight <1000) that are able to diffuse across membranes in their uncharged state.

pH

Since most drugs are either weak bases, weak acids, or amphoteric, the pH of the environment in which they dissolve, as well as the pK_a value of the drug, will be important in determining the fraction in the un-ionized form that is in solution and able to diffuse across cell membranes. The pK_a of a drug is defined as the pH at which 50% of the molecules in solution are in the ionized form, and is characterized by the Henderson–Hasselbalch equation:

For acidic molecules: HA $\leftrightarrow$ H$^+$ + A$^-$
pK_a = pH + log [HA] / [A$^-$]

For basic molecules: BH$^+$ $\leftrightarrow$ B + H$^+$
pK_a = pH + log [BH$^+$] / [B]

Drugs will tend to exist in the ionized form when exposed to an environment with a pH opposite to their own state. Therefore, acids become increasingly ionized with increasing pH (i.e. basic).

It is useful to consider three important body compartments—plasma (pH = 7.4), stomach (pH = 2.0), and urine (pH = 8.0)—in relation to drugs. Thus:

- Aspirin is a weak acid (pK_a = 3.5) and its absorption will therefore be favoured in the stomach, where it is uncharged, and not in the plasma or the urine, where it is highly charged; aspirin in high doses may even damage the stomach.
- Morphine is a weak base (pK_a = 8.0) that is highly charged in the stomach, quite charged in the plasma, and half charged in the urine. Morphine is able to cross the blood–brain barrier but is poorly and erratically absorbed from the stomach and intestines, and metabolized by the liver, and must

therefore be given by injection or delayed-release capsules. Some drugs, such as quaternary ammonium compounds (e.g. suxamethonium, tubocurarine), are always charged, and must therefore be injected.

Drug distribution

Once drugs have reached the circulation, they are distributed around the body. As most drugs are of a very small molecular size, they are able to leave the circulation by capillary filtration to act on the tissues.

The half-life of a drug ($t_{1/2}$) is the time taken for the plasma concentration of that drug to fall to half of its original value.

Bulk transfer in the blood is very quick. Drugs:
- Exist either dissolved in blood or bound to plasma proteins such as albumin. Albumin is the most important circulating protein for binding many acidic drugs.
- That are basic tend to be bound to a globulin fraction that increases with age. A drug that is bound is confined to the vascular system and is unable to exert its actions; this becomes a problem if more than 80% of the drug is bound.
- Interact and one drug may displace another. For example, aspirin can displace the anxiolytic diazepam from albumin.

The apparent volume of distribution (V_d) is the calculated pharmacokinetic space into which a drug is distributed.

$$V_d = \frac{\text{dose administered}}{\text{initial apparent plasma concentration}}$$

V_d values:
- That amount to less than a certain body compartment volume indicate that the drug is contained within that compartment. For example, when the volume of distribution is less than 5 L, it is likely that the drug is restricted to the vasculature.
- Less than 15 L, imply that the drug is restricted to the extracellular fluid.
- Greater than 15 L, suggest distribution within the total body water. Some drugs (usually basic) have a volume of distribution that exceeds body weight, in which case tissue binding is occurring. These drugs tend to be contained outside the circulation and may accumulate in certain tissues. Very lipid-soluble substances, such as thiopentone, can build up in fat;

lead accumulates in bone; and mepacrine, an anti-malarial drug, has a concentration in the liver 200 times that in the plasma because it binds to nucleic acids. Some drugs are even actively transported into certain organs.

Drug metabolism

Before being excreted from the body, most drugs are metabolized. A small number of drugs exist in their fully ionized form at physiological pH (7.4) and, owing to this highly polar nature are metabolized to only a minor extent, if at all. The sequential metabolic reactions that occur have been categorized as phases 1 and 2.

Sites of metabolism

The liver is the major site of drug metabolism although most tissues are able to metabolize specific drugs. Other sites of metabolism include the kidney, the lung, and the gastrointestinal tract.

Orally administered drugs, which are usually absorbed in the small intestine, reach the liver via the portal circulation. At this stage, or within the small intestine, the drugs may be extensively metabolized; this is known as first-pass metabolism and means that considerably less drug reaches the systemic circulation than enters the portal vein. This causes problems because it means that higher doses of drug must be given and, owing to individual variation in the degree of first-pass metabolism, the effects of the drug can be unpredictable. Drugs that are subject to a high degree of first-pass metabolism, such as the local anaesthetic lignocaine, cannot be given orally and must be administered by some other route.

Phase 1 metabolic reactions

Phase 1 metabolic reactions include oxidation, reduction, and hydrolysis. These reactions introduce a functional group, such as -OH or NH_2, which increases the polarity of the drug molecule and provides a site for phase 2 reactions.

Oxidations

Oxidations are the most common type of reaction and are catalysed by an enzyme system known as the microsomal mixed function oxidase system, which is located on the smooth endoplasmic reticulum. The enzyme system forms small vesicles known as microsomes when the tissue is homogenized.

Cytochrome P_{450}:
- Is the most important enzyme, although other

enzymes are involved. This enzyme is a haemoprotein that requires the presence of oxygen, reduced nicotinamide adenine dinucleotide phosphate (NADPH) and NADPH cytochrome P_{450} reductase in order to function.
- Exists in several hundred isoforms, some of which are constitutive while others are synthesized in response to certain signals. The substrate specificity of this enzyme depends on the isoform but tends to be low, meaning that a whole variety of drugs can be oxidized.

Although oxidative reactions usually result in inactivation of the drug, sometimes a metabolite is produced that is pharmacologically active and may have a duration of action exceeding that of the original drug. In these cases the drug is known as a prodrug, e.g. codeine which is demethylized to morphine.

Reductions

Reduction reactions also involve microsomal enzymes but are much less common than oxidation reactions. Examples of drugs subject to reduction include prednisone, which is given as a prodrug and reduced to the active glucocorticoid prednisolone, and warfarin, an anticoagulant, which is inactivated by the transformation of a ketone group to a hydroxyl group.

Hydrolysis

Hydrolysis is not restricted to the liver and occurs in a variety of tissues. Aspirin is spontaneously hydrolysed to salicylic acid in moisture.

Phase 2 metabolic reactions

Drug molecules that possess a suitable site that was either present before phase 1 or is the result of the phase 1 reaction, are susceptible to phase 2 reactions. Phase 2 reactions involve conjugation—the attachment of a large chemical group to a functional group on the drug molecule. Conjugation results in the drug being more hydrophilic and thus more easily excreted from the body. In conjugation:
- It is mainly the liver that is involved, although conjugation can occur in a wide variety of tissues.
- Chemical groups involved are endogenous activated moieties such as glucuronic acid, sulphate, methyl, acetyl, and glutathione.
- The conjugating enzymes exist in many isoforms and show relative substrate and metabolite specificity.

Unlike the products of phase 1 reactions, the conjugate is almost invariably inactive. An important exception is morphine, which is converted to morphine-6-glucuronide, which has an analgesic effect lasting longer than that of its parent molecule.

Factors affecting metabolism

Enzyme induction is the increased synthesis or decreased degradation of enzymes and occurs as a result of the presence of an exogenous substance. For example:

- Some drugs are able to increase the activity of certain isoenzyme forms of cytochrome P_{450} and thus increase their own metabolism, as well as that of other drugs.
- Smokers can show increased metabolism of certain drugs because of the induction of cytochrome P_{448} by a constituent of tobacco smoke.
- In contrast, some drugs inhibit microsomal enzyme activity and therefore increase their own activity as well as that of other drugs.

Competition for a metabolic enzyme may occur between two drugs, in which case there is a decreased metabolism of one or both drugs. This is known as inhibition.

Enzymes that metabolize drugs are affected by many aspects of diet, such as the ratio of protein to carbohydrate, flavonoids contained in cruciferous vegetables, and polycyclic aromatic hydrocarbons found in barbecued foods.

Paracetamol poisoning

Paracetamol is a classic example of a drug that can be lethal at high doses (2–3 times the maximum therapeutic dose), owing to the accumulation of its metabolites.

In phase 2 of the metabolic process, paracetemol is conjugated with glucuronic acid and sulphate. When high doses of paracetemol are taken, these pathways become saturated and the drug is metabolised by the mixed function oxidases. This results in the formation of the toxic metabolite N-acetyl-p-benzoquinone which is inactivated by glutathione. However, when glutathione is depleted, this toxic metabolite reacts with nucleophilic constituents in the cell leading to necrosis in the liver and kidneys.

N-Acetylcysteine or methionine can be administered in cases of paracetamol overdose, since they increase liver glutathione formation and the conjugation reactions, respectively.

Drug excretion

Drugs are excreted from the body in a variety of different ways. Excretion can occur by the kidneys into urine, by the gastrointestinal tract into bile and faeces, and by the lungs into exhaled air. Drugs may also leave the body through breast milk and sweat. The most important routes for drug excretion are through the urine and faeces.

The volume of plasma cleared of drug per unit time is known as the clearance.

Renal excretion

Glomerular filtration, tubular reabsorption (passive and active), and tubular secretion all determine the extent to which a drug will be excreted by the kidneys.

Glomerular capillaries allow the passage of molecules with a molecular weight <20 000. The glomerular filtrate thus contains most of the substances in plasma except proteins. In the glomerular capillaries:

- The negative charge of the corpuscular membrane also repels negatively charged molecules, including plasma proteins.
- Drugs that bind to plasma proteins such as albumin will not be filtered.

Most of the drug in the blood does not pass into the glomerular filtrate, but passes into the peritubular capillaries of the proximal tubule where, depending on its nature, it may be transported into the lumen of the tubule by either of two transport mechanisms. One transport mechanism deals with acidic molecules, the other with basic molecules. In the peritubular capillaries:

- Tubular secretion is responsible for most of the drug excretion carried out by the kidneys and, unlike glomerular filtration, allows the clearance of drugs bound to plasma proteins. Competition between drugs that share the same transport mechanism may occur, in which case the excretion of these drugs will be reduced. Probenecid is a drug that was designed to compete with penicillin for excretion and therefore increase the duration of action of penicillin.
- Reabsorption of a drug will depend upon the fraction of molecules in the ionized state which is in turn dependent on the pH of the urine. Intoxification with aspirin (weak acid, $pK_a = 3.5$) can be treated by administering bicarbonate which makes the urine more alkaline; this ionizes aspirin and renders it less prone to reabsorption.

• Renal disease will affect the excretion of certain drugs. The extent to which excretion is impaired can be deduced by measuring 24-hour creatinine clearance.

Gastrointestinal excretion
Some drug conjugates are excreted into the bile and subsequently released into the intestines where they are hydrolysed back to the parent compound and reabsorbed. This 'enterohepatic circulation' prolongs the effect of the drug.

Mathematical aspects of pharmacokinetics
Kinetic order
Two types of kinetics, related to the plasma concentration of a drug, describe the rate at which a drug leaves the body:
• Zero-order kinetics (Fig. 1.8) describes a decrease in drug levels in the body that is independent of the plasma concentration. When the plasma concentration is plotted against time, the decrease is a straight line. Alcohol is an example of a drug that displays zero-order kinetics.
• First-order kinetics (Fig. 1.9) is displayed by most drugs. It describes a decrease in drug levels in the body that is dependent on the plasma concentration. When the plasma concentration is plotted against time, the decrease is exponential.

One-compartment model
The one-compartment model considers the body to be a single compartment. Within this single compartment a drug is absorbed, immediately distributed (e.g. by intravenous injection), and subsequently eliminated by metabolism and excretion.

If the volume of the compartment is V_d and the dose administered D, then the initial drug concentration, C_o, will be:

$$C_o = D / V_d$$

The time taken for the plasma drug concentration to fall to half of its original value is the half-life of that drug. The decline in concentration may be exponential, but this situation expresses itself graphically as a straight line when the log plasma concentration is plotted against the time after intravenous dose (Fig. 1.10).

Half-life is related to the elimination rate constant (K_{el}) by the following equation:

$$t_{1/2} \times K_{el} = 0.693$$

Half-life is related to V_d, but does not determine the ability of the body to remove the drug from the circulation, since both V_d and half-life change in the same direction. The body's ability to remove a drug from the blood is termed clearance (Cl_p) and is constant for individual drugs:

$$Cl_p = V_d \times K_{el}$$

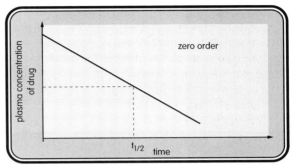

Fig. 1.8 Plasma drug concentration versus time plot for a drug displaying zero-order kinetics.

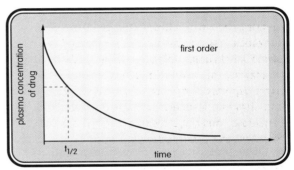

Fig. 1.9 Plasma drug concentration versus time plot for a drug displaying first-order kinetics.

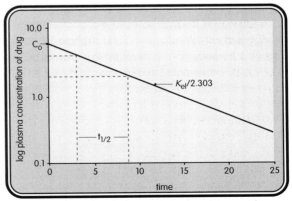

Fig. 1.10 Log plasma drug concentration versus time plot compatible with the one-compartment open pharmacokinetic model for drug disposition after a parenteral dose.

Introduction to Pharmacology

If the drug is not administered parenterally, plotting the log plasma drug concentration against time will require the consideration of both absorption and elimination from the compartment (Fig. 1.11).

The one-compartment model is widely used to determine the dose of drug to be administered.

Two-compartment model

The distribution of drugs between the peripheral compartment (i.e. tissues) and the central compartment (i.e. plasma) occurs at rates varying from rapid to insignificant.

Some drugs distribute slowly or extensively, and in these cases a curvilinear relationship between the log of the plasma concentration and time is seen. Two phases can be observed (Fig. 1.12):

- An early, rapid, α-phase, which represents the redistribution of the drug to the peripheral compartment and a modest component of elimination.
- A later, slower, β-phase, which is a combination of elimination and return of the drug from the peripheral compartment to the central compartment, in which the drug then distributes rapidly.

Model-independent approach

For drugs displaying first-order kinetics, the level of the drug in the body increases until it is equal to the level excreted, at which point steady-state is reached (Fig. 1.13), such that:

- The time to reach steady-state is usually equal to four to five half-lives.
- The amount of drug in the body at steady-state will depend upon the frequency of drug administration—the greater the frequency, the greater the amount of drug and the less the variation between peak and trough plasma concentrations. If the frequency of administration is greater than the half-life, then accumulation of the drug will occur.

The loading dose can be calculated according to the desired plasma concentration at steady-state (C_{ss}) and the volume of distribution (V_d) of the drug:

Loading dose (mg/kg) = V_d (L/kg) × C_{ss} (mg/L)

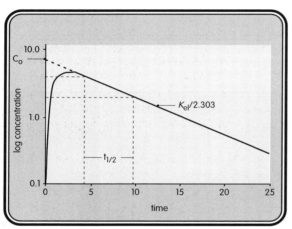

Fig. 1.11 Log plasma drug concentration versus time plot for a drug compatible with the one-compartment open pharmacokinetic model for drug disposition after an oral dose.

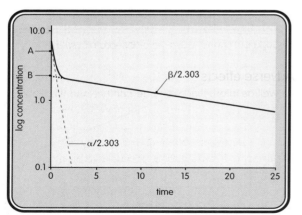

Fig. 1.12 Log plasma drug concentration versus time plot that requires a two-compartment open model to account for its disposition after a parenteral dose.

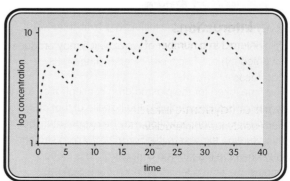

Fig. 1.13 Log plasma drug concentration versus time plot for a drug administered by mouth every 6 hours when its terminal disposition half-life is 6 hours.

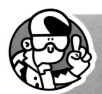

Highly charged and
water-soluble drugs are
termed hydrophilic,
whereas uncharged and
lipid-soluble drugs are
termed lipophilic or
hydrophobic.

○ **Why is compliance
important?**
○ **Describe the
advantages and
disadvantages of the three
main routes through which
drugs are administered.**
○ **What factors affect drug
absorption and distribution?**
○ **Describe the sites and
mechanisms of drug
metabolism and excretion.**
○ **Summarize the three
approaches to drug
distribution within the body.**

DRUG INTERACTIONS AND ADVERSE EFFECTS

Drug interactions

Drugs interact in a number of ways which may produce
unwanted effects. Two types of interactions exist,
pharmacodynamic and pharmacokinetic.

Pharmacodynamic interactions

Pharmacodynamic interactions involve a direct conflict
between the effects of drugs. This conflict results in the
effect of one of the two drugs being enhanced or
reduced. For example:

- Propranolol, a β-adrenoceptor antagonist given for
  angina and hypertension, will reduce the effect of
  salbutamol, a β_2-adrenoceptor agonist given for the

treatment of asthma. The administration of β-blockers
to asthmatics should therefore be avoided.
- Administration of monoamine oxidase inhibitors,
  which inhibit the metabolism of catecholamines,
  enhances the effects of drugs such as ephedrine.
  This enhancement causes the release of
  noradrenaline from stores in the nerve terminal and
  is known as 'potentiation'.

Pharmacokinetic interactions

Absorption, distribution, metabolism, and excretion all
affect the pharmacokinetic properties of drugs. Thus
any drug that interferes with these processes will be
altering the effect of other drugs. For example:

- If administered with diuretics, non-steroidal anti-
  inflammatory drugs (NSAIDs) will reduce the
  antihypertensive action of these drugs. NSAIDs bring
  about this effect by reducing prostaglandin synthesis
  in the kidney, thus impairing renal blood flow and
  consequently decreasing the excretion of waste and
  sodium. This results in an increased blood volume
  and a rise in blood pressure.
- Enzyme induction, which occurs as a result of the
  administration of certain drugs, can affect the
  metabolism of other drugs served by that enzyme (p. 14).

In some cases, however, drugs are used together so
that their interaction can bring about the desired effect.

- For example, carbidopa prevents the conversion of
  levodopa (L-dopa) to dopamine and is therefore used
  with L-dopa in the treatment of Parkinson's disease.
  L-Dopa is able to cross the blood–brain barrier and
  enter the brain, where it is converted to dopamine.
  Carbidopa reduces the peripheral side effects of L-
  dopa but cannot cross the blood–brain barrier.

Adverse effects

As well as interacting with one another and with their
target tissue, drugs will also interact with other tissues
and organs and alter their function. No drug is
without side effects, although the severity and
frequency of these will vary from drug to drug and
from person to person.

Adverse drug reactions tend to be more severe
where cell division occurs frequently, such as in the
lining of the gastrointestinal tract, the skin and the
haematopoietic system.

The liver and the kidneys are susceptible to the

adverse effects of drugs, as these are the sites of drug metabolism and excretion. Some drugs cause hepatotoxicity or nephrotoxicity.

Those who are more prone to the adverse effects of drugs, include:

- Pregnant women, who must be careful about taking drugs as certain drugs are teratogenic, i.e. cause fetal malformations (e.g. thalidomide taken in the 1960s for morning sickness).
- Breast-feeding women, who must also be careful about which drugs they take, as many drugs can be passed on in the breast milk and consumed by the developing infant.
- Patients with an underlying illness other than the one being treated, such as liver or kidney disease. These illnesses will result in decreased metabolism and excretion of the drug and will produce the side effects of an increased dose of the same drug.
- The elderly, who tend to take a large number of drugs, greatly increasing the risk of drug interactions and the associated side effects. In addition, elderly patients have a reduced renal clearance, and a nervous system that is more sensitive to drugs. The dose of drug initially given is usually 50% of the adult dose, and certain drugs are contraindicated.

- Patients with genetic enzyme defects, such as glucose-6-phosphate dehydrogenase deficiency. The deficiency will result in haemolysis if an oxidant drug, e.g. aspirin, is taken.

Certain drugs are carcinogenic, i.e. induce cancer. Genotoxic carcinogens cause mutations, either directly (primary carcinogens) or through their metabolites (secondary carcinogens). Epigenetic carcinogens, such as phorbol esters, do not induce mutations themselves, but increase the likelihood that a mutagen will do so.

Allergic reactions to certain drugs are common, occurring in 2–25% of cases. Most of these are not serious, e.g. skin reactions; however, rarely, reactions such as anaphylactic shock (type 1 hypersensitivity) occur that may be lethal, unless treated with intravenous adrenaline. The most common allergic reaction is to penicillin, which produces anaphylactic shock in approximately 1 in 50 000 people.

Some drugs, e.g. the vasodilator hydralazine, induce autoimmune reactions similar to systemic lupus erythematosus. Stopping the drug usually puts an end to this reaction, although in some cases glucocorticoid therapy may be needed.

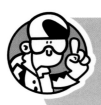

The 'risk' of the drug is the probability that the drug will cause some specified harm.

- Distinguish between pharmacodynamic and pharmacokinetic interactions.
- Give an example of a wanted drug interaction and an unwanted drug interaction.
- Which tissues are more at risk of the adverse effects of drugs, and why?
- Which people are more at risk of the adverse effects of drugs, and why?
- What is meant by teratogenic and carcinogenic?

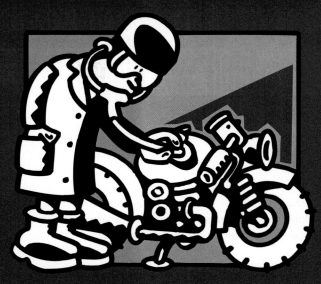

PHARMACOLOGY OF THE MAJOR ORGAN SYSTEMS

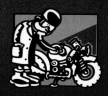

2. Peripheral and Autonomic Nervous Systems

Local anaesthetics

History

Local anaesthetics are drugs used to inhibit pain. These drugs work by reversibly blocking nerve conduction.

South American Indians have been chewing the leaves of the coca plant, *Erythroxylon coca,* for thousands of years. When they chewed the plant, they found that their mouth and tongue went numb, and that euphoria and excitement were induced. Cocaine was found to be the active ingredient, and it was first isolated from the coca plant in 1860.

Freud was the first to use cocaine clinically to treat his patients, but this was unsuccessful. In 1884, however, Koller obtained some cocaine from Freud and was able to demonstrate its local anaesthetic effects on the cornea.

Procaine was first synthesized in 1905 as a synthetic substitute for cocaine.

Nerve conduction

Conduction of impulses through nerves occurs as an all-or-none event called the action potential. The action potential is caused by voltage-dependent opening of sodium and potassium channels.

The sodium equilibrium potential (Eq Na^+) is +60 mV and the potassium equilibrium potential (Eq K^+) is –90 mV. Since a resting nerve has 50–75 more K^+ channels open than Na^+ channels the resting membrane potential is –70 mV.

Fig. 2.1 shows the concentrations of sodium and potassium inside and outside a resting nerve. The Na^+/K^+ pump (Na^+/K^+ ATPase) is an energy-dependent pump that functions to maintain the concentration gradient across the membrane. Three sodium ions are pumped out of the cell for every two potassium ions pumped in, and thus the excitability of the cell is retained.

Figs. 2.2 and 2.3 summarize the events that occur during a nerve action potential. During a nerve action potential:

- The rate of sodium entry into the nerve axon becomes greater than the rate of potassium out of the axon, at which point the membrane becomes depolarized.
- Depolarization sets off a sodium-positive feedback whereby more voltage-gated sodium channels open and the membrane becomes more depolarized.
- A threshold, which is usually 15 mV greater than the resting membrane potential, must be reached if an action potential is to be generated.
- The membrane repolarizes when the sodium channels become inactivated; a special set of potassium channels open and potassium leaves the axon.
- The sodium channels eventually regain their resting excitable state and the Na^+/K^+ ATPase restores the membrane potential back to –70 mV.

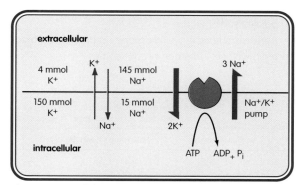

Fig. 2.1 Intracellular and extracellular sodium and potassium concentrations. The Na^+/K^+ ATPase pump maintains these concentration gradients.

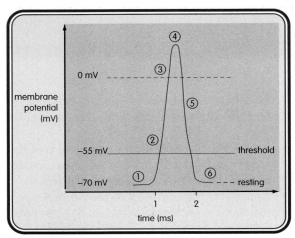

Fig. 2.2 Nerve action potential. For explanation of points 1–6, see Fig. 2.3.

Fig. 2.4 shows the voltage-operated sodium channels in their inactivated, activated, and resting states. Two types of gate exist within the channel, the m-gates and the h-gates. These gates are open or closed according to the state of the channel.

Sodium channel

The sodium channel is present in all excitable tissues. It is:

- Sensitive to membrane potential and selectively passes sodium ions.
- A transmembrane protein made up of four domains each with six transmembrane regions.

Local anaesthetics block the sodium channel and thus nerve conduction by binding to the sixth transmembrane region of the fourth domain.

Size of the nerve fibre

Small nerve fibres are preferentially blocked because of their high surface-area to volume ratio. This results in a differential block whereby the small nocioceptive (pain) and autonomic fibres are blocked but not the larger fibres responsible for the mediation of movement and touch.

Chemistry of local anaesthetics

All local anaesthetics have the same basic structure:

- An aromatic group (lipophilic end) linked to a basic side chain (hydrophilic end) by an ester or amide bond (Fig. 2.5).
- The basic side chain (usually a secondary or tertiary amine) is important since only the uncharged molecule can enter the nerve axoplasm.

Potency and duration of action are correlated with high lipid solubility.

Pharmacokinetics

Elimination of local anaesthetics is dependent upon the nature of the chemical bond:

- Local anaesthetics with ester bonds are inactivated by plasma cholinesterases.
- Local anaesthetics with amide bonds are degraded by N-dealkinylation in the liver.

Metabolites can often be pharmacologically active.

	Sodium channels	Potassium channels	Membrane potential
State of sodium and potassium channels and membrane potential at different stages of the nerve action potential			
1	closed resting	closed resting	resting (–70 mV)
2	open	closed resting	depolarization (action potential upstroke)
3	more channels open	closed resting	more depolarization
4	channels close (inactive)	special set of channels start opening	peak of action potential reached
5	all inactivated	more channels open	hyperpolarization
6	closed resting	channels close	resting membrane potential re-established

Fig. 2.3 State of sodium and potassium channels and membrane potential at different stages of the nerve action potential.

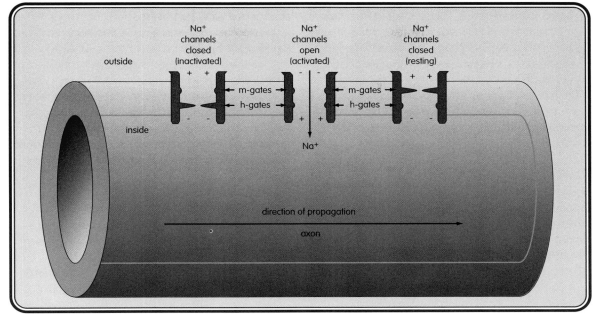

Fig. 2.4 Voltage-operated sodium channels in their inactivated, activated, and resting states. The m-gates and h-gates open or close according to the state of the channel.

Mechanism of block

Importance of pH and ionization

Local anaesthetics are weak bases (pK_a = 8–9). Only the uncharged form can penetrate lipid membranes; thus, quaternary ammonium compounds, which are fully protonated, must be injected directly into the nerve axon if they are to work.

The proportion of uncharged local anaesthetic is governed by the pH, the pK_a, and the Henderson–Hasselbalch equation (see Chapter 1):

$$B + H^+ = BH^+$$
$$pK_a = pH + \log [BH^+] / [B]$$

A local anaesthetic with a pK_a of 8.0 will be 10% uncharged at pH 7.0, 50% uncharged at pH 8.0, and 5% uncharged at pH 6.0.

Routes of block

The majority of local anaesthetics block by two routes (Fig. 2.6):

- By the hydrophobic route, the uncharged form enters the membrane and blocks the channel from a site in the protein membrane interface.

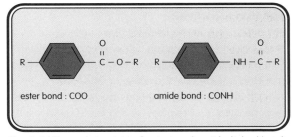

Fig. 2.5 General structure of ester- and amide-linked local anaesthetics.

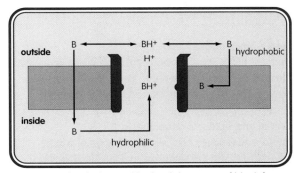

Fig. 2.6 Hydrophobic and hydrophilic routes of block for local anaesthetics.

- By the hydrophilic route, the uncharged form crosses the membrane to the inside where the charged form blocks the channel. This pathway depends on the channel being open and therefore this type of block is use dependent. Use dependency is especially important in the antiarrhythmic action of local anaesthetics.

Nerve block occurs when the number of non-inactivated channels is insufficient to bring about depolarization to threshold.

Routes of administration
Surface anaesthesia
In surface anaesthesia, the local anaesthetic is applied directly to the mucous membranes, e.g. cornea, bronchial tree, oesophagus, and genitourinary tract. The local anaesthetic, e.g. lignocaine, must be able to penetrate the tissues easily. For skin:

- A non-crystalline eutetic mixture of local anaesthetics (EMLA) consisting of lignocaine and prilocaine is used; this takes about an hour to work.
- Benzocaine as a dry powder, which is slow release and long lasting, is used for skin ulcers.

Problems occur when large areas, e.g. the bronchial tree, are anaesthetized.

Infiltration anaesthesia
Infiltration anaesthesia involves direct injection of a local anaesthetic into tissue. Often, a vasoconstrictor such as adrenaline or felypressin is used with the local anaesthetic to prevent the spread of the local anaesthetic into the circulation. Vasoconstrictors must never be used at extremities as ischaemia could result.

Intravenous regional anaesthesia (IVRA) involves the injection of the local anaesthetic distal to a cuff inflated above arterial pressure. It is important that the cuff is not released prematurely as this could cause the release of a potentially toxic bolus into the circulation.

Nerve block anaesthesia
In nerve block anaesthesia, local anaesthetic is injected close to the appropriate nerve trunk, e.g. the brachial plexus. The injection must be accurate in location.

Spinal and epidural anaesthesia
Spinal anaesthesia involves the injection of a local anaesthetic into the cerebrospinal fluid (CSF) in the subarachnoid space. A certain amount of spread can be controlled by increasing the specific gravity of the solution and tilting the patient.

In epidural anaesthesia, the local anaesthetic is injected into the space between the dura mater and the spinal cord.

In both spinal and epidural anaesthesia, the local anaesthetic acts by blocking mainly spinal roots, as opposed to the spinal cord itself. Problems arise from the block of preganglionic sympathetic fibres causing vasodilatation and bradycardia and leading to hypotension. Rostral spread can lead to the blocking of intercostal and phrenic nerves and result in respiratory depression.

Unwanted effects
Unwanted effects of local anaesthetics are mainly associated with the spread of the drug into the systemic circulation. These include:

- Effects on the central nervous system (CNS) such as restlessness, tremor, confusion, and agitation. At high doses, CNS depression can occur. Procaine is worse than lignocaine or prilocaine for causing CNS depression. The exception is cocaine which, owing to its monoamine-uptake blocking activity, produces euphoria.
- Respiratory depression.
- Possible effects on the cardiovascular system, including myocardial depression and vasodilatation.
- Visual disturbances and twitching. Severe toxicity causes convulsions and coma.

Properties and uses
Fig. 2.7 shows the properties and uses of the main local anaesthetics, and Fig. 2.8 lists other compounds that block sodium channels.

Neuromuscular junction
Physiology of transduction
Skeletal (voluntary) muscle is innervated by motor neurons, the axons of which are able to propagate action potentials at high velocities.

The area of muscle that lies below the axon terminal is known as the motor end-plate, and the chemical synapse between the two is known as the neuromuscular junction (NMJ).

The axon terminal incorporates membrane-bound vesicles containing the neurotransmitter acetylcholine (ACh). Depolarization of the presynaptic terminal of the nerve by an action potential (generated by sodium influx) causes voltage-sensitive calcium channels to open, allowing calcium ions into the terminal.

Normally, the level of calcium ions inside the nerves is very low, 10 000 times lower than the external concentration. This calcium influx causes the release of ACh by exocytosis from vesicles. ACh diffuses across to the muscle membrane where it binds to the nicotinic acetylcholine receptor (nicAChR) and/or is inactivated

Properties and uses of the main local anaesthetics					
	Rate of onset	Duration	Tissue penetration	Chemistry	Common use
cocaine	rapid	moderate	rapid	ester bond	little used due to its side effects. Never inject
procaine	moderate	short	slow	ester bond	little used, CNS effects
amethocaine (tetracaine)	slow	long	moderate	ester bond	surface, ophthalmology
oxybuprocaine (benoxinate)	rapid	short	rapid	ester bond	surface, ophthalmology
benzocaine	very slow	very long	rapid	ester bond, no basic side chain	surface
lignocaine (lidocaine)	rapid	moderate	rapid	amide bond	widely used in all applications, EMLA
prilocaine	moderate	moderate	moderate	amide bond	many uses, IVRA, EMLA. Low toxicity
bupivacaine	slow	long	moderate	amide bond	epidural and spinal anaesthesia

Fig. 2.7 Properties and uses of the main local anaesthetics.

Fig. 2.8 Sodium channel blockers.

Sodium channel blockers		
Compound	Source	Type of block
tetrodotoxin	puffer fish	outside only
saxitoxin	plankton	outside only
μ-conotoxins	piscivorous marine snail	affects inactivation
μ-agatoxins	funnel web spider	affects inactivation
α-, β-, and γ-toxins	scorpions	complex
QX314 and QX222	synthetic, permanently charged local anaesthetics	inside only (hydrophilic pathway)
benzocaine	synthetic, uncharged local anaesthetic	from within the membrane (hydrophobic pathway)
local anaesthetics	plant (cocaine), others synthetic	inside and from within the membrane

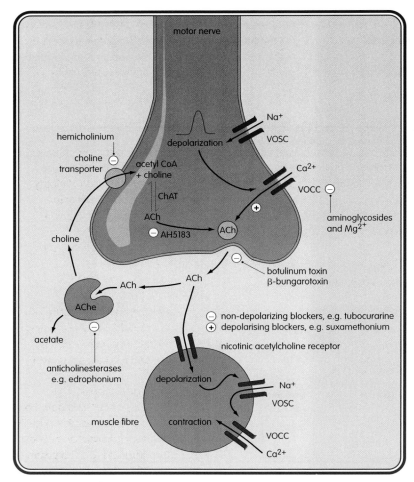

Fig. 2.9 Physiology of transduction at the neuromuscular junction (NMJ) showing the site of action of drugs used in conjunction with the NMJ. (VOSC, voltage-operated sodium channel; VOCC, voltage-operated calcium channel; AChe, acetylcholinesterase; ChAT, cholineacetyl transferase.)

by acetylcholinesterase (Fig. 2.9). Several events then occur:

- During association, ACh binds to the nicAChR, which is an ion channel that allows cations into the muscle (mainly sodium but also potassium to a lesser extent).
- During the conformational change, the pore of the ion channel is open for 1 ms, during which approximately 20 000 sodium ions enter the cell. The resulting depolarization, called an end-plate potential (EPP), depolarizes the adjacent muscle fibre.
- If the cellular response is large enough, an action potential is generated in the rest of the muscle fibre (sodium influx), resulting in the opening of voltage-operated calcium channels, but this time the calcium influx mediates contraction.
- ACh is rapidly inactivated by an enzyme called acetylcholinesterase (AChe) which hydrolyses ACh

into the inactive metabolites choline and acetic acid.
- In the synthesis of ACh, the choline generated is taken up by the nerve terminal where another enzyme, choline acetyl transferase (ChAT), converts it back to ACh to be re-used.

Nicotinic acetylcholine receptor

The nicAChR is made up of five subunits (two α, one β, one γ, and one δ) which traverse the membrane and surround a central pore. The four different subunits show high sequence homology.

ACh must bind to both of the α-subunits in order to open a channel.

Each subunit has four membrane-spanning regions (helices), i.e. each receptor has a total of 20. One of the transmembrane helices (M_2) from each subunit forms the lining of the channel pore (see Fig. 1.1).

Pharmacological targets of the NMJ

There are three major targets for clinically useful drugs (Fig. 2.10):

- The presynaptic release.
- The nicotinic acetylcholine receptor.
- Acetylcholinesterase.

Drugs used in association with the NMJ

Presynaptic agents

Drugs inhibiting ACh synthesis: The rate-limiting step in the synthesis of ACh is the uptake of choline into the nerve terminal.

Hemicholinium is an analogue of choline that blocks the choline transporter and causes a depletion of ACh stores. Because of the time taken for the stores to run down, the onset of this drug is slow. This, and the frequency-dependent nature of the block (depletion of stores is related to release of ACh), means that it is not useful clinically. The block is reversed by the addition of choline.

Drugs inhibiting vesicular packaging of ACh: AH5183 inhibits the active transport of ACh into storage vesicles and results in neuromuscular block.

Drugs inhibiting ACh release: Calcium entry into the nerve terminal is necessary for the release of ACh; thus, agents such as aminoglycoside antibiotics (e.g. streptomycin) that prevent this step will cause neuromuscular blockade. Muscle paralysis is

occasionally a side effect of aminoglycoside antibiotics, but can be reversed by the administration of calcium salts.

Botulinum toxin is a neurotoxin produced by the anaerobic bacillus *Clostridium botulinum*. The toxin is very potent and is believed to inhibit ACh release by inactivating actin which is necessary for exocytosis. In botulism, a serious type of food poisoning caused by this toxin, victims experience progressive parasympathetic and motor paralysis. Botulinum toxin type A is sometimes used clinically in the treatment of excessive muscle contraction disorders (dystonias) such as strabismus (squint), spasticity, and tremors.

β-Bungarotoxin contained in snake venom acts in a similar manner to botulinum toxin.

Postsynaptic agents

Non-depolarizing blockers: These act as competitive antagonists by binding to the nicAChR but not activating it, and producing motor paralysis. Details of the most commonly used non-depolarizing blockers are given in Fig. 2.11.

Approximately 80–90% of receptors must be blocked to prevent transmission, since the amount of ACh released by nerve terminal depolarization usually greatly exceeds that required to generate an action potential in the muscle. The drugs are all quaternary ammonium compounds and therefore do not cross the blood–brain barrier or the placenta. They are poorly absorbed orally and must be administered by intravenous injection. 'Tetanic fade' (i.e. non-maintained muscle tension during brief nerve stimulation) is seen with some of these drugs. This can be explained by the blocking of presynaptic autoreceptors which usually maintain the release of ACh during repeated stimulation.

The block can be reversed by anticholinesterases and depolarizing drugs. It is also enhanced in patients with myasthenia gravis. The main side effect from these drugs is hypotension caused by the blocking of ganglionic transmission. Histamine release from mast cells, resulting in bronchospasm, may be a problem in certain individuals (Fig. 2.11).

Depolarizing (non-competitive) blockers: Depolarizing blockers initially activate receptors, causing depolarization, but in doing so block further activation.

Targets for clinically useful drugs at the neuromuscular junction		
Site	**Action**	**Use**
nicAChR	block transmission	neuromuscular blockers for surgery
AChe	enhance transmission	peripheral neuropathy, e.g. myasthenia gravis
release	block transmission	spasms, e.g. squints, tics, tremors, etc.

Fig. 2.10 Targets for clinically useful drugs at the neuromuscular junction. Myasthenia gravis is an autoimmune disease in which there are decreased numbers of receptors at the end-plate. To allow normal neuromuscular function, drugs that increase the amount of acetylcholine in the cleft are given. (AChe, acetylcholine esterase; nicAChR, nicotinic acetylcholine receptor.)

Non-depolarizing blockers of postsynaptic receptors at the neuromuscular junction					
Drug	Approximate duration (mins)	Side effects			Elimination
		Ganglion block	Histamine release	Other	
tubocurarine	30–40	partial	sometimes	hypersensitivity (rare)	mainly hepatic
pancuronium	40–60	X	minimal	block of muscarinic receptors in the heart → tachycardia	mainly renal
gallamine	15	X	X	block of muscarinic receptors in the heart → tachycardia	mainly renal: avoid in patients with renal disease
alcuronium	20	X	X	dose dependency	mainly hepatic
vecuronium	20–30	X	X		mainly hepatic
atracurium	15–30	X	sometimes		degradation in plasma at body pH (Hofmann elimination)

Fig. 2.11 Non-depolarizing blockers of postsynaptic receptors at the neuromuscular junction.

Depolarizing blockers act on the motor end-plate in the same manner as ACh, i.e. they are agonists and increase the cation permeability of the end-plate. However, unlike ACh, which is released in brief spurts and rapidly hydrolysed, depolarizing blockers remain associated with the receptors long enough to cause a sustained depolarization and a resulting loss of electrical excitability (phase I).

Repeated or continuous administration of depolarizing blockers leads to the block becoming more characteristic of non-depolarizing drugs. This is known as phase II and is probably due to receptor desensitization, whereby the end-plate becomes less sensitive to ACh. The block starts to show tetanic fade and is partly reversed by anticholinesterase drugs.

Suxamethonium is the only depolarizing blocker used clinically because of its rapid onset time and short duration of action (approximately 4 minutes).

Suxamethonium:
- Is a quaternary ammonium compound and must be given by intravenous injection.
- Is rapidly hydrolysed by plasma cholinesterase, although certain people with a genetic variant of this enzyme may experience a neuromuscular block which may last for hours.

Depolarizing blockers have no effect in patients with myasthenia gravis, since these patients have a decreased number of receptors at the end-plate. In this instance, the blocking potency of depolarizing blockers is reduced.

The side effects of depolarizing blockers include:
- Initial spasms, which occur prior to paralysis, often resulting in postoperative muscle pain.
- Muscarinic receptor activation resulting in bradycardia. Bradycardia can be prevented by the administration of atropine.
- Potassium release from muscle resulting in elevated plasma potassium levels. This is usually a problem only in the case of trauma.

Anticholinesterases

Anticholinesterases inhibit AChe and thus increase the amount of ACh in the synaptic cleft and enhance cholinergic transmission.

Most of the anticholinesterases used are quaternary ammonium compounds and thus do not penetrate the blood–brain barrier.

Short-acting anticholinesterases include edrophonium. This is selective for the NMJ and clinically relevant in the diagnosis of myasthenia gravis. Edrophonium's duration of action is only 2–10 minutes because it binds by electrostatic forces (no covalent bonds) to the active site of the enzyme. Edrophonium is therefore not used therapeutically.

Intermediate-acting anticholinesterases include neostigmine, pyridostigmine, and physostigmine.

Neostigmine is used intravenously to reverse the effects of non-depolarizing blockers. It's duration of action is 2–4 hours, and it is used orally in the treatment of myasthenia gravis. Although neostigmine shows some selectivity for the NMJ, atropine is sometimes co-administered to block the muscarinic effects of the drug.

Pyridostigmine has a duration of action of 3–6 hours, and is also used orally in the treatment of myasthenia gravis. It has few parasympathetic actions.

Physostigmine: shows selectivity for the postganglionic parasympathetic junction. It is a tertiary amine and its use is therefore associated with central effects such as initial excitation followed by depression and possibly respiratory depression and unconsciousness. The central effects can be antagonized by atropine. Physostigmine is used in the form of eye drops to constrict the pupil and contract the ciliary muscle in the treatment of glaucoma.

Most of the long-lasting or irreversible anticholinesterases are organophosphorous compounds. For example sarin and tabun were developed as nerve gases, and parathion was developed as an insecticide, as well as for clinical use. These drugs have many adverse effects, such as bradycardia, hypotension, breathing problems, depolarizing neuromuscular block, central effects, and possible death from peripheral nerve demyelination. Ecothiopate shows selectivity for the postganglionic parasympathetic junction and is used in the treatment of glaucoma.

A simple mnemonic for the main local anaesthetics is Cocaine Potentially Allows Ordinary Beings Lasting Pain Block (cocaine, procaine, amethocaine, oxybuprocaine, benzocaine, lignocaine, prilocaine and bupivacaine).

A simple mnemonic for the main non-depolarizing blockers is Vercuronium Prevents Absolute Transmission At Ganglia (vercuronium, pancuronium, alcuronium, tubocurarine, atracurium, and gallamine).

- How does the size of a nerve fibre affect its potential to be blocked?
- Summarize the mechanism of action of local anaesthetics, the importance of pH, and the two routes by which block occurs.
- Describe how presynaptic agents can be used to block transmission at the NMJ. Give examples and describe their clinical use.
- What are the distinguishing characteristics between non-depolarizing and depolarizing postsynaptic blockers? Give examples and describe their clinical use.
- Discuss, and give examples of, the effects of anticholinesterases and how these are used clinically.

AUTONOMIC NERVOUS SYSTEM

Basic concepts

The autonomic nervous system is the means by which all tissues other than skeletal muscle are innervated (Fig. 2.12.)

The axons of the autonomic nervous system leave their cell body, which is located in the CNS, as preganglionic fibres, synapse in the appropriate ganglion, and leave as postganglionic fibres. These postganglionic fibres reach the effector cells.

The neurotransmitter released by preganglionic fibres at autonomic ganglia, regardless of whether sympathetic or parasympathetic, is ACh.

The ACh receptors located on postganglionic fibres are of the nicotinic type.

In general, the sympathetic and parasympathetic systems mediate opposite effects (see Fig. 2.20).

Autonomic ganglia

Fig. 2.13 summarizes the differences between ganglionic nicAChR and those found on skeletal muscle at the NMJ.

Ganglion-stimulating drugs
Nicotinic agonists

There are few agonists that act selectively on the nicAChR without affecting muscarinic receptors. Carbachol is the best example of a drug that shows preference for the nicotinic receptor, but its action is not selective. Nicotine and lobeline both show preference for ganglionic nicotinic receptors, but at slightly higher concentrations than those needed to affect ganglionic transmission. Nicotine and lobeline are able to stimulate the NMJ.

These drugs have no clinical use, since their range of effects is vast, affecting both sympathetic and parasympathetic transmission:

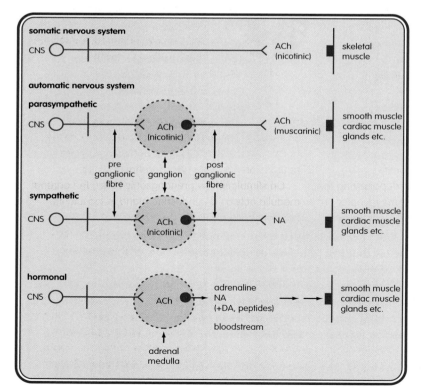

Fig. 2.12 Somatic and autonomic nervous systems: organization and neurotransmitters. (ACh, acetylcholine; CNS, central nervous system; DA, dopamine; NA, noradrenaline.)

Distinguishing features of nicotinic acetylcholine receptors		
	Skeletal muscle	**Neurons**
structure	2α 1β 1γ or ϵ 1δ	2α 3β
specific agonists	suxamethonium	DMPP
specific antagonists	gallamine tubocurarine α-bungarotoxin	hexamethonium mecamylamine κ-bungarotoxin
function	end-plate region depolarization at NMJ	neuronal depolarisation in ganglia and CNS

Fig. 2.13 Distinguishing features of the ganglionic nicotinic acetylcholine receptors and those found on skeletal muscle at the neuromuscular junction. (DMPP, dimethylphenyl-piperazinium.)

- Sympathetic effects include tachycardia and vasoconstriction leading to hypertension.
- Parasympathetic effects include increased gastrointestinal motility and glandular secretions.

Ganglion-blocking drugs

Autonomic ganglia can be blocked presynaptically by inhibiting ACh synthesis, vesicular packaging, or release (p. 27), or postsynaptically by blocking the nicotinic receptors.

Non-depolarizing ganglion blockers

A few of these drugs act solely as competitive antagonists, blocking receptors without depolarizing the ganglion. However, most block not only the receptor but also the ion channel associated with the receptor, and produce their action through this latter mechanism. For example:

- Some ganglion blockers such as tubocurarine are not antagonists at the ganglionic nicotinic receptor, but produce ganglion block through channel blockade.
- Tubocurarine also blocks transmission at the NMJ but does this through receptor antagonism.
- Hexamethonium was initially developed for use against hypertension, but is no longer in clinical use.

- Trimetaphan is the only clinically useful ganglion blocker. It is used where controlled hypotension is needed, such as in anaesthesia. It has a short duration of action and can be administered intravenously.

Ganglion-blocking drugs have a wide range of complex effects, although the sympathetic and parasympathetic systems tend to oppose one another. (Paton describes the 'hexamethonium man.') The effects of ganglion-blocking drugs include:

- Arteriolar vasodilatation leading to a marked reduction in blood pressure (block of sympathetic ganglia).
- Postural and postexercise hypotension (loss of cardiac reflexes).
- Slight reduction in cardiac output.
- Inhibition of gastrointestinal secretions and motility, leading to constipation, urinary retention, impotence, and failure of ejaculation.

Sympathetic nervous system

The fibres of the sympathetic nervous system leave the CNS from the thoracolumbar regions of the spinal cord (T1–L3). They synapse in ganglia located close to the spinal cord. These ganglia form a chain along each side of the spinal cord and are thus known as sympathetic trunks.

The major transmitter released by postganglionic fibres at the junction with effector cells is noradrenaline (NA).

Adrenal medulla

Some postganglionic neurons in the sympathetic division do not have axons, but instead release their transmitters directly into the bloodstream. These neurons are located in the adrenal medulla.

On stimulation by preganglionic fibres, the adrenal medulla acts as an endocrine gland, releasing its hormones/transmitters which consist of ~80% adrenaline, ~20% noradrenaline, as well as small amounts of dopamine, neuropeptides, and ATP.

Adrenoceptors

In 1913 Henry Dale observed that adrenaline constricted some blood vessels but relaxed others, while in 1948 Ahlquist defined two receptor subtypes based on the rank order of potency of three agonists, namely isoprenaline, adrenaline, and noradrenaline. The two receptor subtypes were α and β. Potency at:

- α-receptors is noradrenaline > adrenaline > isoprenaline.
- β-receptors is isoprenaline > adrenaline > noradrenaline.

Effects mediated by α-adrenoreceptors
α₁-Receptors
α_1-Receptors are located postsynaptically. Their activation causes smooth muscle contraction (except for the non-sphincter part of the gastrointestinal tract, where activation causes relaxation), glycogenolysis in the liver, and potassium release from the liver and salivary glands. Transduction is via G-proteins and an increase in the second messengers inositol (1,4,5) triphosphate (IP_3) and diacylglycerol (DAG).

α₂-Receptors
α_2-Receptors are located mainly presynaptically, but also postsynaptically on liver cells, platelets, and the smooth muscle of blood vessels. The activation of presynaptic α_2-receptors inhibits noradrenaline release and therefore provides a means of end-product negative feedback. Activation of postsynaptic α_2-receptors causes blood vessel constriction and platelet aggregation. Transduction is via G-proteins and a decrease in the second messenger cyclic adenosine monophosphate (cAMP).

Effects mediated by β-adrenoceptors
β₁-Receptors
β_1-Receptors are mainly postsynaptic and located in the heart, platelets, and non-sphincter part of the gastrointestinal tract. They can, however, be found presynaptically. Activation causes an increase in the rate and force of contraction of the heart, relaxation of the non-sphincter part of the gastrointestinal tract, aggregation of platelets, an increase in the release of noradrenaline, lipolysis in fat, and amylase secretion from the salivary glands. Presynaptically, their activation causes an increase in noradrenaline release. Transduction is via G-proteins and an increase in the second messenger cAMP.

β₂-Receptors
β_2-Receptors are located postsynaptically. Their activation causes smooth muscle relaxation, glycogenolysis in the liver, inhibition of histamine release from mast cells, and tremor in skeletal muscle. Transduction is via G-proteins and an increase in the second messenger cAMP.

Drugs acting on the sympathetic system
Fig. 2.14 summarizes the drugs acting on the sympathetic system.

Presynaptic agents
Noradrenaline synthesis: The precursor to noradrenaline is L-tyrosine, which is taken by adrenergic neurons.
Drugs decreasing noradrenaline synthesis: The rate-limiting step (RLS) is the conversion of tyrosine to dihydroxyphenylalanine (dopa), which is catalyzed by tyrosine hydroxylase and inhibited by a methyltyrosine. Noradrenaline provides a negative feedback upon this step. Carbidopa inhibits dopa decarboxylase and is used in Parkinson's disease to increase dopamine levels. Because this is not the RLS, drugs that inhibit dopa decarboxylase do not greatly affect noradrenaline synthesis. Administering α-methyldopa (used in hypertension) results in the formation of a false transmitter, α-methylnoradrenaline.
Drugs increasing noradrenaline synthesis: Levodopa (L-dopa) administration bypasses the RLS and is used in Parkinson's disease.

Noradrenaline is stored in vesicles as a complex with ATP and a protein called chromogranin A.
Drugs inhibiting noradrenaline storage: Reserpine is a drug used in the treatment of hypertension and schizophrenia. It reduces stores of noradrenaline by preventing the accumulation of noradrenaline in vesicles. Its action is effectively irreversible since it has a very high affinity for the noradrenaline storage site. The displaced noradrenaline is immediately broken down by monoamine oxygenase (MAO) and is therefore unable to exert sympathetic effects.
Drugs inhibiting the breakdown of leaked noradrenaline stores: These include monoamine oxidase inhibitors (MAOIs), which are used in the treatment of depression and Parkinson's disease. They prevent the breakdown of leaked catecholamines so that noradrenaline that leaves the vesicles is protected and eventually leaks out from the nerve ending.
Drugs inhibiting noradrenaline release: These include guanethidine and bretylium. These are adrenergic neuron-blocking drugs that prevent the exocytosis of noradrenaline from nerve terminals and are used as

hypotensive drugs. They are taken up by uptake 1 (see p. 34) and concentrated in nerve terminals where they have a local anaesthetic effect on impulse conduction. The tricyclic antidepressants, which inhibit uptake 1, prevent these drugs from exerting their effects. Clonidine is an α_2-receptor agonist and therefore inhibits noradrenaline release.

Drugs promoting noradrenaline release: These include: amphetamines, tyramine, and ephedrine, which are sympathomimetic drugs that act indirectly. They are taken up by uptake 1 and displace noradrenaline from the vesicles. Because they also inhibit MAO, the displaced noradrenaline is not broken down and is able to exert sympathetic effects. These drugs act in part through a direct agonist effect on adrenoceptors.

Yohimbine is an α_2-receptor antagonist and therefore prevents noradrenaline from exerting a negative feedback effect on noradrenaline release.

Postsynaptic agents

Adrenoceptor agonists: These are termed 'sympathomimetics'. They activate postsynaptic receptors, eliciting a response (Fig. 2.15).

Adrenoceptor antagonists: These are termed 'sympatholytics. They block postsynaptic receptors (Fig. 2.16).

Inactivation

Uptake 1: This is located on neuronal terminals and is the main mechanism for noradrenaline inactivation.

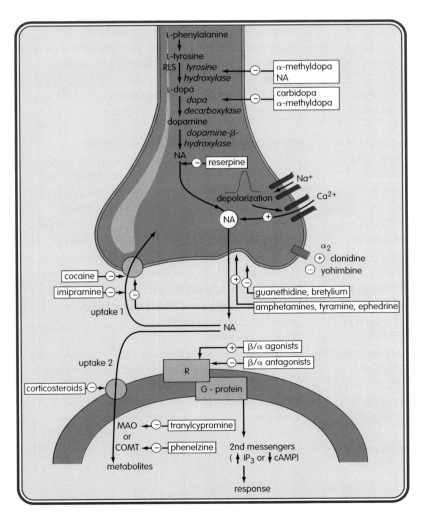

Fig. 2.14 Drugs affecting adrenergic transmission. (cAMP, cyclic adenosine monophosphate; COMT, catechol-*O*-methyltransferase; IP$_3$, inositol triphosphate; MAO, monoamine oxidase; NA, noradrenaline.)

Uptake 1 has a high affinity for the uptake of noradrenaline (K = 0.3 mmol/L in the rat) but the maximum rate of uptake is low (V_{max} = 1.2 nmol/g/min in the rat). It has a specificity rank of noradrenaline > adrenaline> isoprenaline; and is blocked by cocaine, amphetamines, and tricyclic antidepressants (e.g. imipramine), which therefore potentiate the actions of noradrenaline.

Uptake 2: This is located outside neurons, e.g. in smooth muscle, cardiac muscle, and endothelium, and is the main mechanism for the removal of circulating adrenaline from the bloodstream. It has a low affinity for the uptake of noradrenaline (K = 250 mmol/L in the rat) but a high maximum rate of uptake (V_{max} = 100 nmol/g/min in the rat). Uptake 2 has a specificity rank of adrenaline > noradrenaline > isoprenaline and is blocked by corticosteroids.

Metabolism of catecholamines by monoamine oxidase: MAO is found on the surface of mitochondria, principally within adrenergic nerve terminals but also in other cells, such as those of the liver and intestines. MAO metabolizes catecholamines into their corresponding aldehydes. It comprises two major forms: MAOA and MAOB. Noradrenaline is mainly broken down by MAOA in nerve terminals.

Inhibitors of MAO increase the releasable store of noradrenaline but do not greatly potentiate sympathetic transmission, since catecholamines are mainly inactivated by reuptake. MAOIs include the antidepressant drugs phenelzine and tranylcypromine.

Metabolism of catecholamines by catechol-O-methyltransferase: Catechol-*O*-methyltransferase (COMT) is found in all tissues and breaks down most catecholamines and the byproducts of the actions of MAO. COMT metabolizes catecholamines to give a methoxy derivative.

Parasympathetic nervous system

The fibres of the parasympathetic nervous system leave the CNS from the sacral region (S3 and S4) of the spinal cord and via cranial nerves 3, 7, 9, and 10. The fibres synapse in ganglia, which, unlike the sympathetic system, are located within the innervated organs themselves.

The major transmitter released by postganglionic fibres at the junction with effector cells is ACh.

Parasympathetic receptors

The ACh released by postganglionic nerve fibres acts on muscarinic receptors, of which between three and five subtypes exist.

'Neuroparietal' M_1 receptors

M_1 'neuroparietal' receptors are principally found in the CNS, peripheral neurons, and gastric parietal cells. Their effects tend to be excitatory, depolarizing membranes through a decrease in potassium conductance. Activation causes central excitation and gastric acid secretion, while transduction is via G-proteins and an increase in the second messengers IP_3 and DAG through stimulation of phospholipase C.

'Neurocardiac' M_2 receptors

M_2 'neurocardiac' receptors are found in the heart and on peripheral neurons. Their effects are inhibitory, increasing potassium conductance and inhibiting calcium channels. In the heart, their activation causes a decrease in the rate (via potassium) and force of contraction (via calcium). Transduction is via G-proteins and a decrease in the second messenger cAMP through inhibition of adenylyl cyclase.

'Smooth muscle–glandular' M_3 receptors

M_3 'smooth muscle–glandular' receptors are found in smooth muscle and glands. Their effects tend to be excitatory, increasing sodium conductance. Activation causes glandular secretions such as saliva and sweat, and smooth muscle contraction. Transduction is via G-proteins and an increase in the second messengers IP_3 and DAG. M_3 receptors are also located on vascular endothelium, activation of which causes vasodilatation through the release of endothelium-derived relaxing factor (EDRF).

'Eye' M_4 receptors

M_4 'eye' receptors are believed to be exclusive to the eye. Their activation causes constriction of the pupil and accommodation for near vision. Transduction is via G-proteins and an decrease in the second messenger cAMP through inhibition of adenylyl cyclase.

Adrenoceptor agonists				
Drug	**Receptor**	**Uses**	**Side effects**	**Phamacokinetics**
noradrenaline	α/β	no use clinically	hypertension, tachycardia ventricular arrhythmias	poor oral absorption, metabolized by MAO and COMT, $t_{1/2} \sim$ 2 min
adrenaline	α/β	anaphylactic shock cardiac resuscitation with local anaesthetics	hypertension, tachycardia ventricular arrhythmias	poor oral absorption, metabolized by MAO and COMT, $t_{1/2} \sim$ 2 min given intravenously or intramuscularly
oxymetazoline	α	nasal decongestant	rebound congestion	given intranasally
phenylephrine	$α_1$	hypotension nasal decongestant	hypertension reflex bradycardia	metabolized by MAO $t_{1/2} <$ 1 min, given intramuscularly or intranasally
clonidine	$α_2$	hypertension migraine	drowsiness, hypotension	good oral absorption, $t_{1/2} \sim$ 12 h
isoprenaline	β	asthma cardiac resuscitation	arrhythmias, tachycardia	metabolized by COMT, given sublingually or as aerosal $t_{1/2} \sim$ 2 h
dobutamine	$β_1$	heart failure	tachycardia	
salbutamol	$β_2$	asthma premature labour	arrhythmias, tachycardia, vasodilatation	given by aerosol $t_{1/2} \sim$ 4 h

Fig. 2.15 Adrenoceptor agonists. (COMT, catechol-*O*-methyltransferase; MAO, monoamine oxidase.)

Adrenoceptor antagonists				
Drug	**Receptor**	**Uses**	**Side effects**	**Pharmacokinetics**
labetalol	α/β	hypertension	postural hypotension	oral absorption $t_{1/2} \sim$ 4 h
phentolamine	α	no clinical use	hypotension tachycardia nasal congestion	metabolized by the liver, given intravenously $t_{1/2} \sim$ 2 h
prazosin	$α_1$	hypertension	hypotension tachycardia nasal congestion drowsiness	oral absorption, metabolized by the liver $t_{1/2} \sim$ 4 h
yohimbine	$α_2$	no clinical use	hypertension excitement	oral absorption, metabolized by the liver $t_{1/2} \sim$ 4 h
propranolol	β	hypertension angina arrhythmias	bronchoconstriction heart failure	oral absorption, first-pass metabolism, 90% plasma-protein-bound $t_{1/2} \sim$ 4 h
practolol	$β_1$	hypertension angina arrhythmias	bronchoconstriction heart failure	oral absorption $t_{1/2} \sim$ 4 h
butoxamine	$β_2$	no clinical use		

Fig. 2.16 Adrenoceptor antagonists. (COMT, catechol-*O*-methyltransferase; MAO, monoamine oxidase.)

Drugs acting on the parasympathetic system

Fig. 2.17 summarizes the drugs that act on the parasympathetic system.

Presynaptic agents

For information regarding presynaptic agents, see p. 27.

Anticholinesterases

For information regarding anticholinesterases, see pp. 29–30.

Postsynaptic agents

Muscarinic-receptor agonists: These are termed 'parasympathomimetic', they activate postsynaptic receptors (Fig. 2.18).

Muscarinic-receptor antagonists: These are termed 'parasympatholytic' and block postsynaptic receptors (Fig. 2.19).

Non-selective antagonists can be used in anaesthesia to prevent bronchial secretions and vagal slowing of heart rate.

Different tissues respond differently to muscarinic antagonists (Fig. 2.20). Salivary, sweat, and bronchial glands are the most sensitive and can be blocked by very low doses of atropine. In contrast, the parietal cells are the most resistant, and the block of gastric acid secretion requires high doses of atropine.

The side effects of muscarinic antagonists include:

- Dry mouth and skin, and increased body temperature (inhibition of salivary and sweat glands).
- Blurred vision and pupil no longer responsive to light (dilatation of pupil).
- Paralysis of accommodation: cycloplegia (relaxation of ciliary muscle).
- Urinary retention.
- Central excitation: irritability and hyperactivity.
- Sedation (hyoscine).

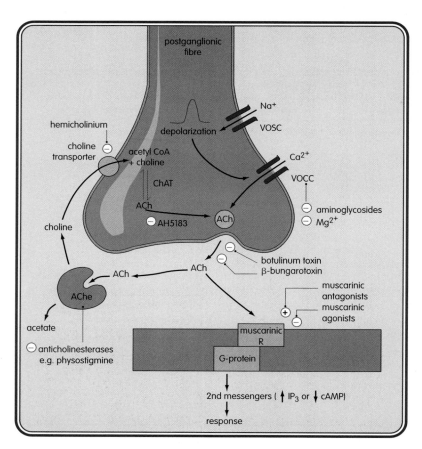

Fig. 2.17 Drugs acting on the parasympathetic nervous system. (VOSC, voltage-operated sodium channel; VOCC, voltage-operated calcium channel; AChe, acetylcholinesterase; ChAT, cholineacetyl transferase.)

Drugs acting on the parasympathetic nervous system			
Drug	Muscarinic receptors	Nicotinic receptors	Uses
carbachol	++	+	gut and bladder stimulation postoperatively
methacholine	+++	+	
bethanechol	+++	—	gut and bladder stimulation postoperatively
muscarine	+++	—	
pilocarpine	++	—	to decrease intraocular pressure in glaucoma

Fig. 2.18 Muscarinic agonists.

Sympathetic transmission is enhanced under conditions of stress, known as the 'fight–or–flight response'.

Fig. 2.19 Muscarinic antagonists.

Muscarinic antagonists		
Drug	Muscarinic receptor	Specific uses
atropine	non-selective	reduces gastrointestinal motility
hyoscine	non-selective	motion sickness
ipratropium	non-selective	bronchodilator
cyclopentolate	M_4	dilation of pupil
tropicamide	M_4	dilation of pupil
pirenzipine	M_1	reduces gastric acid secretion
benzhexol	M_1	Parkinson's disease

- What distinguishes nicotinic receptors found at the NMJ from those found at autonomic ganglia?
- Summarize the different ways in which ganglia can be stimulated or blocked, and state whether these are of clinical use. Give examples of drugs.
- How do drugs interfere with NA synthesis, storage, release, receptors, and inactivation? How are these drugs used clinically? Give examples of each.
- How do drugs interfere with ACh synthesis, storage, release, receptors, and inactivation? How are these drugs used clinically? Give examples of each.

Effects of sympathetic and parasympathetic nerve stimulation					
Target tissue	**Sympathetic**		**Parasympathetic**		**Overall effect**
nerve terminals	α_2	decreased release	M_2	decreased release	decreased transmission
smooth muscle					
blood vessels	$\alpha_{1/2}$ β_2	contraction relaxation	M_3	relaxation (via EDRF)	vasoconstriction vasodilation
bronchi	β_2 α_1	relaxation contraction	M_3 M_3	contraction secretion	bronchodilatation bronchoconstriction bronchsecretion
gastrointestinal tract: non-sphincter sphincter secretions	β_1/α_1 α_1	relaxation contraction	M_3 M_3 M_3	contraction relaxation secretion	increased/decreased motility and tone GI secretions
parietal cells			M_1	contraction	gastric acid secretion
pancreas			M_3	contraction	increased secretions
uterus	α_1 β_2	contraction relaxation	M_3 M_3		
bladder: detrusor sphincter	β_2 α_1	relaxation contraction	M_3 M_3	contraction relaxation	micturition urine retention
seminal tract vas deferens penis venous sphincter	α_1 β_2 α_1	contraction relaxation contraction	 M_3	 vasodilation	ejaculation ejaculation erection
radial muscle (iris) ciliary muscle lacrimal gland	α_1 β_2	contraction relaxation	M_4 M_4 M_4	relaxation contraction contraction	pupil relaxation/constriction accommodation tear secretion
heart	β_1	increased rate and force	M_2	decreased rate and force	
liver	α_1/β_2	glycogenolysis			
fat	β_1	lipolysis			
salivary glands	α_1/β_1	secretion of thick saliva	M_3	abundant secretion of watery saliva	
platelets	α_2	platelet aggregation			
mast cells	β_2	inhibition of histamine release			

Fig. 2.20 Summary table of the opposing effects of sympathetic and parasympathetic nerve stimulation on body tissues.

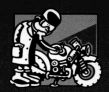
PARKINSONISM

Parkinson's disease and parkinsonism

Definitions

Parkinson's disease is a progressive neurological disorder of the basal ganglia that occurs most commonly in the elderly.

Parkinsonism is the condition caused by Parkinson's disease. Parkinsonism is characterized by a resting tremor, slow initiation of movements (bradykinesia), and muscle rigidity known collectively as the 'parkinsonian triad'. A patient with parkinsonism will present with characteristic signs including:

- A shuffling gait.
- A blank 'mask-like' facial expression.
- Speech impairment.
- An inability to perform skilled tasks.

Pathogenesis

Analysis of brains of parkinsonian patients post mortem shows a substantially reduced concentration of dopamine (less than 10% of normal) in the basal ganglia. The basal ganglia exert an extrapyramidal neural influence that normally acts to maintain smooth voluntary movement.

The main pathology in Parkinson's disease is a progressive degeneration of the dopaminergic neurons of the substantia nigra, which project in the nigrostriatal pathway to the corpus striatum (Fig. 3.1). The inhibitory dopaminergic activity of the nigrostriatal pathway is therefore considerably reduced (by 20–40%) in people with Parkinson's disease.

The reduction in the inhibitory dopaminergic activity of the nigrostriatal pathway results in cholinergic neuron hyperactivity from the corpus striatum, which contributes to the pathological features of parkinsonism. Frank symptoms of parkinsonism appear only when more than 80% of the dopaminergic neurons of the substantia nigra have degenerated.

Parkinsonism is progressive, with continued loss of dopaminergic neurons in the substantia nigra correlating well with worsening of clinical symptoms. Untreated Parkinson's disease is progressive, leading eventually to dementia and death.

Aetiology

The cause of Parkinson's disease is unknown in most cases ('idiopathic') although both endogenous and environmental neurotoxins have been sought (Fig. 3.2).

The possibility of a neurotoxic cause has been strengthened by the finding that 1-methyl-4-phenyl-1,2,3,6-tetrahydropyridine (MPTP), which is a chemical contaminant produced in the synthesis of heroin substitutes, causes irreversible damage to the nigrostriatal dopaminergic pathway. This damage can lead to the development of symptoms similar to those of idiopathic Parkinson's disease, and has been seen in Californian drug addicts and induced in experimental primates.

Parkinsonism can also be induced by drugs that block dopamine receptors. Neuroleptic drugs (p. 52) used in the treatment of schizophrenia can produce a parkinsonian-like disease as an adverse effect.

Aetiology of parkinsonism
• mostly unknown (idiopathic)
• toxin induced: MPTP; carbon monoxide, manganese
• drug induced: neuroleptics (dopamine antagonists)
• rare causes: cerebral ischaemia; viral encephalitis and others?

Fig. 3.2 Aetiological mechanisms in the development of Parkinson's disease. (MPTP, methyl-4-phenyl-1,2,3,6-tetrahydropyridine.)

Fig. 3.1 Basal ganglia systems involved in Parkinson's disease. (DA, dopamine; GABA, γ-aminobutyric acid.)

corpus striatum   thalamus   motor cortex

GABA

ACh

degenerates in Parkinson's disease   DA   GABA   impulse travels via the spinal cord to muscles

substantia nigra

Rare causes of parkinsonism are cerebral ischaemia (progressive atheroschlerosis or stroke), viral encephalitis, or other pathological damage.

Treatment of parkinsonism

The treatment of parkinsonism is based on correcting the imbalance between the dopaminergic and cholinergic systems at the basal ganglia (Fig. 3.3). Two major groups of drugs are used: drugs that increase dopaminergic activity between the substantia nigra and the corpus striatum, and anticholinergic drugs that inhibit striatal cholinergic activity. The former drugs include:

- Dopamine precursors.
- Dopamine agonists.
- Drugs stimulating the release of dopamine.
- Monoamine oxidase B (MAO_B) inhibitors.

Drugs that increase dopaminergic activity

Dopamine precursors

An example of a dopamine precursor is levodopa (L-dopa).
Mechanism of action: L-dopa is the immediate precursor of dopamine and is able to penetrate the blood–brain barrier to replenish the dopamine content of the corpus striatum. L-dopa is decarboxylated to dopamine in the brain by dopa decarboxylase and has beneficial effects produced through the actions of dopamine on D_2 receptors (Fig. 3.3). Dopamine itself is not used, owing to its inability to cross the blood–brain barrier.
Route of administration: L-dopa is administered orally. It reaches peak plasma concentrations after 1–2 h, and only 1% reaches the brain, owing to peripheral metabolism.
Indications: L-dopa is used in the treatment of parkinsonism.
Contraindications: Should not be used in people with closed-angle glaucoma.
Adverse effects: The extensive peripheral metabolism of L-dopa means that large doses have to be given to produce therapeutic effects in the brain. However, large doses produce several adverse effects. These include:

- Nausea and vomiting.
- Psychiatric side effects.
- Cardiovascular effects.
- Dyskinesias.

Nausea and vomiting are caused by stimulation of dopamine receptors in the chemoreceptor trigger zone in the area postrema, which lies outside the blood–brain barrier.

Psychiatric side effects are common limiting factors in L-dopa treatment and include vivid dreams, confusion, and psychotic symptoms more commonly seen in schizophrenia. These effects are probably due to increased dopaminergic activity in the mesolimbic area of the brain, possibly similar to that found pathologically in schizophrenia (dopaminergic overactivity is implicated in schizophrenia, p. 52).

Hypotension is common but usually asymptomatic. Cardiac arrhythmias are due to increased catecholamine stimulation following the excessive peripheral metabolism of L-dopa.

Dyskinesias can often develop and tend to involve the face and limbs. They usually reflect over-treatment and respond to simple dose reduction.

Three strategies have been developed to optimize L-dopa treatment, that is to maximize the central effects of L-dopa and minimize its unwanted peripheral effects. These strategies involve co-administration of:

- Carbidopa, an inhibitor of dopa decarboxylase in the periphery, that cannot penetrate the blood–brain barrier. Hence, extracerebral conversion of L-dopa to dopamine is inhibited.
- Domperidone, a dopamine antagonist, that does not penetrate the blood–brain barrier and can therefore block the stimulation of dopamine receptors in the periphery.
- Selegiline, a MAO_B inhibitor that inhibits dopamine degradation in the central nervous system (CNS).

Therapeutic notes: Initially, treatment with L-dopa is effective in 80% of patients with possible restoration of near-normal motor function, but although L-dopa restores dopamine levels in the short term, therapy has no effect on the underlying degenerative disease process.

As progressive neuronal degeneration continues, the capacity of the corpus striatum to buffer fluctuating L-dopa levels becomes reduced. This affects the majority of patients within 5 years and manifests itself as 'end of dose deterioration'—a shortening of duration of each dose of L-dopa, and the 'on–off effect', rapid fluctuations in clinical state, varying from increased mobility and a general improvement to increased rigidity and hypokinesia. The latter effect occurs suddenly and for short periods from a few minutes to a few hours, tending to worsen with length of treatment.

Dopamine agonists

Examples of dopamine agonists include bromocriptine, lysuride, and apomorphine.

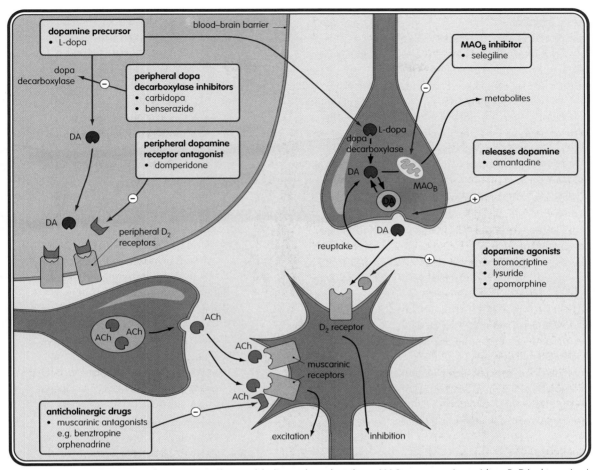

Fig. 3.3 Drugs used to treat parkinsonism. (ACh, acetylcholine; L-dopa, levodopa; MAO_B, monoamine oxidase B; DA, dopamine.)

Mechanism of action: Bromocriptine, lysuride, and apomorphine are dopamine agonists selective for the D_2 receptor (Fig. 3.3). Apomorphine also has agonist action at D_1 receptors.

Indications: Dopamine agonists are used in combination with L-dopa in an attempt to reduce the late adverse effects of L-dopa therapy ('end of dose deterioration' and 'on–off effect') or when L-dopa alone does not adequately control the symptoms.

Adverse effects: The adverse effects of dopamine agonists are essentially similar to those of L-dopa (i.e. nausea, postural hypotension, psychiatric symptoms), but tend to be more common and more severe.

Therapeutic notes: Currently, bromocriptine is the most clinically used of the dopamine agonists in the treatment of Parkinson's disease. A new drug, pergolide, which relieves symptoms as effectively as bromocriptine with fewer adverse effects, is undergoing clinical evaluation.

Drugs stimulating release of dopamine

Amantadine is an example of a drug that stimulates the release of dopamine (Fig. 3.3).

Mechanism of action: Facilitation of neuronal dopamine release and inhibition of its reuptake into nerves, and additional muscarinic blocking actions.

Route of administration: Amantadine is administered orally.

Indications: Amantidine has a synergistic effect when used in conjunction with L-dopa therapy in Parkinson's disease.

Adverse effects: Side effects of amantadine include anorexia, nausea, and hallucinations.

Therapeutic notes: Amantadine has modest antiparkinsonian effects but is only of short-term benefit, since most of its effectiveness is lost within 6 months of initiating treatment.

41

MAO$_B$ inhibitors

Selegiline is an example of a MAO$_B$ inhibitor.

Mechanism of action: Selegiline selectively inhibits the MAO$_B$ enzyme in the brain that is normally responsible for the degradation of dopamine (Fig. 3.3). By reducing the catabolism of dopamine, the actions of L-dopa are potentiated, thus allowing the dose to be reduced by up to one-third. There is evidence to suggest that selegiline may slow the progression of the underlying neuronal degeneration in Parkinson's disease.

Indications: MAO$_B$ inhibitors can be used on their own in mild cases of parkinsonism or in conjunction with L-dopa to reduce 'end-of-dose' deterioration in severe parkinsonism.

Adverse effects: The adverse effects of MAO$_B$ inhibitors are those that might be expected by potentiation of L-dopa.

Drugs that inhibit striatal cholinergic activity

Anticholinergic agents

Benztropine and orphenadrine are examples of anticholinergic agents.

Mechanism of action: Benztropine and orphenadrine are antagonists at the muscarinic receptors that mediate striatal cholinergic excitation (Fig. 3.3). Their major action in the treatment of Parkinson's disease is to reduce the excessive striatal cholinergic activity that characterizes the disease.

Adverse effects: Typical peripheral anticholinergic effects, such as a dry mouth and blurred vision, are less common. More often, patients experience a variety of CNS effects, ranging from mild memory loss to acute confusional states.

Therapeutic notes: Termination of anticholinergic treatment should be gradual, as parkinsonism can worsen when these drugs are withdrawn. Anticholinergic drugs are more effective in controlling tremor than other symptoms of Parkinson's disease.

Transplantation

The transplantation of cells from the substantia nigra of human fetuses into the putamen of patients with Parkinson's disease has shown some success, with graft survival and modest improvement in parkinsonian symptoms.

Transplantation in the treatment of Parkinson's disease is still experimental and its role is not yet clear.

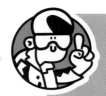

Note that with the possible exception of selegiline, none of the drugs used in Parkinson's disease affect the inevitable progressive degeneration of nigrostriatal dopaminergic neurons. The disease process is unaffected, just compensated for by drug therapy.

○ **Describe the signs and symptoms of Parkinson's disease and the neural pathology responsible.**

○ **How do the different classes of drug used in Parkinson's disease correct the neurotransmitter imbalances found in patients with this condition?**

○ **Describe the different ways in which dopaminergic activity can be increased in the basal ganglia.**

○ **What is the rationale for optimizing L-dopa treatment and reducing adverse effects; name the drugs used.**

ANXIOLYTICS AND HYPNOTICS

Anxiety and anxiolytics

Anxiety is a state characterized by psychological symptoms such as a diffuse, unpleasant and vague feeling of apprehension, often accompanied by physical symptoms of autonomic arousal such as headache, palpitations, perspiration, 'butterflies', and, in some people, restlessness.

While occasional anxiety is perfectly normal, it is a common and disabling symptom in a variety of mental illnesses including phobias, panic disorders, and obsessive compulsive disorders. Drugs used to treat such anxiety disorders are called anxiolytics.

Sleep disorders and hypnotics

Insomnia is a common and non-specific disorder and may be reported by 40–50% of people at any given time.

Causes of insomnia include medical illness, alcohol or drugs, periodic limb movement disorder, sleep apnoea, and psychiatric illness. Without an obvious underlying cause, it known as primary or psychophysiological.

Hypnotics are drugs used to treat psychophysiological (primary) insomnia. The distinction between the treatment of anxiety and that of sleep disorders is not clear-cut, particularly if anxiety is the main impediment to sleep.

γ-Aminobutyric acid (GABA) receptor

The γ-aminobutyric (GABA) receptors of the $GABA_A$ type are involved in the actions of some classes of hypnotic/anxiolytic drugs, notably:

- The benzodiazepines (BDZs), which are currently the most commonly used clinically.
- Newer non-benzodiazepine hypnotics, e.g. zoplicone.
- The now obsolete barbiturates (BARBs).

The $GABA_A$ receptor belongs to the superfamily of ligand-gated ion channels. It consists of several subunits—α, β, γ, and δ—which form the $GABA/Cl^-$ channel complex, as well as containing benzodiazepine and barbiturate modulatory receptor sites. The GABA site appears to be located on the α- and β-subunits while the benzodiazepine modulatory site is distinct and located on the γ-subunit.

GABA released from nerve terminals binds to postsynaptic $GABA_A$ receptors, the activation of which increases the Cl^- conductance of the neuron.

Occupation of the benzodiazepine sites by benzodiazepine receptor agonists enhances the actions of GABA on the Cl^- conductance of the neuronal membrane. The barbiturates similarly enhance the action of GABA but by occupying a distinct modulatory site (Fig. 3.4).

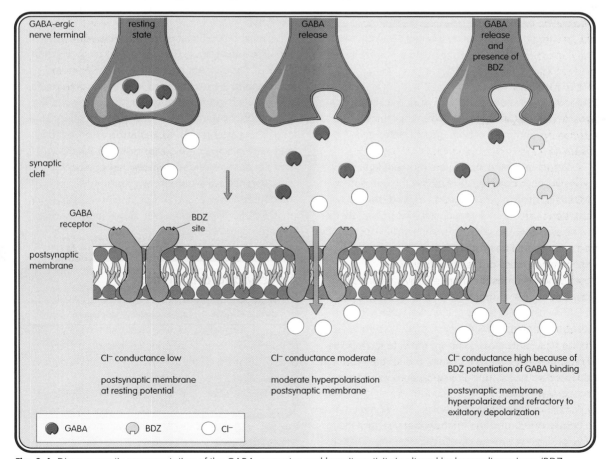

Fig. 3.4 Diagrammatic representation of the $GABA_A$ receptor and how its activity is altered by benzodiazepines. (BDZ, benzodiazephine; GABA γ-aminobutyric acid; CL⁻, chlonde ion.)

Anxiolytic and hypnotic drugs

The pharmacotherapy of anxiety and sleep disorders involves several different classes of drug, as shown in Fig. 3.5, with the benzodiazepines dominant in current therapeutics.

Anxiolytics and hypnotics	
Anxiolytics	**Hypnotics**
benzodiazepines (act on GABA$_A$ receptors) e.g. diazepam, lorazepam	benzodiazepines (act on GABA$_A$ receptors) e.g. triazolam, temazepam lormetazepam, nitrazepam
acting on serotonergic receptors (act on 5HT$_{1A}$ or 5HT$_3$ receptors) e.g. buspirone	non-benzodiazepine hypnotics (act on GABA$_A$ receptors e.g. zoplicone and zolpidem
autonomic suppression (act by β-adrenoreceptor antagonism) e.g. propranolol	other drugs e.g. choral hydrate chlormethiazole barbiturates (obsolete) sedative antidepressants sedative antihistamines

Fig. 3.5 Drugs used to treat anxiety and sleep disorders.

Benzodiazepines

Benzodiazepines are drugs with anxiolytic, hypnotic, muscle relaxant, and anticonvulsant actions that are used in the treatment of both anxiety states and insomnia.

Different benzodiazepines are marketed as hypnotics and anxiolytics. It is mainly the duration of action that determines the choice of drug (see below).

Mechanism of action: Benzodiazepines potentiate the action of GABA, the primary inhibitory neurotransmitter in the CNS. They do this by binding to a site on GABA$_A$ receptors, increasing their affinity for GABA. This results in an increased opening frequency of these ligand-gated Cl$^-$ channels, thus potentiating the effect of GABA release in terms of inhibitory effects on the postsynaptic cell (Fig. 3.4).

Indications: Benzodiazepines are used clinically in the short-term relief of severe anxiety and severe insomnia, preoperative sedation, status epilepticus, and acute alcohol withdrawal.

Contraindications: Benzodiazepines should not be given to people with bronchopulmonary disease, and they have additive or synergistic effects with other central depressants such as alcohol, barbiturates, and antihistamines.

Adverse effects: Benzodiazepines have several adverse effects:

- Drowsiness, ataxia, and reduced psychomotor performance which are common; thus care is necessary when driving or operating machinery.
- Dependence becomes apparent after 4–6 weeks, and is both physical and psychological. The withdrawal syndrome (in 30% of patients) comprises rebound anxiety and insomnia, tremulousness and twitching. Withdrawal is more severe after taking a short-acting benzodiazepine.

Although in overdose benzodiazepines alone are relatively safe when compared with other sedatives (e.g. barbiturates), if benzodiazepines are taken in combination with alcohol the CNS-depressant effects are potentiated and fatal respiratory depression can result. Treatment is with the benzodiazepine antagonist flumazenil.

Therapeutic notes: Benzodiazepines are active orally, and differ mainly in respect of their duration of action (Fig. 3.6). Short-acting agents (e.g. lorezapam and temazepam) are metabolized to inactive compounds, and are used mainly as sleeping pills because of the relative lack of 'hangover' effects in the morning. Some long-acting agents (e.g. diazepam) are converted to long-lasting active metabolites with half-lives longer than the administered parent drug. With others (e.g. nitrazepam) it is the parent drug itself that is metabolized slowly. Such drugs are more suitable for an anxiolytic effect maintained all day long, or when early morning waking is the problem.

Approximate elimination half–lives of benzodiazepines	
Benzodiazepine	**Approximate half-life (hours)**
triazolam	5
temazepam	6
lormetazepam	10
lorazepam	12
nitrazepam	24
diazepam	32 (one metabolite is active for up to 200 hours)

Fig. 3.6 Approximate elimination half-lives of benzodiazepines.

Non-benzodiazepine hypnotics

Zoplicone and zolpidem are new-generation hypnotics that both have a short duration of action with little or no hangover effect. Zoplicone is a cyclopyrrolone and zolpidem is an imidazopyridine.

Although neither of these drugs is a benzodiazepine, both act in a comparable manner on the $GABA_A$ receptor as benzodiazepines, although (it is thought) at a slightly different site.

Anxiolytic drugs acting at serotonergic receptors

The serotonergic theory of anxiety suggests that serotonergic transmission is involved in anxiety because, in general, stimulation of this system causes anxiety while a reduction in serotonergic neuronal activity reduces anxiety.

The serotonergic theory prompted the development of anxiolytic drugs that act to moderate serotonergic neurotransmission while not causing sedation and incoordination.

$5-HT_{1A}$ agonists

Buspirone is a serotonergic (5-hydroxytryptamine 1A; $5-HT_{1A}$) agonist.

Mechanism of action: In the raphe nucleus the dendrites of serotonergic neurons possess inhibitory presynaptic autoreceptors of the $5-HT_{1A}$ type that, when stimulated, decrease the firing of 5-HT neurons. A new class of anxiolytic agents called azapirones are thought to reduce 5-HT transmission by acting as partial agonists at these $5-HT_{1A}$ receptors. Buspirone is the first of this new class of anxiolytics. Isapirone and sumatriptan are similar.

Indications: Buspirone is indicated for the short-term relief of generalized anxiety disorder.

Contraindications: $5-HT_{1A}$ agonists should not be used in people with epilepsy.

Adverse effects: The adverse effects of $5-HT_{1A}$ agonists include nervousness, dizziness, headache, and light-headedness.

In contrast to benzodiazepines, buspirone does not cause significant sedation or cognitive impairment and carries only a minimal risk of dependence and withdrawal. It does not potentiate the effects of alcohol.

Therapeutic notes: The anxiolytic effect of buspirone gradually evolve over 1–3 weeks.

$5-HT_3$ antagonists

Ondansetron is a $5-HT_3$ receptor antagonist that is well established for use as an antiemetic drug.

Ondansetron also has anxiolytic properties by virtue of its antagonism at the excitatory postsynaptic $5-HT_3$ receptor.

β-Adrenoreceptor blockers

β-Adrenoreceptor blockers or β-blockers, e.g. propranolol, can be very effective in alleviating the somatic manifestations of anxiety caused by marked sympathetic arousal, such as palpitations, tremor, sweating, and diarrhoea.

Mechanism of action: β-Blockers act by antagonism at β-adrenoreceptors so that excessive catecholamine release does not produce the physiological responses of tachycardia, sweating, etc.

Indications: β-Blockers are indicated in patients with predominantly somatic symptoms; this, in turn, may prevent the onset of worry and fear. Patients with predominantly psychological symptoms may obtain no benefit. β-Blockers can be useful in social phobias and to reduce performance anxiety in musicians, for whom fine motor control may be critical.

Contraindications: β-Blockers should not be used in people with asthma or heart failure.

Adverse effects: β-Blockers can cause bradycardia, heart failure, bronchospasm, and peripheral vasoconstriction.

Barbiturates

Barbiturates are non-selective CNS depressants that produce effects ranging from sedation and reduction of anxiety to unconsciousness and death from respiratory and cardiovascular failure. Barbiturates increase GABA-mediated inhibition by acting on the same receptor as benzodiazepines, though at a different site.

At low doses, barbiturates prolong the *duration* of individual Cl^- channel openings triggered by a given GABA stimulus (benzodiazepines increase the *frequency* of Cl^- channel openings). At high doses, they are far more depressant than benzodiazepines because they start to increase Cl^- conductance directly, thus decreasing the sensitivity of the postsynaptic membrane to excitatory transmitters.

While very popular until the 1960s as sedative/hypnotic agents, they are now obsolete since they

readily lead to psychological and physical dependence, and a relatively small overdose can be fatal. Conversely, benzodiazepines, which have largely replaced barbiturates as sedative/ hypnotics, have been taken in huge overdoses without serious long-term effects.
Barbiturates are still important in anaesthesia (p. 63) and in the treatment of epilepsy (p. 61).

Miscellaneous hypnotics

There are a number of miscellaneous hypnotic agents that have been used historically and are still prescribed under certain circumstances.

Chloral hydrate and derivatives

Chloral hydrate is metabolized to trichloroethanol, which is an effective hypnotic. It is cheap but causes gastric irritation and there is no convincing evidence that it has any advantage over the newer benzodiazepines.

Chloral hydrate and its derivatives were previously popular hypnotics for children. Current thinking does not justify the use of hypnotics in children and these drugs now have very limited uses.

Chlormethiazole

Chlormethiazole may be a useful hypnotic in the elderly because of the relative freedom from hangover effects. It has no advantage over benzodiazepines in younger adults.

Chlormethiazole is also indicated for intravenous use to attenuate the symptoms of alcohol withdrawal.

Sedative antidepressants

If the underlying cause of insomnia is associated with depression, or particularly in depressed patients exhibiting anxiety and agitation, then tricyclic anti-depressants (TCAs) with sedative actions (p. 48), e.g. amitriptyline, may be useful, as they act as a hypnotic when given at bedtime.

Sedative antihistamines

The older antihistamine drugs, e.g. diphenhydramine, have antimuscarinic actions and pass the blood–brain barrier, commonly causing drowsiness and psycho-motor impairment.

Proprietary brands of diphenhydramine are on sale to the public to relieve temporary sleep disturbances, as these drugs are relatively safe.

An understanding of the GABA$_A$ GABA/Cl$^-$ channel complex is central to the mechanism of action of several classes of hypnotic/anxiolytic drugs. You should be aware which these are.

Anxiolytics and hypnotics
- Relate the action of benzodiazepines on the GABA$_A$ receptor to their clinical effectiveness.
- How do differences in elimination half-life make some benzodiazepines suitable as anxiolytics and others more as hypnotics?
- What are the side effects of benzodiazepine use?

Anxiolytics
- What are the psychological and somatic symptoms of anxiety?
- Name the different classes of anxiolytic drug and their mechanisms of action.
- What is the rationale for using 5-HT modulatory drugs and β-adrenoreceptor blockers in anxiety?

Hypnotics
- Under what circumstances are the different hypnotics suitable for prescription?
- Name the different classes of sedative/hypnotic drugs and explain their mechanism of action.
- Which hypnotics are currently used and why are they favoured over obsolete drugs?

AFFECTIVE DISORDERS AND ANTIDEPRESSANTS

Affective disorders

Affective disorders involve a disturbance of mood (cognitive/emotional symptoms) associated with changes in behaviour, energy, appetite, and sleep (biological symptoms).

Affective disorders can be thought of as pathological extremes of the normal continuum of human moods, from extreme excitement and elation (mania) to severe depressive states.

There are two types of affective disorder, unipolar affective disorders and bipolar affective disorders (BPADs).

Unipolar affective disorders

Unipolar affective disorders (UPAD) present with either of the following:
- Mania, which is characterized by euphoria, increased motor activity, flight of ideas, and grandiose self-confidence.
- Depression, which is characterized by misery, malaise, despair, guilt, apathy, indecisiveness, low energy and fatigue, changes in sleeping pattern, loss of appetite, and suicidal thoughts.

Of these, unipolar depression is much more common. Attempts have been made to classify types of depression as either 'reactive' or 'endogenous' in origin, such that:
- Reactive depression is where there is a clear psychological cause, e.g. bereavement. It involves less-severe symptoms and less likelihood of biological disturbance. It affects 3–10% of the population, with the incidence increasing with age, and is more common in females.
- Endogenous depression is where there is no clear cause and more severe symptoms, e.g. suicidal thoughts, and a greater likelihood of biological disturbance, e.g. insomnia, anorexia. It affects 1% of the population, usually starting in early adulthood, and affecting both sexes equally.

The distinction between reactive and endogenous depression is of importance since there is some evidence that depressions with endogenous features tend to respond better to drug therapy.

Bipolar affective disorders

Bipolar affective disorder (BPAD) presents with mood and behaviour oscillating between depression and mania, and is thus is also known as manic–depressive disorder.

Bipolar affective disorder develops earlier in life than unipolar depressive disorders, and tends to be inherited. It affects 1% of the population and can have associated elements of psychotic phenomena.

Monoamine theory of depression

The aetiology of major depressive disorders is not clear. Genetic, environmental, and neurochemical influences have all been examined as possible aetiological factors.

The most widely accepted neurochemical explanation of endogenous depression involves the monoamines [noradrenaline (NA), serotonin (5-HT), and dopamine (DA)]. The original hypothesis of depression, 'the monoamine theory', stated that depression was due to a functional deficit of these transmitter amines, while conversely mania was caused by an excess.

The monoamine theory explains why:
- Drugs that deplete monoamines are depressant, e.g. reserpine and methyldopa.
- A wide range of drugs that increase the functional availability of monoamine neurotransmitters improve mood in depressed patients, e.g. tricyclic antidepressants (TCAs) and monoamine oxidase inhibitors (MAOIs).
- The concentration of monoamines and their metabolites is reduced in the cerebrospinal fluid (CSF) of depressed patients.
- In some post mortem studies the most consistent finding is an elevation in cortical 5-HT$_2$ binding.

The theory cannot explain why:
- A number of compounds that increase the functional availability of monoamines, e.g. amphetamines, cocaine, and L-dopa, have no effect on the mood of depressed patients.
- Atypical antidepressants e.g. iprindole, work without manipulating monoaminergic systems.
- There is a 'therapeutic delay' of 2 weeks between the full neurochemical effects of antidepressants and the start of their therapeutic effect.

It is unlikely, therefore, that monoamine mechanisms alone are responsible for the symptoms of depression.

Other systems that may be involved in depression include:
- The GABA system.
- The neuropeptide systems, particularly vasopressin and the endogenous opiates.
- Secondary-messenger systems also appear to have a crucial role in some treatments.

Treatment of unipolar depressive disorders

The major classes of drug that are used to treat depression, and their mechanisms of action, are summarized in Fig. 3.7.

Although the monoamine theory in its simplest form is no longer plausible as a full explanation of depression, pharmacological manipulation of monoamine transmission remains the most successful therapeutic approach.

Major classes of antidepressant drug and mechanism of action		
Class of antidepressant drug	Examples	Mode of action
tricyclic antidepressants (TCAs)	amitriptyline imipramine	non–specific blockers of monoamine uptake
specific serotonin reuptake inhibitors (SSRIs)	fluoxetine paroxetine sertraline	selective blockers of 5-HT reuptake
serotonin–noradrenaline reuptake inhibitors (SNRIs)	venlafaxine	selective blockers of 5-HT and noradrenaline uptake
monoamine oxidase inhibitors (MAOIs)	phenelzine tranylcypromine	non–competitive, non–selective irreversible blockers of MAO_A and MAO_B
reversible inhibitors of MAO_A (RIMAs)	moclobemide brofarmine	reversibly inhibit MAO_A selectively
atypical	mianserin trazodone	act by various mechanisms that are poorly understood

Fig. 3.7 Major classes of antidepressant drug and their mechanism of action.

Tricyclic antidepressants and related drugs

Examples of TCAs and related drugs include amitriptyline, imipramine, nortriptyline, and clomipramine.

Mechanism of action: TCAs act by blocking 5-HT and noradrenaline uptake into the presynaptic terminal from the synaptic cleft (Fig. 3.8). They have a certain affinity for H_1 and muscarinic receptors, and for α_1- and α_2-receptors.

Contraindications: TCAs and related drugs should not be used in:
- Recent myocardial infarction or arrhythmias (especially heart block) since TCAs increase the risk of conduction abnormalities.
- Manic phase.
- Severe liver disease.
- Epilepsy, where TCAs lower the seizure threshold.
- Patients taking other anticholinergic drugs, alcohol, and adrenaline as TCAs potentiate the effects of these. Lignocaine is contraindicated in combination with TCAs, owing to a potentially fatal drug interaction.

Adverse effects: While TCAs are an effective therapy for depression, the adverse effects can reduce patient compliance and acceptability. Side effects include:
- Muscarinic blocking effects such as a dry mouth, blurred vision, and constipation.
- α-Adrenergic blocking effects such as postural hypotension.
- Noradrenaline uptake block in the heart, increasing the risk of arrhythmias.
- Histamine-blocking effects leading to sedation.
- Weight gain.

TCAs are relatively dangerous in overdose. Patients present with confusion, mania, and potentially fatal arrhythmias due to the cardiotoxic nature of the drug.

Therapeutic notes: No individual TCA has superior antidepressant activity, and the choice of drug is usually determined by the most acceptable or desired side effects. For example drugs with sedative actions, such as amitriptyline or trimipramine, are the TCAs of choice for patients in agitated or anxious states. Trazodone is a TCA-related drug that is commonly used in the elderly and may be the antidepressant of choice in epilepsy.

Therapeutic effects take 2–3 weeks to develop. TCA-related antidepressants should be withdrawn slowly.

Specific serotonin reuptake inhibitors

Specific serotonin reuptake inhibitors (SSRIs) are a novel class of agents that have recently been developed and are increasingly being prescribed as antidepressants. Fluoxetine (Prozac) is an SSRI. Other examples include citalopram, fluvoamine, paroxetine, sertraline, and nefazodone.

Mechanism of action: SSRIs act with a high specificity for potent inhibition of serotonin reuptake into nerve terminals from the synaptic cleft, while having only minimal effects on noradrenaline uptake (Fig. 3.8). They block serotonin transporters, which belong to a class of Na^+/Cl^--coupled transporters.

Contraindications: Contraindications with SSRIs are few. They should not be used with MAOIs as the combination can cause a potentially fatal serotonergic syndrome of hyperthermia and cardiovascular collapse.

Adverse effects: The side effect profile of SSRIs is much better than that of TCAs and MAOIs as there are no amine interactions, anticholinergic actions, adrenergic blockade, or toxic effects in overdose. However, adverse effects, caused by their effect on serotonergic nerves throughout the body, include nausea, diarrhoea, insomnia, anxiety, and agitation. Sexual dysfunction is sometimes a problem; nefazodone rarely causes this effect.

Therapeutic notes: SSRIs have a similar efficacy to that of TCAs. It is their clinical advantages and lack of side effects that have led to their popularity. These include no anticholinergic effects, no toxicity in overdose, and no cardiotoxic effects. SSRIs are now the most widely prescribed antidepressants.

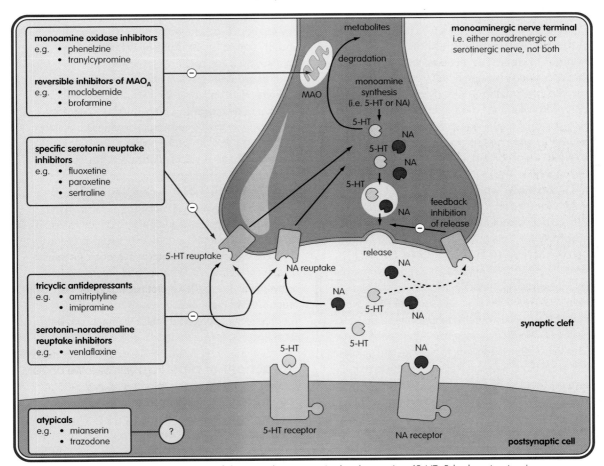

Fig. 3.8 Site of action of the major classes of drug used to treat unipolar depression. [5-HT, 5-hydroxytryptamine (serotonin); MAO, monoamine oxidase; NA, noradrenaline.]

Serotonin–noradrenaline reuptake inhibitors

The only drug currently in the serotonin–noradrenaline reuptake inhibitor (SNRIs) new class of antidepressants is venlafaxine, a phenyethylamine derivative.

Mechanism of action: SNRIs cause potentiation of neurotransmitter activity in the CNS, probably by inhibiting reuptake of serotonin and noradrenaline (Fig. 3.8).

Contraindications: The drug interactions of SNRIs are much like those of SSRIs; however, extra care must be taken with hypertensive patients as venlafaxine raises blood pressure.

Adverse effects: The adverse effects of SNRIs are similar to those of SSRIs, but they occur with lower frequency.

Therapeutic notes: The pharmacological effects of venlafaxine are similar to those of the TCAs, but adverse effects are reduced because it has little affinity for cholinergic and histaminergic receptors or α-adrenoreceptors.

Monoamine oxidase inhibitors

Examples of irreversible monoamine oxidase inhibitors (MAOIs) include phenelzine, tranylcypromine, and isocarboxazid, and examples of reversible inhibitors of MAO_A (RIMAs) include moclobemide and brofarmine.

Mechanism of action: MAOIs block the action of MAO_A and MAO_B, which are neuron enzymes that metabolize (degrade) the monoamines (noradrenaline, serotonin, and dopamine) (Fig. 3.8). MAO has two main isoforms, MAO_A and MAO_B, which differ in terms of substrate preference; inhibition of the MAO_A form correlates best with antidepressant efficacy. Both non-selective irreversible blockers of MAO_A and MAO_B, and drugs that reversibly inhibit MAO_A are available.

Adverse effects: Dietary interactions may occur, such as the 'cheese reaction'. MAO in the gut wall and liver normally breaks down ingested tyramine. When the enzyme is inhibited, tyramine reaches the circulation and causes the release of noradrenaline from sympathetic nerve terminals; this can lead to a severe and potentially fatal rise in blood pressure. Patients on MAOIs must therefore avoid foods rich in tyramine, which include cheese, game, and alcoholic drinks. Preparations containing sympathomimetic amines (e.g. cough mixtures and nasal decongestants) should also be avoided. MAOIs are not specific and reduce the metabolism of barbiturates, opioids, and alcohol. Side effects include CNS stimulation causing excitement and tremor, sympathetic blockade causing postural hypotension, and muscarinic blockade causing a dry mouth and blurred vision. Phenelzine can be hepatotoxic.

Therapeutic notes: Response to treatment with MAOIs may be delayed for 3 weeks or more. Phobic and depressed patients with atypical, hypochondriacal, or hysterical features are said to respond best to MAOIs. Because of the dietary and drug restrictions outlined above, MAOIs are largely reserved for depression refractory to other antidepressants and treatment.

Atypical antidepressants

Examples of atypical antidepressants include mianserin and trazodone.

Mechanism of action: Atypical antidepressant drugs have little or no activity on amine uptake and act by various mechanisms (receptor antagonism) that are poorly understood (Fig. 3.8). Examples include mianserin (which has α_2-adrenoreceptor-, $5\text{-}HT_2$-, and H_2-blocking activity and which, by acting on inhibitory α_2-autoreceptors on central noradrenergic nerve endings, may increase the amount of noradrenaline in the synaptic cleft) and trazodone, which is a weak 5-HT-blocker and antagonizes $5\text{-}HT_2$- and α_2-receptors.

Contraindications: The contraindications for atypical antidepressants are similar to those for TCAs.

Adverse effects: Atypical antidepressants generally cause less autonomic side effects and are less dangerous in overdose, owing to their lower cardiotoxicity compared with TCAs. Mianserin may cause agranulocytosis and aplastic anaemia (especially in the elderly) and trazodone may cause postural hypotension and, rarely, priapism (persistent penile erection).

Therapeutic notes: Mianserin and trazodone are both sedative and are therefore used in depression when a degree of sedation is desirable. Neither is currently a first-line drug for the treatment of depression.

Treatment of bipolar affective disorders

Bipolar affective disorder (BPAD) is treated with a combination of mood stabilizers and antidepressants, and sometimes antipsychotics (p. 52). Mood stabilizers include lithium and carbamazepine.

Lithium

Lithium is administered as lithium carbonate and is the

most widely used mood stabilizer, with antimaniac and antidepressant activity.

Mechanism of action: The mechanism of action of lithium is unclear, but probably involves modulation of secondary-messenger pathways of cAMP and inositol triphosphate (IP_3). It is known that lithium inhibits the pathway for recapturing inositol for the resynthesis of polyphosphoinositides. It may exert its effect by reducing the concentrations of lipids important in secondary signal transduction in the brain.

Indications: Lithium salts are mainly used in the prophylaxis and treatment of BPAD, but also in the prophylaxis and treatment of acute mania and in the prophylaxis of resistant recurrent depression.

Contraindications: Some drugs may interact, causing a rise in plasma lithium concentation and thus should be avoided. Such drugs include antipsychotics, non-steroidal anti-inflammatory drugs (NSAIDs), diuretics, and cardioactive drugs.

Adverse effects: Lithium has a long plasma half-life and a narrow therapeutic window; therefore side effects are common and plasma concentration monitoring is essential. Early side effects include thirst, nausea, diarrhoea, tremor, and polyuria; late side effects include weight gain, oedema, acne, nephrogenic diabetes insipidus, and hypothyroidism. Toxicity/overdose (serum level >2–3 mmol/L) effects include vomiting, diarrhoea, tremor, ataxia, confusion, and coma.

Therapeutic notes: The decision to give prophylactic lithium requires specialist advice, and careful monitoring after initiation of treatment is essential.

Carbamazepine

Carbamazepine is as effective as lithium in the prophylaxis of BPAD and acute mania, particularly in rapidly alternating bipolar illness.

Mechanism of action: Carbamazepine is a GABA agonist and this may be the basis of its antimaniac properties. The relevance of its effect in stabilizing neuronal sodium, and on calcium channels, is unclear.

Adverse effects: Side effects of carbamazepine include drowsiness, diplopia, nausea, ataxia, rashes, and headache; blood disorders such as agranulocytosis and leucopenia; and drug interactions with lithium, antipsychotics, TCAs, and MAIOs. Many other drugs can be affected by the effect of carbamazepine on inducing hepatic enzymes. Diplopia, ataxia, clonus, tremor, and sedation are associated with acute carbamazepine toxicity.

Therapeutic notes: At the start of treatment with carbamazepine, plasma concentrations should be monitored to establish a maintenance dose.

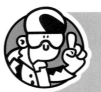

Although almost certainly flawed and incomplete, the monoamine theory is probably the best way to rationalize your thinking about affective disorders, and to understand the mechanism of action of the drugs used in their treatment.

- What is an affective disorder and how are they classified?
- List the evidence for and against the monoamine theory.
- Describe the action and major side effects of drugs used to treat depression: TCAs, SSRIs, SNRIs, MAOIs, and atypicals.
- Describe the action and major side effects of the drugs used to treat bipolar affective disorder: the mood stabilizers lithium and carbamazepine.
- Name some examples of each of the classes of drug used in the treatment of affective disorders.

NEUROLEPTICS

Basic concepts of psychotic disorders

Psychotic disorders are characterized by a mental state that is out of touch with reality, involving a variety of abnormalities of perception, thought, and ideas.

Psychotic illnesses include:
- Schizophrenia.
- Schizoaffective disorder.
- Delusional disorders.
- Some depressive and manic illnesses.

Schizophrenia is the most important of these psychotic illnesses, because of its prevalence, young age of onset, and chronic and disabling nature.

Neuroleptics are drugs used in the treatment of psychotic disorders.

Schizophrenia

Epidemiology

Schizophrenia characteristically develops in people aged 15–45; it has a relatively stable cross-cultural incidence affecting 1% of the population; 64% of cases are male.

Symptoms and signs

Schizophrenia is a psychotic illness characterized by multiple symptoms affecting thought, perceptions, emotion, and volition.

Symptoms fall into two groups—positive and negative—which may have different underlying causes.

Positive symptoms include:
- Delusions, which are false personal beliefs held with absolute conviction.
- Hallucinations, which are false perceptions in the absence of a real external stimulus; most commonly, these are auditory (hearing voices) and occur in 60–70% of schizophrenics but they can be visual, tactile, or olfactory.
- Thought alienation and disordered thought, which is the belief that one's thoughts are under the control of an outside agency (e.g. aliens, MI5). This type of belief is common, and thought processes are often incomprehensible.

Negative symptoms include:
- Poverty of speech, which is a restriction in the amount of spontaneous speech.
- Flattening of affect, which is a loss of normal experience and expression of emotion.
- Social withdrawal.
- Anhedonia, which is an inability to experience pleasure.
- Avolition/apathy, involving reduced drive, energy, and interest.
- Attention deficit, manifested by inattentiveness at work or on interview.

The distinction between the positive and negative symptoms found in schizophrenia is of importance as neuroleptic drugs tend to have most effect on positive symptoms, while negative symptoms are fairly refractory to treatment and carry a worse prognosis.

Theories of schizophrenia

The cause of schizophrenia remains mysterious. Any theory of the cause of schizophrenia must take into account the strong, though not invariable, hereditary tendency (50% concurrence in monozygotic twins), as well as the environmental factors known to predispose towards its development.

Many hypotheses have been suggested to explain the manifestations of schizophrenia at the level of neurotransmitters in the brain. The potential role of excessive dopaminergic activity, in particular, has attracted considerable attention. Evidence for this theory includes the following:
- Most antipsychotic drugs block dopamine receptors, the clinical dose being proportional to the ability to block D_2 receptors.
- Single positive electron tomography ligand scans show that there are increased D_2 receptors in the nucleus accumbens of schizophrenic patients.
- Psychotic symptoms can be induced by drugs that increase dopaminergic activity.

However, there is much evidence that the dopaminergic theory fails to explain. Current research indicates a likely role for other neurotransmitters in schizophrenia, including 5-HT, GABA, and glutamate. Although the dopamine theory cannot explain many of the features and findings in schizophrenia, most current pharmacological treatment (typical neuroleptics) is aimed at dopaminergic transmission (Fig. 3.9).

Neuroleptic drugs

The treatment of schizophrenia and all other psychotic illnesses involves the use of antipsychotic medication, the neuroleptic drugs. Neuroleptic drugs produce a general improvement in all the acute positive symptoms of schizophrenia, but it is less clear how effective they are in the treatment of chronic schizophrenia and negative symptoms.

Mechanism of action: Antipsychotic drugs have a variety of structures and fall into various classes (Fig. 3.10). There is a strong correlation between clinical potency and affinity for D_2-receptors among the typical neuroleptics.

Neuroleptics take days or weeks to work, suggesting that secondary effects (e.g. increase in number of D_2 receptors in limbic structure) may be more important than a direct effect of D_2-receptor block. It was once thought, therefore, that neuroleptics exerted their antipsychotic effect by interfering with dopamine transmission at D_2-receptors in the mesocortical and mesolimbic systems. The development of newer atypical neuroleptics that are not very active at the D_2-receptor but are still clinically effective has challenged this hypothesis.

Most neuroleptics also block other monoamine receptors and this is often the cause of some of the side effects of these drugs.

The distinction between typical and atypical groups is not clearly defined, but rests partly on the incidence of extrapyramidal motor side effects and partly on receptor specificity. Atypical neuroleptics are less prone to producing motor disorders than other drugs and tend to have different pharmacological profiles with respect to dopamine and other receptor specificity.

Typical neuroleptics
Phenothiazines
This class of compounds is subdivided into three groups by the type of side chain attached to the mother structure (phenothiazine ring) (Fig. 3.10). Side-effect patterns vary with the different side chains. Thus:

- Propylamine side chains, e.g. in chlorpromazine, produce strong sedation, a moderate muscarinic block, and moderate motor disturbance. Indicated for violent patients, owing to their sedative effect.
- Piperidine side chains, e.g. in thioridazine, produce moderate sedation, strong muscarinic block, and low motor disturbance. Favoured for use in the elderly.
- Piperazine side chains, e.g. in fluphenazine, produce low sedation, low muscarinic block, and strong motor disturbance. Contraindicated for use in the elderly, owing to the motor effects.

Butyrophenones and thioxanthenes
The butyrophenone and thioxanthine groups of compounds have the same profile of low sedation, low muscarinic block, and high incidence of motor disturbance.

Examples of butyrophenone compounds include haloperidol and droperidol; the thioxanthenes include flupenthixol and clopenthixol.

Dopamine receptors		
Type	**2nd messengers + cellular effects**	**Location in CNS and postulated function**
D_1	cAMP increase	• mainly postsynaptic inhibition • functions unclear
D_2	cAMP decrease K^+ conductance up Ca^{++} conductance down	• mainly presynaptic inhibition of dopamine synthesis/release in nigrostriatal, mesolimbic, and tuberoinfundibular systems • affinity of neuroleptics for D_2 receptors correlates with antipsychotic potency
D_3	unknown	• localized mainly in limbic and cortical structures concerned with cognitive functions and emotional behaviour • not clear whether antipsychotic effects of neuroleptics are mediated by the D_3 type
D_4	unknown	• similar to D_3 type; clozapine has particular affinity for D_4 receptors

Fig. 3.9 Classes of dopamine receptor.

Neuroleptic drugs		
Class	**Chemical classification**	**Examples**
typical anti-psychotics	phenothiazines: • propylamine side chains • piperidine side chains • piperazine side chains	chlorpromazine thioridazine fluphenazine, trifluoperazine
	butyrophenones	haloperidol, droperidol
	thioxanthines	flupenthixol, clopenthixol
	dibenzodiazepines	clozapine, olanzepine
atypical anti-psychotics	dopamine/5-HT blockers: • diphenylbutylpiperidines • substituted benzamides • benzixasoles	pimozide sulpiride risperidone

Fig. 3.10 Classes of neuroleptic drugs.

Atypical neuroleptics
Dibenzodiazepines
Dibenzodiazepines such as clozapine have a low affinity for the D_2 receptor and a higher affinity for D_1 and D_4 receptors.

Indications: In the UK and US, atypical neuroleptics are indicated only in chronic cases refractory to other drugs, or with severe motor disturbance. This is because of the risk of potentially fatal neutropenia in 1% of cases treated.

Adverse effects: Clozapine has a low incidence of adverse motor effects due to its low affinity for the D_2-receptor. Side effects of dibenzodiazepines include hypersalivation, sedation, weight gain, tachycardia, and hypotension.

Dopamine/5-HT blockers
Examples of dopamine/5-HT blockers include the diphenylbutylpiperidines and the benzixasoles. Examples of the former include pimozide and substituted benzamides (e.g. sulpiride); examples of the latter include risperidone.

Sulpiride, and the newer agent pimozide, show high selectivity for D_2 receptors compared with D_1 or other neurotransmitter receptors. Both drugs are effective in treating schizophrenia but, sulpiride is claimed to have less tendency to cause adverse motor effects. Pimozide appears to be similar to conventional neuroleptic agents, but has a longer duration of action, allowing once-daily medication.

Benzixasoles such as risperidone show a high affinity for 5-HT receptors and a lower affinity for D_2 receptors.

With this class of drugs, extrapyramidal motor side effects occur with less frequency than with 'classic' neuroleptics.

Adverse effects of neuroleptics
Neuroleptic drugs cause a variety of adverse effects (Fig. 3.11).

The majority of the unwanted effects of neuroleptics can be inferred from their pharmacological actions, such as the disruption of dopaminergic pathways—the major action of most neuroleptics—and the blockade of monoamine and other receptors, including:
- Muscarinic receptors.
- α-Adrenoreceptors.
- Histamine receptors.

In addition, individual drugs may cause immunological reactions or have their own characteristic side-effect profile.

Adverse effects on the dopaminergic pathways
There are three main dopaminergic pathways in the brain (Fig. 3.12):
- Mesolimbic and/or mesocortical dopamine pathways running from groups of cells in the midbrain to the nucleus accumbens and amygdala. This pathway affects thoughts and motivation.
- Nigrostriatal dopamine pathways running from the midbrain to the caudate nuclei. This pathway is important in smooth motor control.
- Tuberoinfundibular neurons running from the hypothalamus to the pituitary gland, the secretions of which they regulate.

Antagonism of dopamine receptors leads to interference with the normal functioning of these pathways, bringing about unwanted side effects as well as the desired antipsychotic effect. This antagonism is the cause of the most serious side effects associated with neuroleptic use, which include:
- Psychological effects due to D_2-receptor blockade of the mesolimbic/mesocortical pathway.
- Movement disorders due to D_2-receptor blockade of the nigrostriatal pathways.
- Neuroendocrine disorders due to D_2 blockade of the tuberoinfundibular pathway.

Adverse effects of neuroleptics

- Acute neurologic effects: acute dystonia, akathisia, parkinsonism
- Chronic neurologic effects: tardive dyskinesia, tardive dystonia
- Neuroendocrine effects: amenorrhea, galactorrhea, infertility
- Idiosyncratic: neuroleptic malignant syndrome
- Anticholinergic: dry mouth, blurred vision, constipation, urinary retention, ejaculatory failure
- Antihistaminergic: sedation
- Antiadrenergic: hypotension, arrhythmia
- Miscellaneous: photosensitivity, heat sensitivity, cholestatic jaundice, retinal pigmentation

Fig. 3.11 Adverse effects of neuroleptics.

It is by dopaminergic antagonism of the mesolimbic mesocortical pathway that it is thought that typical neuroleptics exert their antipsychotic effects. However, as a side effect of mesolimbic and mesocortical dopaminergic inhibition, sedation and impaired performance are common.

Blocking of dopamine receptors in the basal ganglia (corpus striatum) frequently results in distressing and disabling movement disorders. Two main types of movement disorder occur. Acute reversible parkinsonian-like symptoms (tremor, rigidity, and akinesia), are treated by dose reduction, anticholinergic drugs, or switching to an atypical neuroleptic. Slowly developing tardive dyskinesia, often irreversible, and manifesting as involuntary movements of the face, trunk, and limbs, appears months or years after the start of neuroleptic treatment. It may be due to proliferation or sensitization of dopamine receptors. Incidence is unpredictable and affects approximately 20% of long-term users of neuroleptics. Treatment is generally unsuccessful. The newer atypical neuroleptics may be less likely to induce tardive dyskinesia.

By reducing the negative feedback on the anterior pituitary, oversecretion of prolactin can result

Fig. 3.12 Effect of D_2 dopamine receptor blockade on the dopaminergic pathways in the brain.

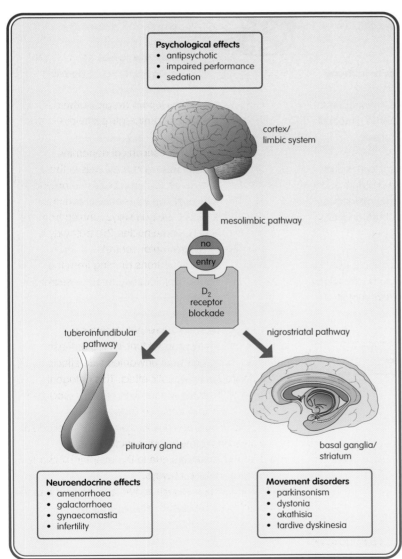

Psychological effects
- antipsychotic
- impaired performance
- sedation

cortex/limbic system

mesolimbic pathway

no entry

D_2 receptor blockade

tuberoinfundibular pathway

nigrostriatal pathway

pituitary gland

basal ganglia/striatum

Neuroendocrine effects
- amenorrhoea
- galactorrhoea
- gynaecomastia
- infertility

Movement disorders
- parkinsonism
- dystonia
- akathisia
- tardive dyskinesia

55

(hyperprolactinaemia). This can lead to gynaecomastia, galactorrhoea, menstrual irregularities, impotence, and weight gain in some patients.

Adverse effects from unselective receptor blockade
The adverse effects of neuroleptics from unselective receptor blockade include:
- Anticholinergic effects due to muscarinic-receptor blockade, such as dry mouth, urinary retention, constipation, blurred vision, etc.
- Adverse effects due to α-adrenoreceptor blockade. Many neuroleptics have the capacity to block α-adrenoreceptors and cause postural hypotension.
- Adverse effects due to histamine-receptor blockade. Antagonism of central histamine H_1 receptors may contribute to sedation.

Adverse effects due to individual drugs or immune reactions
The neuroleptic drug clozapine can cause neutropenia due to toxic bone marrow suppression, while pimozide can cause sudden death secondary to cardiac arrhythmia.

Immune reactions to neuroleptic drugs can include dermatitis, rashes, photosensitivity, and urticaria. Such reactions are more common with the phenothiazines, which can also cause deposits in the cornea and lens.

Neuroleptic malignant syndrome:
- Is the most lethal adverse effect of neuroleptic use. It is an idiosyncratic reaction of unknown pathophysiology.
- Symptoms include fever, extrapyramidal motor disturbance, muscle rigidity, and coma. Urgent treatment is indicated.

Neuroleptics have many side effects, some related to their principal mechanism of action (dopamine receptor antagonism) and some unrelated to this. Learn these well as they are a popular examination topic.

- Outline the concept of psychotic disorders (schizophrenia) and the two types of symptoms, positive and negative.
- Summarize the theories of schizophrenia, and the relevance of dopaminergic activity in schizophrenia, and relate this to the mechanism of action of antipsychotic drugs.
- Name the three chemical classes of typical antipsychotics, and an example of a drug from each class.
- Name the classes of atypical antipsychotic drugs, and give an example from each class.
- List the range of adverse effects that neuroleptics cause under the following headings:
  - Adverse effects due to blockade of dopaminergic pathways in the brain (three pathways involved).
  - Adverse effects due to unselective receptor blockade.
  - Adverse effects due to individual drugs or immune reactions.

EPILEPSY AND ANTICONVULSANTS

Epilepsy, seizures, and epileptic syndromes

Epilepsy is a chronic disease in which seizures result from the abnormal discharge of cerebral neurons.

A seizure is a particular behaviour produced by an abnormal high-frequency discharge of a group of neurons, starting focally and spreading to a varying extent to affect other parts of the brain. According to the focus and spread of discharges, seizures may be classified as:

- Partial (focal), which originate at a specific locus and do not spread to involve other cortical areas.
- Generalized, which usually have a focus (often in the temporal lobe) and then spread to other areas.

Different epileptic syndromes can be classified on the basis of seizure type and pattern, with other clinical features (such as age of onset), anatomical location of focus, and aetiology taken into account.

Common types of epileptic syndrome

Epileptic syndromes result from either generalized seizures or focal seizures (Fig. 3.13).

Generalized seizure involves loss of consciousness and may be convulsive or non-convulsive:

- Tonic–clonic or grand-mal epilepsy, is a convulsive generalized seizure characterized by periods of tonic muscle rigidity followed later by massive jerking of the body (clonus).
- Absence, or petit-mal, seizures are generalized seizures characterized by changes in consciousness lasting less than 10 seconds. They occur most commonly in children, where they can be confused with day-dreaming.

The effect on the body of focal seizures depends on the location of the abnormal signal focus: e.g. involvement of the motor cortex will produce convulsions whereas involvement of the brainstem can produce unconsciousness. Psychomotor or temporal lobe epilepsy results from a partial seizure with cortical activity localized to the temporal lobe. Such seizures are characterized by features which include Impaired consciousness or confusion, amnesia, emotional instability, atypical behaviour, outbursts.

Partial motor seizures have their focus in cortical motor regions and present with convulsive or tonic activity corresponding to the neurons involved.

Another type of epileptic syndrome is status epilepticus. This is a state in which fits follow each other without consciousness being regained. Status epilepticus constitutes a medical emergency because of possible exhaustion of vital centres.

Causes of epilepsy

The aetiology of epilepsy is unknown in 60–70% of cases, but heredity is an important factor.

Damage to the brain, for example by tumours, head injury, infections, or cerebrovascular accident, may subsequently cause epilepsy.

The neurochemical basis of the abnormal discharges in epilepsy are not known, but may involve altered GABA metabolism.

Treatment of epilepsy

Drugs used to treat epilepsy are termed antiepileptics; the term anticonvulsant is also used.

The aim of pharmacological treatment of epilepsy is to control seizures without producing adverse drug effects.

Classification of common epileptic syndromes	
Partial (local, focal) seizures	**Generalised seizures**
• psychomotor (temporal lobe) epilepsy	• tonic–clonic seizure or grand-mal epilepsy
• partial motor epilepsy	• absence seizure or petit-mal epilepsy

Fig. 3.13 Classification of common epileptic syndromes.

Drug treatment can control, but not cure, 60–90% of recurrences of epileptic seizures, but treatment is necessarily long term.

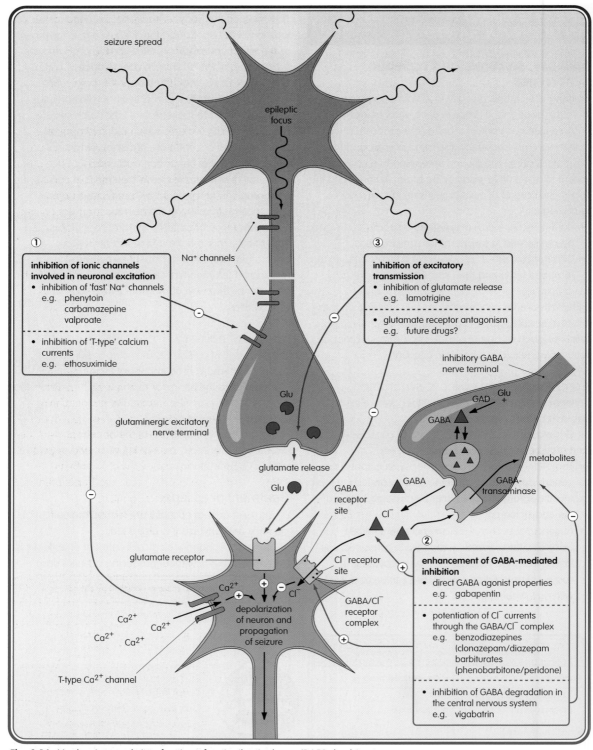

Fig. 3.14 Mechanism and site of action of antiepileptic drugs. (BARB, barbituates; BZDs, benzodiazepines, GAD, glutamic acid decarboxylase; Glu, glutamate.)

Mechanisms of action of antiepileptics

Antiepileptic drugs act generically to inhibit the rapid, repetitive neuronal firing that characterizes seizures. There are three established mechanisms of action by which the antiepileptic drugs achieve this. These mechanisms are numbered as follows in Fig. 3.14:
1. Inhibition of ionic channels involved in neuronal excitability.
2. Enhancement of GABA-mediated inhibition.
3. Inhibition of excitatory transmission.

1. Drugs such as phenytoin, carbamazepine, and valproate inhibit the 'fast' sodium current. These drugs bind preferentially to inactivated (closed) sodium channels, preventing them from opening. The high-frequency repetitive depolarization of neurons during a seizure increases the proportion of sodium channels in the inactivated state susceptible to blockade. Eventually, sufficient sodium channels become blocked so that the 'fast' neuronal sodium current is insufficient to cause a depolarization. Note that neuronal transmission at normal frequencies is relatively unaffected because a much smaller proportion of the sodium channels are in the inactivated state.

Ethosuximide, for example, inhibits 'T-type' low-threshold, fast-inactivating calcium. Absence seizures involve oscillatory neuronal activity between the thalamus and the cerebral cortex. The oscillation involves 'T-type' calcium channels, which produce low-threshold spikes, thus allowing groups of cells to fire in bursts. It appears that the antiabsence drug ethosuximide reduces this fast-inactivating calcium current, dampening the thalamocortical oscillations that are critical in the generation of such absence seizures.

2. Enhancement of GABA-mediated inhibition can take any of the following forms:
- Enhancement by direct GABA agonist properties, e.g. by gabapentin, which is a new antiepileptic agent that has been designed to mimic GABA in the CNS.
- Potentiation of chloride currents through the $GABA_A/Cl^-$ channel complex, e.g. by benzodiazepines and barbiturates. The increased postsynaptic inhibitory chloride current at $GABA_A$ receptors, hyperpolarizes neurons and makes them refractory to excitation (Fig. 3.4).
- Inhibition of GABA degradation in the CNS, e.g. by

vigabatrin, which is an irreversible inhibitor of GABA transaminase ($GABA_T$), the enzyme normally responsible for metabolism of GABA in the neuron. Inhibition of $GABA_T$ therefore leads to an increase in synaptic levels of GABA and thus enhances GABA-mediated inhibition.

3. Drugs that block excitatory amino acid receptors [N-methyl-D-aspartate (NMDA) antagonists] have been shown to be antiepileptic in animal models. Such drugs may prove useful in the clinical treatment of epilepsy in the future. Lamotrigine, a new antiepileptic agent, inhibits the release of glutamate as one of its actions, and this may contribute to its antiepileptic activity.

Drugs used in the treatment of epilepsy

Antiepileptic drugs can be classified according to their mechanism of action, but in clinical practice it is useful to think of the drugs according to their use (Figs 3.14 and 3.15).

Phenytoin

Mechanism of action: This involves use-dependent block of voltage-gated sodium channels. Phenytoin reduces the spread of a seizure. Electroencephalographic (EEG) recordings show that phenytoin does not stop the 'spiking' at a focus (i.e. it does not prevent the ignition of an epileptic discharge), but it does stop it spreading and causing overt clinical symptoms.
Route of administration: Phenytoin is administered orally, although absorption is variable.
Indications: Phenytoin is indicated in all forms of epilepsy except absence seizures.

Drugs used for epilepsy classified by clinical use		
Seizure type	Primary drugs	Secondary drugs
partial and/or generalized tonic–clonic seizures	• phenytoin • carbamazepine	• phenobarbital • primidone • valproate
absence seizures	• ethosuximide • valproate	• clonazepam
status epilepticus	• diazepam (i/v)	• clonazepam, lorazepam • barbiturates and anaesthesia if refractory

Fig. 3.15 Drugs used for epilepsy, classified by clinical use.

Contraindications: Phenytoin has many contraindications, mainly because it induces the hepatic P_{450} oxidase system, increasing the metabolism of oral contraceptives, anticoagulants, dexamethasone, and pethidine.

Adverse effects: The adverse effects of phenytoin may be dosage- or non-dosage-related. The dosage-related effects of phenytoin affect the cerebrovestibular system, leading to ataxia, blurred vision, and hyperactivity. Acute toxicity causes sedation and confusion. The non-dosage-related effects include collagen effects such as gum hypertrophy and coarsening of facial features; allergic reactions such as rash, hepatitis, and lymphadenopathy; haematological effects, e.g. megoblastic anaemia; endocrine effects, e.g. hirsutism (hair growth); and teratogenic effects (it may cause congenital malformations).

Therapeutic notes: The use of phenytoin is complicated by its zero-order pharmacokinetics, characteristic toxicities, and necessity for long-term administration. Phenytoin has a narrow therapeutic index and the relationship between dose and plasma concentration is non-linear. This is due to the fact that phenytoin is metabolized by a hepatic enzyme system that is saturated at therapeutic levels. Small dosage increases may therefore produce large rises in plasma concentrations with acute side effects. Monitoring of plasma concentration greatly assists dosage adjustment.

Carbamazepine

Mechanism of action: Like phenytoin, carbamazepine causes use-dependent block of voltage-gated sodium channels.

Route of administration: Carbamazepine is administered orally.

Indications: Carbamazepine can be used in all forms of epilepsy except absence seizures.

Contraindications: Like phenytoin, carbamazepine is a strong enzyme inducer and thus causes similar drug interactions.

Adverse effects: The adverse effects of carbamazepine are really limited to the nervous system—ataxia, nystagmus, dysarthria, vertigo, and sedation.

Therapeutic notes: Carbamazepine is well absorbed orally with a long half-life (25–60 hours) when first given. Enzyme induction subsequently reduces this half-life.

Sodium valproate

Mechanism of action: Sodium valproate has two mechanisms of action: like phenytoin, it causes use-dependent block of voltage-gated sodium channels; it also increases the GABA content of the brain when given over a long term.

Route of administration: Sodium valproate is administered orally.

Indications: Sodium valproate is useful in reducing the frequency of tonic–clonic and (particularly) absence seizures.

Contraindications: Sodium valproate should not be given to people with acute liver disease or a history of hepatic dysfunction.

Adverse effects: Sodium valproate has much fewer side effects than other antiepileptics, the main problems being gastrointestinal upset and, more importantly, liver failure. Hepatic toxicity appears to be more common when sodium valproate is used in combination with other antiepileptics.

Therapeutic notes: Sodium valproate is well absorbed orally and has a half-life of 10–15 hours.

Ethosuximide

Mechanism of action: Ethosuximide exerts its effects by inhibition of low-threshold calcium currents ('T-currents').

Route of administration: Ethosuximide is administered orally.

Indications: Ethosuximide is the drug of choice in simple absence seizures and is particularly well-tolerated in children.

Contraindications: Ethosuximide may make tonic–clonic attacks worse.

Adverse effects: The adverse effects of ethosuximide include gastrointestinal upset, drowsiness, mood swings, and skin rashes. Rarely, it causes serious bone marrow depression.

Vigabatrin

Mechanism of action: Vigabatrin exerts its effects by irreversible inhibition of GABA transaminase.

Route of administration: Vigabatrin is administered orally.

Indications: Vigabatrin is indicated in epilepsy not satisfactorily controlled by other drugs.

Contraindications: Vigabatrin should not be used in people with a history of psychosis because of the side effect of hallucinations.

Adverse effects: Vigabatrin's side effects include drowsiness, dizziness, depression, and visual hallucinations.

Therapeutic notes: Vigabatrin is a new drug, used as an adjunct to other therapies.

Barbiturates

Examples of barbiturates include phenobarbitone and primidone.

Mechanism of action: Barbiturates cause potentiation of chloride currents through the $GABA_A/Cl^-$ channel complex.

Route of administration: Barbiturates are usually administered orally, but intravenously in status epilepticus.

Indications: Barbiturates are used in all forms of epilepsy (except absence seizures), including status epilepticus.

Contraindications: Barbiturates should not be used in children, the elderly, and people with respiratory depression

Adverse effects: The main side effect of barbiturates is sedation, which limits their use clinically, along with the danger of potentially fatal CNS depression in overdose. Phenobarbitone is a good inducer of cytochrome P_{450} and so can be involved in drug interactions.

Therapeutic notes: Only the long-acting barbiturates are antiepileptic. Phenobarbitone has a plasma half-life of 10 hours.

Benzodiazepines

Examples of benzodiazepines include clonazepam, diazepam, and lorezapam.

Mechanism of action: Benzodiazepines cause potentiation of chloride currents through the $GABA_A/Cl^-$ channel complex (see Fig. 3.4).

Route of administration: Benzodiazepines are usually administered orally, but intravenously in status epilepticus.

Indications: Clonazepam is useful for absence seizures and other forms of epilepsy. Diazepam and lorezapam are effective in the management of status epilepticus.

Contraindications: Benzodiazepines should not be used in people with respiratory depression.

Adverse effects: The most common adverse effect of the benzodiazepines is sedation. Intravenous diazepam can depress respiration.

Therapeutic notes: The repeated seizures of status epilepticus can damage the brain and be potentially life threatening, so should be controlled by administration of intravenous diazepam.

New antiepileptic agents

The role of the new antiepileptic agents gabapentin, lamotrigine, and topiramate in the treatment of epilepsy has yet to be fully defined.

Gabapentin is a lipophilic drug that is designed to act like GABA in the CNS (agonist). It seems to be useful as an adjunct therapy for patients with partial seizures. It is relatively free of side effects other than sedation and dizziness.

Lamotrigine appears to act via an effect on sodium channels. It is used both as the sole therapy in partial seizures and as an adjunct. Adverse effects include dizziness, ataxia, blurred vision, gastrointestinal upset, and drug interactions.

- **Outline the neuronal basis of a seizure.**
- **Describe the different types of epilepsy.**
- **Outline the three broadly different mechanisms by which antiepileptics inhibit the neuronal activity that characterizes seizures and relate these activities to their ability to inhibit seizures.**
- **List examples of each of the major classes of antiepileptic drug, and when they are used clinically.**
- **List the major side effects of the important drugs.**

GENERAL ANAESTHETICS

Concepts of general anaesthesia

General anaesthesia is the absence of sensation associated with a reversible loss of conciousness.

General anaesthetics are used as an adjunct to surgical procedures in order to render the patient unaware of, and unresponsive to, painful stimuli. Modern anaesthesia is characterized by the so-called balanced technique in which drugs and anaesthetic agents are used specifically to produce:

- Analgesia.
- Sleep.
- Muscle relaxation.
- Abolition of reflexes.

No one drug or anaesthetic agent can produce all these effects and so a combination of agents is used in the three clinical stages of surgical general anaesthesia. The three stages are:

- Premedication.
- Induction.
- Maintenance.

Premedication

Premedication is often given on the ward before the patient is taken to the operating theatre (Fig. 3.16), and has four component aims:

- Relief from anxiety.
- Reduction of parasympathetic bradycardia and secretions.
- Analgesia.
- Prevention of postoperative emesis.

Relief from anxiety

Oral benzodiazepines, e.g. diazepam and lorazepam (see p. 44), are most effective and perform three useful functions:

- To relieve apprehension and anxiety before anaesthesia.
- To lessen the amount of general anaesthetic required to achieve and to maintain unconsciousness.
- Possibly, to sedate postoperatively.

Reduction of parasympathetic bradycardia and secretions

Muscarinic antagonists, e.g. atropine and hyoscine (see Chapter 2), are used to prevent salivation and bronchial secretions, and more importantly to protect the heart from arrhythmias, particularly bradycardia caused by some inhalation agents and neuromuscular blockers.

Analgesia

Opioid analgesics, e.g. morphine (see pp. 67–71), are often given prior to an operation: although the patient is unconscious during surgery, adequate analgesia is important to stop physiological stress reactions to pain.

Postoperative antiemesis

Drugs that provide postoperative antiemesis include metoclopramide, droperidol, and prochlorperazine. Nausea and vomiting are common after general anaesthesia, often because of the administration of opioid drugs peri- and postoperatively. Antiemetic drugs can be given with the premedication to inhibit this.

Induction

Intravenous agents are used to produce a rapid induction of unconsciousness. Intravenous agents are preferred by patients, since injection lacks the menacing quality of having a mask placed over the face (Fig. 3.16).

Maintenance

Inhalation anaesthetic agents are used to maintain a state of general anaesthesia after induction (Fig. 3.16).

Anaesthetic agents

Anaesthetic agents depress all excitable tissues including central neurons, cardiac muscle, and smooth and striated muscle. Different parts of the CNS have different sensitivities to anaesthetics, and the reticular activating system (RAS), which is responsible for consciousness, is among the most sensitive. Hence, it is possible to use anaesthetics at a concentration that produces unconsciousness without unduly depressing the cardiovascular or respiratory centres of the brain, or the myocardium. However, for the majority of anaesthetics the margin of safety is small.

Intravenous anaesthetics

Intravenous anaesthetics, e.g. thiopentone, propofol, and ketamine, are all CNS depressants. They produce anaesthesia by relatively selective depression of the RAS of the brain. They may be used alone for short surgical procedures, but are used mainly for the induction of anaesthesia, and thus it is rapidity of onset that is the desirable feature.

Intravenous anaesthetics are all highly lipid-soluble agents and cross the blood–brain barrier rapidly; their rapid onset (<30 seconds) is due to this rapid transfer into the brain, and high cerebral blood flow. Duration of action is short (minutes) and terminated by redistribution of the drug from the CNS into less-well-perfused tissues (Fig. 3.17); drug metabolism is irrelevant to recovery.

Thiopentone

Mechanism of action: Thiopentone is a highly lipophilic member of the barbiturate group of CNS depressants that act to potentiate the inhibitory effect of GABA on the $GABA_A/Cl^-$ receptor channel complex.

Route of administration: Thiopentone is administered intravenously.

Indications: Thiopentone causes rapid induction of general anaesthesia.

Contraindications: Thiopentone should not be given to patient with a previous allergy to it.

Adverse effects: The side effects of thiopentone include respiratory depression, myocardial depression (bradycardia), vasodilatation, and anaphylaxis. There is a risk of severe vasospasm if it is accidently injected into an artery.

Therapeutic notes: Thiopentone is a widely used induction agent, but it has no analgesic properties. It provides smooth and rapid (<30 seconds) induction but, owing to its narrow therapeutic margin, overdosage with consequent cardiorespiratory depression can occur. Thiopentone is given as the sodium salt, which is unstable in solution and must be made up immediately before use.

Propofol

Mechanism of action: Propofol is similar to thiopentone in its mechanism of action.

Route of administration: Propofol is administered intravenously.

Indications: Propofol causes rapid induction of general anaesthesia.

Contraindications: Propofol should not be given to patients with a previous allergy to it.

Adverse effects: Convulsions, anaphylaxis, and

delayed recovery from anaesthesia, have occasionally been reported as side effects.

Therapeutic notes: Propofol is associated with rapid recovery without nausea or hangover and is very widely used.

General anaesthetics		
Premedication	**Induction/ intravenous agents**	**Maintenance/ inhalation agents**
• relief from anxiety e.g. diazepam, lorazepam • reduction of parasympathetic bradycardia and secretions e.g. atropine, hyoscine • analgesia e.g. morphine • postoperative antiemesis e.g. metoclopramide, droperidol, prochlorperazine	• barbiturates e.g. thiopentone • non-barbiturates e.g. propofol, ketamine	nitrous oxide halothane enflurane isoflurane

Fig. 3.16 General anaesthetics.

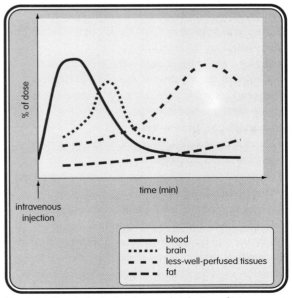

Fig. 3.17 Graph illustrating how redistribution of intravenous anaesthetic agents causes a short central duration of action. (Adapted from *Pharmacology* by H Rang, M. Dale, J. Ritter, Churchill Livingstone, 1995.)

Etomidate

Mechanism of action: The mechanism of action of etomidate is similar to that of thiopentone.

Route of administration: Etomidate is administered intravenously.

Indications: Etomidate causes rapid induction of general anaesthesia.

Contraindications: Etomidate should not be given to patients with a previous allergy to it.

Adverse effects: Side effects of etomidate include extraneous muscle movement and pain on injection, and possible adrenocortical suppression.

Therapeutic notes: Etomidate is an induction agent that gained favour over thiopentone because of its larger therapeutic margin and faster metabolism leading to fewer hangover effects. Etomidate is more prone to causing extraneous muscle movement and pain on injection compared to other agents.

Ketamine

Mechanism of action: Ketamine produces full surgical anaesthesia but the form of the anaesthesia is known as disassociative anaesthesia, as the patient may remain conscious though amnesic and insensitive to pain. This effect is probably related to an action on NMDA-type glutamate receptors.

Ketamine is a derivative of the street drug phencyclidine (PCP/'angel dust').

Route of administration: Ketamine is administered intravenously or intramuscularly.

Indications: Ketamine is used in the induction and maintenance of anaesthesia, especially in children.

Contraindications: Ketamine should not be given to people with hypertension or psychosis.

Adverse effects: These include:
- Cardiovascular stimulation, tachycardia, and raised arterial blood pressure.
- Transient psychotic sequelae such as vivid dreams and hallucinations.

Therapeutic notes: Ketamine is not often used as an induction agent, owing to the high incidence of dysphoria, and hallucinations during recovery in adults. These effects are much less marked in children, and ketamine, in conjunction with a benzodiazepine, is often used for minor procedures in paediatrics.

Inhalation anaesthetics

Examples of inhalation anaesthetics include nitrous oxide, halothane, enflurane, and isoflurane.

Inhalation anaesthetics may be gases or volatile liquids. They are commonly used for the maintenance of anaesthesia after induction with an intravenous agent.

Mechanism of action

It is not known exactly how inhalation anaesthetic agents produce their effects. Unlike most drugs, inhalation anaesthetics do not all belong to one recognizable chemical class. The shape and electronic configuration of the molecule are evidently unimportant. A distinct anaesthetic 'receptor' is therefore unlikely, and it would seem that the pharmacological action of inhalation anaesthetics is dependent on the physicochemical properties of the molecule.

Three theories of anaesthesia have received the most attention—the lipid, hydrate, and protein theories.

The lipid theory arose because a close correlation was noticed between anaesthetic potency and lipid solubility. It has been suggested that anaesthetics dissolve in membrane lipid and affect its physical state by two possible mechanisms. These are:
- Volume expansion, which is supported by pressure reversal of anaesthesia, but qualitative inconsistencies exist.
- Membrane fluidization, although the high concentrations required and weak effect of temperature make this difficult to accept.

The hydrate theory arose because anaesthetic molecules stabilize water molecules in their vicinity. It has been suggested that this alteration of the membrane accounts for the effects of anaesthetics.

While there is some correlation between potency and the ability to form hydrates, anomalous compounds

A positive correlation between lipid solubility and anaesthetic potency exists for many homologus series of anaesthetics. However, at a certain point, potency sharply decreases despite a continuing increase in lipid solubility—know as the 'cut-off phenomenon'. This is not consistent with the lipid theory but may be explained by the protein theory of anaesthesia.

such as sulphur hexafluoride do not form hydrates but do have anaesthetic properties.

The protein theory arose because there is increasing evidence that anaesthetics may act by binding to discrete hydrophobic domains of membrane proteins. This would explain the 'cut-off' phenomenon, and stereoselectivity of anaesthetics. The protein theory is currently popular, but the nature of the target protein(s) in the CNS has not been identified. Possible targets include voltage-operated channels, receptor-operated channels, or secondary-messenger systems.

Pharmacokinetic aspects

The depth of anaesthesia produced by inhalation anaesthetics is directly related to the partial pressure (tension) of the agent in the arterial blood, as this determines the concentration of agent in the CNS. The concentration of anaesthetic in the blood is in turn determined by:

- The concentration of anaesthetic in the inspired gas (alveolar concentration).
- The solubility of the anaesthetic in blood (blood:gas partition coefficient).
- Cardiac output.
- Alveolar ventilation.

Rapid induction and recovery are important properties of an anaesthetic agent, allowing flexible control over the arterial tension (and hence brain tension) and therefore the depth of anaesthesia. The speed at which induction of anaesthesia occurs is determined by two properties of the anaesthetic: its solubility in blood (blood:gas partition coefficient) and its solubility in fat (lipid solubility). Thus:

- Agents of low blood solubility (e.g. nitrous oxide, enflurane) produce rapid induction and recovery because relatively small amounts are required to saturate the blood, and so the arterial tension (and hence brain tension) rises and falls quickly (Fig. 3.18).
- Agents of high blood solubility (e.g. halothane) have much slower induction and recovery times because much more anaesthetic solution is required before the arterial anaesthetic tension approaches that of the inspired gas (Fig. 3.18).
- Agents with high lipid solubility (e.g. halothane) accumulate gradually in the body fat during prolonged anaesthesia, and so may produce a prolonged hangover if used for a long operation (Fig. 3.18).

Nitrous oxide

Mechanism of action: See above.

Route of administration: Nitrous oxide is administered by inhalation.

Indications: Nitrous oxide is used for the maintenance of anaesthesia (in combination with other agents), and for analgesia (50% mixture in oxygen: Entonox®).

Contraindications: Pneumothorax: nitrous oxide diffuses into air containing closed spaces resulting in an increased pressure, in the case of pneumothorax, this may compromise breathing.

Adverse effects: Nitrous oxide was thought to be relatively free of side effects—it has little effect on cardiovascular and respiratory systems—but the risk of bone marrow suppression is now a known factor.

Therapeutic notes: Nitrous oxide cannot produce surgical anaesthesia when administered alone, because of a lack of potency. It is commonly used as a non-flammable carrier gas for volatile agents, allowing their concentration to be reduced. As a 50% mixture in oxygen, nitrous oxide is a good analgesic and is used in childbirth and by paramedics.

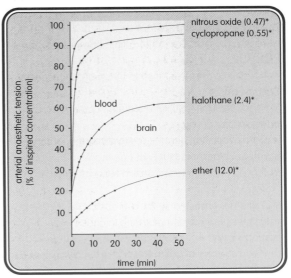

Fig. 3.18 Rate of equilibration of inhalation anaesthetics in humans. (*, blood gas coefficient—larger numbers indicate higher solubility and are associated with longer induction and recovery times.) (Adapted from *Uptake and Distribution of Anaesthetic Agents*, EM Papper and R Kitz, McGraw Hill, 1963.)

Halothane

Mechanism of action: See above.

Route of administration: Halothane is administered by inhalation.

Indications: Halothane is used in the maintenance of anaesthesia.

Contraindications: Halothane should not be given to people with a previous reaction to halothane or exposure to halothane in the past 3 months.

Adverse effects: Like most volatile anaesthetics, halothane causes cardiorespiratory depression. Respiratory depression results in elevated Pco_2 and perhaps ventricular arrhythmias. Halothane also depresses cardiac muscle fibres and may cause bradycardia. The result of this is a concentration-dependent hypotension.

The most significant toxic effect of halothane is severe hepatic necrosis, which occurs in 1 in 35 000 cases. Lesser degrees of liver damage may occur more frequently. The damage is caused by metabolites of the 20% of administered halothane that is biotransformed in the liver (80% of an administered dose is excreted by the lungs).

Therapeutic notes: Halothane is a halogenated hydrocarbon, and is probably the most widely used inhalation agent. It is potent, non-irritant, non-inflammable, and volatile.

Enflurane

Mechanism of action: See above.

Route of administration: Enflurane is administered by inhalation.

Indications: Enflurane is used in the maintenance of anaesthesia.

Contraindications: Enflurane should not be given to people with epilepsy.

Adverse effects: Enflurane causes cardiorespiratory depression similar to that with halothane, although the incidence of arrhythmias is much lower than with halothane.

Enflurane undergoes only 2% metabolism in the liver, so is much less likely than halothane to cause hepatotoxicity.

The disadvantage of enflurane is that it may cause EEG changes and muscle twitching, and special caution is needed in epileptic subjects.

Therapeutic notes: Enflurane is a volatile anaesthetic similar to, but less potent, than halothane, about twice the concentration being necessary for maintenance. Induction and recovery times are faster than for halothane.

Isoflurane

Mechanism of action: See above.

Route of administration: Isoflurane is administered by inhalation.

Indications: It is used in the maintenance of anaesthesia.

Contraindications: None.

Adverse effects: Isoflurane has actions similar to those of halothane but is less cardiodepressant. Hypotension is caused by a dose-related decrease in systemic vascular resistance rather than a marked fall in cardiac output. Less hepatic metabolism (0.2%) occurs than with enflurane, so hepatoxicity is even rarer.

Therapeutic notes: Isoflurane is an isomer of enflurane. It has a potency intermediate between that of halothane and enflurane.

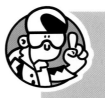

Questions on anaesthetic premedication are popular since they involve knowledge of a number of different classes of drug.

- What are the aims of the three clinical stages of general anaesthesia: premedication, induction, and maintenance?
- Describe the concept of selective depression that underlies the principle by which anaesthetic agents work.
- Discuss the three main theories that propose to explain the mechanism of action of inhalation anaesthetics.
- What are the important pharmacokinetic aspects involved in the use of inhalation anaesthetics?
- List examples of the drugs used in the premedication, induction, and maintenance stages of anaesthesia.

Use of neuromuscular blockers in anaesthesia

For some operations, e.g. intra-abdominal, complete relaxation of skeletal muscle is essential. Some general anaesthetic agents have significant neuromuscular blocking actions but drugs that specifically block the neuromuscular junction are frequently employed, e.g. suxamethonium, rocuronium, vercuronium, atracurium (see Chapter 2).

OPIOID ANALGESICS

Concepts of analgesia

Pain is a common everyday experience that performs an essential defensive function. However, uncontrolled pain can severely diminish quality of life, and may then be amenable to pharmacotherapy.

Pain, which may be acute or chronic, is defined as an unpleasant sensory and emotional experience associated with actual or potential tissue damage. Pain is a subjective experience, not always associated with nociception, which is the process of detecting and signalling the presence of a noxious stimulus to the CNS. This term is frequently reserved to describe the process in experimental animals.

An analgesic drug is one that effectively removes (or at least lessens) the sensation of pain.

Opioid analgesics are drugs (either naturally occurring, e.g. morphine, or chemically synthesized), that interact with specific opioid receptors to produce the pharmacological effect of analgesia.

Pain perception

Pain perception is best viewed as a three-stage process—activation of nociceptors, followed by the transmission, and onward passage, of pain information.

Activation of nociceptors in the peripheral tissues

Noxious thermal, chemical, or mechanical stimuli can trigger the firing of primary afferent fibres (type C/Aδ), through the activation of nociceptors (pain-specific receptors) in the peripheral tissues (Fig. 3.19).

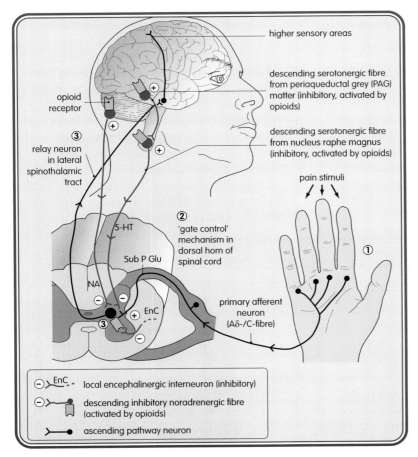

Fig. 3.19 Diagram showing nociceptive pathways and sites of opioid action. (Glu, glutamate; 5-HT, 5-hydroxytryptamine (serotonin); NA, noradrenaline; Sub P, substance P.)

higher sensory areas

descending serotonergic fibre from periaqueductal grey (PAG) matter (inhibitory, activated by opioids)

opioid receptor

descending serotonergic fibre from nucleus raphe magnus (inhibitory, activated by opioids)

③ relay neuron in lateral spinothalamic tract

pain stimuli

5-HT

② 'gate control' mechanism in dorsal horn of spinal cord

Sub P Glu

NA

EnC

③

primary afferent neuron (Aδ-/C-fibre)

①

⊖ EnC - local encephalinergic interneuron (inhibitory)

⊖ descending inhibitory noradrenergic fibre (activated by opioids)

ascending pathway neuron

Transmission of pain information

Transmission of pain information from the periphery to the dorsal horn of the spinal cord is inhibited or amplified by a combination of local (spinal) neuronal circuits and descending tracts from higher brain centres. This constitutes the 'gate-control mechanism'.

In the gate-control mechanism:

- The primary afferent fibres synapse in lamina I and II of the dorsal horn of the spinal cord.
- Transmitter peptides (substance P, calcitonin gene-related peptide, bradykinin, glutamate) and nitric oxide (NO) are involved in the ascending pain pathways, though the interactions are complex and have not yet been fully defined.
- The activity of the dorsal horn relay neurons is modulated by several inhibitory inputs. These include: local inhibitory interneurons, which release opioid peptides; descending inhibitory noradrenergic fibres from the locus ceruleus area of the brainstem, which are activated by opioid peptides; and descending inhibitory serotonergic fibres from the nucleus raphe magnus and periaqueductal grey areas of the brainstem, which are also activated by opioid peptides (Fig. 3.19).

Onward passage of pain information

The onward passage of pain information is via the spinothalamic tract, to the higher centres of the brain. The higher centres of the brain coordinate the cognitive and emotional aspects of pain and control appropriate reactions. Opioid peptide release in both the spinal cord and the brainstem can reduce the activity of the dorsal horn relay neurons and cause analgesia, known as 'shutting the gate' (Fig. 3.19).

Opioid receptors

All opioids, whether endogenous peptides, naturally occurring drugs, or chemically synthesized drugs, interact with specific opioid receptors to produce their pharmacological effects.

Drugs interact with opioid receptors as either full agonists, partial agonists, mixed agonists (full agonists on one opioid receptor, but partial agonists on another), or as antagonists. Opioid analgesics are agonists.

There are three major opioid receptor subtypes—μ, δ, and κ. The existence of a fourth receptor (σ) has been put forward, but recent evidence suggests that its classification as a true opioid receptor may be doubtful.

The distinctions between the actions associated with μ- and δ-receptors are relatively unclear, because selective agonists and antagonists have only recently been discovered. However:

- μ-Receptors are thought to be responsible for most of the analgesic effects of opioids and for some major adverse effects, e.g. respiratory depression. Most of the analgesic opioids in use are μ-receptor agonists.
- δ-Receptors are probably more important in the periphery, but may also contribute to analgesia.
- κ-Receptors contribute to analgesia at the spinal level, and may elicit sedation and dysphoria, but produce relatively few adverse effects, and do not contribute to physical dependence.
- σ-Receptors are not selective opioid receptors, but are the site of action of psychomimetic drugs, such as PCP. They may account for the dysphoria produced by some opioids.

Opioid receptor activation has an inhibitory effect on synapses in the CNS or the gut (Fig. 3.20).

Fig. 3.20 Actions mediated by opioid receptor subtypes.

Action	Receptor subtypes		
	μ/δ	κ	σ
analgesia	supraspinal and spinal	spinal	—
respiratory depression	marked	slight	—
pupil	constricts	—	dilates
GIT mobility	reduced (constipating)	—	—
mood/effect	euphoria inducing but also sedating	dysphoria inducing mildly sedating	marked dysphoric and psychomimetic actions
physical dependence	+++	+	—

Secondary-messenger systems associated with opioid receptor activity include:

- μ/δ-Receptors, the activation of which causes hyperpolarization of a neuron by opening potassium channels and inhibiting calcium channels.
- κ-Receptors, the activation of which inhibits calcium channels.

Activation of all opioid receptors causes a decrease in cAMP production, the functional significance of which is not clear.

Endogenous opioids

Physiologically, the CNS has its own 'endogenous opioids' that are the natural ligands for opioid receptors.

There are three main families of endogenous opioid peptides occurring naturally in the CNS:

- Endorphins.
- Dynorphins.
- Enkephalins.

They are derived from three separate gene products (precursor molecules) but all possess homology at their amino end—either the sequence:

Tyr-Gly-Gly-Phe-Met [Met^5] enkephalin
or: Tyr-Gly-Gly-Phe-Leu [Leu^5] enkephalin .

The expression and anatomical distribution of the products of these three precursor molecules within the CNS is varied, and each has a distinct range of affinities for the different types of opioid receptor (Fig. 3.21).

Endogenous opioid peptides		
Precursor molecules	**Products**	**Relative opioid receptor affinity**
pro-opiomelanocortin (POMC)	endorphins e.g. β-endorphin other non-opioid peptides e.g. ACTH	μ
proenkephalin	enkephalins e.g. [Leu^5] enkephalin, [Met^5] enkephalin, extended [Met^5] enkephalins	δ μ μ
prodynorphin	dynorphins e.g. dynorphin A	κ

Fig. 3.21 Endogenous opioid peptides.

Though it is known that the endogenous opioids possess analgesic activity, their precise function in the CNS and elsewhere is poorly defined. They are not used therapeutically.

Opioid analgesic drugs

Opioid analgesics are drugs, either naturally occurring, e.g. morphine, or chemically synthesized, that interact with specific opioid receptors to produce the pharmacological effect of analgesia.

The first opioid drug was opium, the crude exudate of the seed head of the opium poppy *Papaver somniferum*; simple extraction yields morphine. Subsequently, many synthetic and semi-synthetic opioids have been created by pharmacologists.

Examples of opioid analgesics are given in Fig. 3.22.

Mechanism of action: Opioid analgesic drugs work by agonist action at opioid receptors (see above).

Note that the sense of euphoria produced by strong opioids undoubtedly contributes to their analgesic activity by helping to reduce the anxiety and stress associated with pain. This effect also accounts for the illicit use of these drugs by addicts.

Route of administration: Opioids may be given orally, rectally, intravenously, or intramuscularly. Oral absorption is irregular and incomplete, necessitating larger doses; 70% is removed by first-pass hepatic metabolism.

Indications: Strong opioids are used in moderate to severe pain, particularly visceral, postoperative or cancer related; in myocardial infarction and acute pulmonary oedema; and in perioperative analgesia (p. 62).

Weak opioids are used in the relief of 'mild to moderate' pain, as antitussives (see Chapter 5), and as antidiarrhoeal agents (see Chapter 7), taking advantage of these 'side effects' of opioid analgesics.

Opioid analgesics	
strong opioid analgesics	**weak opioid analgesics**
morphine diamorphine phenazocine pethidine buprenorphine nalbuphine	pentazocine codeine dihydrocodeine dextropropoxyphene

Fig. 3.22 Opioid analgesics.

Contraindications: Opioid analgesics should not be given to people in acute respiratory depression, with acute alcoholism, at risk of paralytic ileus, and with cranial injuries prior to neurological assessment (interferes with pupillary responses).

Adverse effects: Opioid analgesics share many side effects, though qualitative and quantitative differences exist. These can be subdivided into central adverse actions and peripheral adverse actions.

Central adverse actions include the following:

- Drowsiness and sedation, in which initial excitement is followed by sedation and finally coma (on overdose).
- Reduction in sensitivity of the respiratory centre to CO_2, leading to shallow and slow respiration.
- Tolerance and dependence (see later).
- Suppression of cough, which 'adverse' effect is exploited clinically in antitussives (see Chapter 5).
- Vomiting due to stimulation of the chemoreceptor trigger zone (CTZ).
- Pupillary constriction due to stimulation of the parasympathetic third cranial nerve nucleus.
- Hypotension and reduced cardiac output, which are partly due to reduced hypothalamic sympathetic outflow.

Peripheral adverse actions include the following:

- Constipation, which is partly due to stimulation of cholinergic activity in gut wall ganglia that results in smooth wall spasm.
- Contraction of smooth muscle in the sphincter of Oddi and in the ureters, which results in an increase in blood amylase and lipase due to pancreatic stasis.
- Histamine release, which produces bronchospasm, flushing, and arteriolar dilatation.
- Lowered sympathetic discharge and direct arteriolar dilatation, which results in lowered cardiac output and hypotension.

Adverse effects of opioids tend to limit the dose that can be given, and the analgesia that can be maintained. The most serious of all these effects is respiratory depression, which is the most common cause of death from opioid overdose.

Constipation and nausea are also common problems and clinically it is common to co-administer laxatives (see Chapter 7) and an antiemetic.

Tolerance and dependence: Tolerance to opioid analgesics can be detected within 24–48 hours from the onset of administration, and results in larger and larger doses of the drug being needed to achieve the same clinical effect.

Dependence involves μ-receptors and is both physical and psychological in nature.

If physical dependence develops, it is characterized by a definite withdrawal syndrome following cessation of drug treatment. This syndrome comprises a complex mixture of irritable and sometimes aggressive behaviour combined with extremely unpleasant autonomic symptoms such as fever, sweating, yawning, and pupillary dilatation. The withdrawal syndrome is relieved by the administration of μ-receptor agonists, and worsened by the administration of μ-receptor antagonists.

Psychological dependence of opioid analgesics is based on the positive reinforcement provided by euphoria.

In the clinical context, especially in terminal care, where tolerance and dependence can be monitored, they are not inevitably problematic. However, the fear of tolerance and dependence often leads to overcaution in the use of opioid analgesics, and unnecessarily poor pain control in patients.

Therapeutic notes: Strong opioid analgesics include morphine, diamorphine (heroin), phenazocine, pethidine, buprenorphine, and nalbuphine.

- Morphine, remains the most valuable drug for severe pain relief, though it frequently causes nausea and vomiting. It is the drug of choice for severe pain in terminal care. Morphine is the standard against which other opioid analgesics are compared.
- Diamorphine (heroin) is twice as potent as morphine, owing to its greater penetration of the blood–brain barrier. It is metabolized to 6-acetylmorphine and thence morphine in the body. Diamorphine causes less nausea and hypotension than morphine, but more euphoria.
- Phenazocine has a more prolonged action than morphine and can be administered sublingually. It can be useful in biliary colic as it has less of a tendency to increase biliary spasm than other opioids.
- Pethidine is more lipid soluble than morphine and has a rapid onset and short duration of action, making it useful in labour. Pethidine is equianalgesic compared with morphine, but produces less constipation. Interaction with MAOIs is serious, causing fever, delirium, and convulsions or respiratory depression.
- Buprenorphine has both agonist and antagonist actions at opioid receptors, and may precipitate withdrawal symptoms in patients dependent on

other opioids. It has a longer duration of action than morphine and its lipid solubility allows sublingual administration. Vomiting may be a problem. Unlike most opioid analgesics, the effects of buprenorphine are only partially antagonized by naloxone owing to its high-affinity attraction to opioid receptors.

- Nalbuphine is an agonist at κ-receptors and an antagonist at μ-receptors. It is equiananalgesic compared with morphine, but produces less nausea and vomiting. High doses cause dysphoria.

Weak opioid analgesics include pentazocine, codeine, dihydrocodeine, and dextropropoxyphene.

- Pentazocine has both κ/σ-receptor agonist and μ-antagonist actions and may precipitate withdrawal symptoms in patients dependent on other opioids. Pentazocine is weak orally, but by injection has a potency between that of morphine and codeine. It is not recommended, because of the side effects of thought disturbances and hallucinations, which probably are due to its action on σ-receptors.
- Codeine has about one-twelfth of the analgesic potency of morphine. The incidence of nausea and constipation limit the dose and duration that can be used. Codeine is also used for its antitussive and antidiarrhoeal effects.
- Dihydrocodeine has an analgesic efficacy similar to that of codeine. It may cause dizziness and constipation.
- Dextropropoxyphene has an analgesic efficacy about half that of codeine, i.e. very mild, and so is often combined with aspirin or paracetamol. Such mixtures can be dangerous in overdose, with dextropropoxy-phene causing respiratory depression and acute heart failure, while the paracetamol is hepatotoxic.

Opioid antagonists

Examples of opioid antagonists include naloxone and naltrexone.

Mechanism of action: These drugs act by specific antagonism at opioid receptors: μ-, δ-, and κ-receptors are blocked more or less equally. They block the actions of endogenous opioids as well as of morphine-like drugs.

Naloxone is short acting (half-life 2–4 hours) while naltrexone is long acting (half-life 10 hours).

Route of administration: Opioid antagonists are administered intravenously.

Indications: Opioid antagonists are given to reverse opioid-induced analgesia and respiratory depression rapidly, mainly after overdose, or to improve breathing in newborn babies that have been affected by the opioids given to their mother.

Adverse effects: Opioid antagonists have several side effects, including precipitation of withdrawal in those with physical dependence on opioids, increased sensitivity to painful stimuli, and cardiotoxicity.

Heroin addicts are able to tolerate 300–600 mg doses several times per day. This is 30–60 times the normal dose needed to produce an analgesic effect. A non-addict given this would die of respiratory depression.

- What is meant by the terms nociception, pain, and analgesia?
- Describe the pathways and mechanisms involved in the perception of pain and relate the action of opioid analgesics to them.
- List the different types of opioid receptor and describe the actions ascribed to them. Relate the mechanism of action of the opioid analgesics to the opioid receptors and to their clinical effect.
- Discuss the activity of endogenous opioid peptides, natural and synthetic opioid analgesic drugs, and opioid antagonist drugs at opioid receptors in relation to their pharmacological effects.
- List the major side effects of the opioid analgesics.
- Give examples of strong opioid analgesics, weak opioid analgesics, and opioid antagonists.

DRUG MISUSE

Concepts of drug misuse

Introduction

Historically there has been a long relationship between humans and the non-therapeutic use of drugs that act on the mind and body. Virtually all cultures have used drugs for non-therapeutic purposes: for instance, the Incas used psychoactive fungi and the ancient Egyptians (and many other cultures) used alcohol.

It is important to realize that the misuse of drugs is a socially defined concept that has as much to do with the legal, religious, moral, and cultural framework of a society as the pharmacological properties of the drug itself. Drugs now banned in the UK, e.g. opium, were once popular and legal in nineteenth century England, while attitudes to alcohol vary both historically and geographically from total prohibition to deep entrenchment in the culture.

Humans show great ingenuity in creating, harvesting, obtaining, and taking drugs for non-therapeutic reasons, and go to great lengths to do so. The sheer prevalence and associated co-morbidity makes drug misuse an important medical subject.

Drug misuse

Drug misuse is defined as the use of drugs that causes actual physical or mental harm to an individual or to society, or that is illegal. Thus drug misuse includes alcohol, nicotine, and the damaging overprescription of tranquillizers, as well as the more obvious illicit drugs such as LSD.

The term 'drug abuse' is synonymous with 'drug misuse' but is currently less in vogue owing to its negative connotations.

Drug dependence

Drug dependence is defined as the compulsion to take a drug repeatedly, with distress being caused if this is prevented.

Drugs of dependence all have rewarding effects (this is why they are taken), but they also have unpleasant (aversive) effects, often as the drug leaves the brain.

Dependence involves psychological factors as well as physical aspects. These are not exclusive and there is a mixture of both in most people who are dependent on drugs.

Psychological dependence is when the rewarding effects (positive reinforcement) predominate to cause a compulsion to continue taking the drug.

Physical dependence is when the distress on stopping the drug (negative reinforcement) is the main reason for continuing to take it, i.e. avoidance of the 'withdrawal syndrome'.

Drug tolerance

Drug tolerance is the necessity to increase the dose of an administered drug progressively in order to maintain the effect that was produced by the (smaller) original doses. Drug tolerance is a phenomenon that develops with chronic administration of a drug.

Many different mechanisms can give rise to drug tolerance, though they are rather poorly understood. These include:

- Downregulation of receptors.
- Changes in receptors.
- Exhaustion of biological mediators or transmitters.
- Increased metabolic degradation (enzyme induction).
- Physiological adaptation.

Withdrawal

Withdrawal is the term used to describe the syndrome of effects caused by stopping administration of a drug.

Withdrawal results from the change of (neuro)physiological equilibrium induced by the presence of the drug (Fig. 3.23).

Legal aspects of drug misuse (UK)

Misuse of Drugs Act 1971

The Misuse of Drugs Act 1971 prohibits certain activities in relation to 'controlled drugs', in particular their manufacture, supply, and possession. The Act is primarily a legal document for use by the police and judiciary. The penalties applicable to offences involving the different drugs are graded broadly according to the harmfulness attributable to a drug when it is misused, and for this purpose the drugs are categorized into three classes (Fig. 3.24).

Misuse of Drugs Regulations 1985

The Misuse of Drugs Regulations 1985 are a set of working regulations that define the classes of persons who are authorized to supply and possess controlled drugs while acting in their professional capacities, and lay down the conditions under which these activities may be carried out.

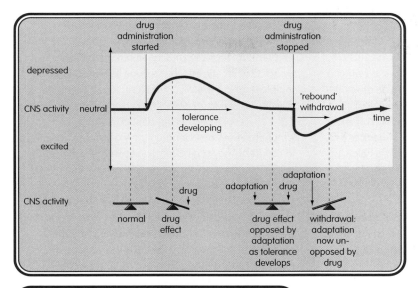

Fig. 3.23 Tolerance to and withdrawal from CNS depressant drugs, e.g. alcohol. The graph for tolerance on and withdrawal from CNS stimulant drugs, e.g. cocaine, would be a mirror image in the x-axis of what is shown.

Classes of controlled drugs		
Class A drugs	**Class B drugs**	**Class C drugs**

cocaine
MDMA ('ecstasy')
diamorphine (heroin)
  and other strong
  opioids
lysergic acid
  diethylamide class B
  (LSD) substances
  when prepared for
  injection
others
	amphetamines
	cannabis
	barbiturates
	some weak
	  opioids
	others
		benzodiazepines
		androgenic and
		  anabolic steroids
		human chorionic
		  gonadotrophin
		others

Fig. 3.24 Classes of controlled drugs.

In these regulations, drugs of addiction or high misuse potential are divided into five schedules, each specifying the requirements governing such aspects as import, export, production, supply, possession, prescription, and record keeping that apply to them (Fig. 3.25).

These regulations are more relevant than the 1971 Act to the clinical practice of health professionals (Fig. 3.25).

Fig. 3.25 Misuse of drugs regulations 1985.

Misuse of drugs regulations 1985	
Classification and example	**Controlled drug requirements**
schedule 1 • drugs that have no medicinal use e.g. cannabis, LSD	possession and supply prohibited without Home Office authority (given e.g. for research)
schedule 2 • medicinal drugs with high misuse potential e.g. heroin, morphine, pethidine, cocaine	drugs subject to full controlled drug requirements, e.g. special prescription requirements, safe custody, register keeping
schedule 3 • medicinal drugs of lesser misuse potential e.g. minor stimulants, barbiturates, some analgesics	drugs subject to some controlled drug requirements, e.g. special prescription requirements, but not safe custody or register keeping
schedule 4 • mainly benzodiazepines with abuse potential e.g. benzodiazepines, anabolic steroids	minimal requirements
schedule 5 • high-strength preparations of non-controlled drugs	virtually no controlled drug requirements other than the retention of invoices for 2 years

Notification and Supply to Addicts Regulations 1973

The Notification and Supply to Addicts Regulations 1973 require that any doctor who attends to a person who he suspects is addicted to any of the 14 notifiable drugs is legally required to furnish details, in writing, of that person's particulars to the Chief Medical Officer. The idea of this is to maintain a confidential 'index of addicts' that can be checked, to safeguard against addicts obtaining supplies simultaneously from two or more doctors.

Drugs of misuse

Drugs with a high potential for misuse fall into many distinct pharmacological categories. They may or may not be used therapeutically, and may be illegal or legal (Fig. 3.26).

Central stimulants

Amphetamines

Streetnames: Speed, Whizz, Billy, Uppers.

Mechanism of action: Amphetamines cause the release of monoamines and the inhibition of monoamine reuptake, especially of dopamine and noradrenaline in neurons.

Route of administration: Amphetamines are administered orally, or 'snorted' as a powder nasally; sometimes used intravenously.

Summary table of drugs with a high misuse potential	
Drug class	**Examples**
central stimulants	cocaine amphetamines MDMA (ecstasy) nicotine
central depressants	alcohol benzodiazepines barbiturates
opioid analgesics	morphine heroin (diamorphine) methadone
cannabinoids	cannabis tetrahydrocannabinoids (THCs)
hallucinogens	LSD mescaline psilocybin
dissociative anaesthetics	ketamine phencyclidine

Fig. 3.26 Drugs with high potential for misuse.

Effects: The effects of amphetamines include the following: increased motor activity; euphoria and excitement; anorexia and insomnia; peripheral sympathomimetic effects, such as hypertension and inhibition of gut motility; and stereotyped behaviour and psychosis, which develop with prolonged usage.

Clinical uses: The (very few) clinical uses of amphetamines are for narcolepsy and for hyperkinesis in children. They are no longer recommended as appetite suppressants, owing to their adverse effects.

Tolerance, dependence, and withdrawal: Tolerance to the peripheral sympathomimetic stimulant effects of amphetamines develops rapidly, but it develops much more slowly to other effects such as locomotor stimulation. Amphetamines cause strong psychological dependence but no real physical dependence. After stopping chronic use, the individual will usually enter a deep, long sleep ('REM rebound') and awake feeling tired, depressed, and hungry. This state may reflect the depletion of the normal monoamine stores.

Adverse effects: Acute amphetamine toxicity causes cardiac arrhythmias, hypertension, and stroke. Chronic toxicity causes paranoid psychosis, vasoconstriction, and tissue anoxia at sites of injection or snorting, and damage to the fetal brain in utero.

Cocaine

Streetnames: Coke, Charlie, Snow, Crack (freebase).

Mechanism of action: Cocaine strongly inhibits the reuptake of catecholamines at noradrenergic neurons, and thus strongly enhances sympathetic activity.

Route of administration: Cocaine hydrochloride is usually snorted nasally. 'Crack' is the freebase, which is more volatile and does not decompose on heating. It can therefore be smoked, producing a brief intense 'rush'.

Effects: The behavioural effects produced by cocaine are similar to those produced by amphetamines, such as euphoria. The euphoric effects may be greater and there is less of a tendency for stereotypical behaviour and paranoid delusions.

The effects of cocaine hydrochloride (lasting about an hour) are not as long lasting as those of amphetamine, while those obtained from crack are brief (minutes).

Clinical uses: Cocaine is occasionally used as a topical anaesthetic in ophthalmology.

Tolerance, dependence, and withdrawal: Cocaine causes strong psychological dependence but no real physical dependence. Withdrawal causes a marked deterioration in motor performance, which is restorable on provision of the drug.

Adverse effects: Acute cocaine toxicity causes toxic psychosis, cardiac arrhythmias, hypertension, and stroke. Chronic toxicity causes paranoid psychosis, vasoconstriction and tissue anoxia at sites of injection or snorting, and damage to the fetal brain.

Methylenedioxymethamphetamine
Streetnames: Ecstasy, E, Disco Biscuits, Pills.
Mechanism of action: Methylenedioxymeth-amphetamine (MDMA) is an amphetamine derivative which has a mechanism of action similar to that of amphetamines (release of monoamines, inhibition of monoamine reuptake). MDMA especially has actions on serotonergic neurons, potentiating 5-HT.

Route of administration: MDMA is usually taken as a pill containing other psychoactive drugs such as amphetamine or ketamine.

Effects: MDMA has mixed stimulant and hallucinogenic properties, especially in its pure form. Euphoria, arousal, and perceptual disturbances are common. Uniquely, MDMA has the effect of creating a feeling of euphoric empathy, so that social barriers are reduced.

Clinical uses: MDMA has no clinical use. Trials have been licensed in the USA for its evaluation as a treatment for people with social avoidant personality disorders.

Tolerance, dependence, and withdrawal: It is not currently known to what extent tolerance and dependence occur with MDMA. The withdrawal syndrome is similar to that with amphetamines.

Adverse effects: The most serious acute consequences of acute MDMA toxicity appear to be hyperthermia, exhaustion, and dehydration caused indirectly by the repetitive locomotor behaviour induced (dancing!). Very rarely this results in fatality. Chronic MDMA toxicity causes neurodegeneration of serotonergic nerves in the brains of experimental primates. The correlation to humans is not known.

Nicotine
Nicotine is found in cigarettes, cigars, pipes, and chewing tobacco.
Mechanism of action: Nicotine exerts its effects by causing nicotinic acetylcholine receptor (nicAChR) excitation leading to neurotransmitter release and nicAChR desensitization.

Route of administration: Nicotine is usually inhaled, although it can be chewed.

Effects: Nicotine has both stimulant and relaxant properties. Physiologically, nicotine increases alertness, decreases irritability, and relaxes skeletal muscle tone.

Peripheral effects due to ganglionic stimulation include tachycardia, increased blood pressure, and decreased gastrointestinal motility.

Clinical uses: Nicotine has no clinical use.

Tolerance, dependence, and withdrawal: Tolerance to nicotine occurs rapidly, first to peripheral effects but later to central effects.

Nicotine is highly addictive, causing both physical and psychological dependence.

Withdrawal from tobacco often leads to a syndrome of craving, irritability, anxiety, and increased appetite for approximately 2–3 weeks.

Adverse effects: Acute nicotine toxicity causes nausea and vomiting. Chronic toxicity caused by smoking leads to more morbidity in the UK than all other drugs combined, predisposing to all of the following diseases, often greatly so:

- Cardiovascular diseases, including atherosclerosis, hypertension, and coronary heart disease.
- Cancer of the lung, bladder, and mouth.
- Respiratory diseases such as bronchitis, emphysema, and asthma.
- Fetal growth retardation.

Central depressants
Ethanol
Mechanism of action: Ethanol, or alcohol, acts in a similar way to volatile anaesthetic agents, as a general CNS depressant. The cellular mechanisms involved may include inhibition of calcium entry, hence reduction in transmitter release, as well as potentiation of inhibitory GABA transmission.

Route of administration: Ethanol is administered orally.

Effects: The familiar effects of ethanol intoxication range from increased self-confidence and motor incoordination through to unconsciousness and coma. Peripheral effects include a self-limiting diuresis and vasodilatation.

Clinical uses: Ethanol is used as an antidote to methanol poisoning.

Tolerance, dependence, and withdrawal: Tolerance, and physical and psychological dependence, all occur with ethanol, such that 15 000 people a year are admitted to psychiatric hospital for alcohol dependence and psychosis, and 20% of males on a medical ward have alcohol-related disabilities.

The alcohol withdrawal syndrome is a rebound of the nervous system after adaptation to the depression caused by alcohol. This syndrome occurs in two stages:

- Early stage ('hangover'), which is common and starts 6–8 hours after cessation of drinking. It involves tremulousness, nausea, retching, and sweating.
- Late stage (delirium tremens), which is much less common and starts 48–72 hours after cessation of drinking. It involves delirium, tremor, hallucinations, and confusion.

Management of these late withdrawal symptoms involves sedation with chlormethiazole or benzodiazepines; clonidine may be useful.

Adverse effects: Acute ethanol toxicity causes ataxia, nystagmus, coma, respiratory depression, and death. Chronic ethanol toxicity causes neurodegeneration (potentiated by vitamin deficiency), dementia, liver damage, pancreatitis, etc., and accompanying psychiatric illness—depression/psychosis is common.

Benzodiazepines

Mechanism of action: Benzodiazepines exert their effects by potentiation of inhibitory GABA transmission (p. 43)

Route of administration: Benzodiazepines are administered orally.

Effects: The effects of benzodiazepines include sedation, agitation, and ataxia.

Clinical uses: Benzodiazepines are heavily prescribed as anxiolytics and hypnotics

Tolerance, dependence, and withdrawal: Benzodiazepines have a potential for misuse—tolerance and dependence are common.

A physical withdrawal syndrome can occur in patients given benzodiazepines, even for short periods. Symptoms include rebound anxiety and insomnia with depression, nausea, and perceptual changes that may last from weeks to months.

Adverse effects: The adverse effects of acute benzodiazepine toxicity include hypotension and confusion.

Cognitive impairment occurs in chronic benzodiazepine toxicity.

Opioid analgesics
Diamorphine (heroin) and other opioids
Streetnames: Smack, Dragon.

Mechanism of action: Opioids, e.g. diamorphine, show agonist action at opioid receptors (p. 67).

Note that the sense of euphoria and wellbeing produced by strong opioids undoubtedly contributes to their analgesic activity by helping to reduce the anxiety and stress associated with pain. This effect also accounts for the illicit use of these drugs by addicts.

Route of administration: Opioids are generally taken intravenously by misusers as this produces the most intense sense of euphoria ('rush').

Effects: Opioids produce feelings of euphoria and wellbeing. Other effects are mentioned on page 70.

Clinical uses: Opioids are used in analgesia for moderate to severe pain.

Tolerance, dependence, and withdrawal: Tolerance to opioid analgesics develops quickly in addicts and results in larger and larger doses of the drug being needed to achieve the same effect.

Dependence involves both psychological factors and physical factors. Psychological dependence is based on the positive reinforcement provided by euphoria.

There is a definite physical withdrawal syndrome in addicts following cessation of drug treatment with opioids. This syndrome comprises a complex mixture of irritable and sometimes aggressive behaviour, combined with extremely unpleasant autonomic symptoms such as fever, sweating, yawning, pupillary dilatation, and piloerection that gives the state its colloquial name of 'cold turkey'. Patients are extremely distressed and restless and strongly crave the drug. Symptoms are maximal at 2 days and largely disappear in 7–10 days.

Treatment of withdrawal: Methadone is a long-acting opiate, active orally, that is used to wean addicts from their addiction. The withdrawal symptoms from this longer-acting compound are more prolonged, but less intense than, for example, those of heroin. Treatment usually involves substitution of methadone followed by a slow reduction in dose over time.

Clonidine, an α_2-adrenoreceptor agonist, inhibits firing of locus coeruleus neurons and is effective in suppressing some components of the opioid withdrawal syndrome, especially the nausea, vomiting, and diarrhoea.

Adverse effects: Acute opioid toxicity causes the following:

- Confusion, drowsiness, and sedation. Initial excitement is followed by sedation and finally coma on overdose.
- Shallow and slow respiration, due to reduction of sensitivity of the respiratory centre to CO_2.
- Vomiting, due to stimulation of the chemoreceptor trigger zone.
- Autonomic effects such as tremor and pupillary constriction.
- Bronchospasm, flushing, and arteriolar dilatation due to histamine release.

Acute toxicity may be countered by use of an opioid antagonist such as naloxone.

The adverse effects of direct chronic toxicity are minor (p. 70).

Cannabinoids
Cannabis
Streetnames: Puff, Weed, Pot, Dope, Gear, Ganja, Blow.
There are two forms of cannabis:
- Marijuana is the dried leaves and flowers of the cannabis plant.
- Hashish is the extracted resin of the cannabis plant.

Mechanism of action: How cannabis exerts its effects is not clearly defined, but includes both depressant, stimulant, and psychomimetic effects.

The active constituent of cannabis is Δ^9-tetrahydro-cannabinol (THC), though metabolites that also have activity may be important.

Route of administration: Cannabis is usually smoked, although it may be eaten.

Effects: Cannabis has several effects:
- Subjectively, users feel relaxed and mildly euphoric.
- Perception is altered, with apparent sharpening of sensory experience.
- Appetite is enhanced.
- Peripheral actions include vasodilatation and bronchodilatation, and a reduction in intraocular pressure.

Clinical uses: Cannabis is not currently licensed for use in the UK. It is being evaluated for palliative or symptomatic relief use in certain conditions in the USA, e.g. for the antiemetic effect of THC, and a possible role in treatment of glaucoma.

Tolerance, dependence, and withdrawal: Tolerance to cannabis occurs to a minor degree. It is not dangerously addictive, with only moderate physical and psychological withdrawal effects noted, such as mild anxiety/dysphoria and sleep disturbances.

Adverse effects: Acute cannabis toxicity causes confusion and hallucinations. Chronic toxicity may cause flashbacks, memory loss, and 'demotivational syndrome'.

Psychotomimetic drugs or hallucinogens
Streetnames: Acid, Trips, Magic mushrooms.
Examples of psychotomimetic drugs include LSD, mescaline, and psilocybin.

Mechanism of action: How LSD, mescaline, and psilocybin produce changes in perception is not well understood but seems to involve serotonin. LSD appears to affect serotonergic systems by acting on 5-HT_2 inhibitory autoreceptors on serotonergic neurons to reduce their firing. Whether LSD is an agonist or an antagonist or both is not clear.

Route of administration: Psychotomimetic drugs are administered orally as a liquid, pills, or paper stamps.

Effects: Psychotomimetic drugs cause a dramatically altered state of perception—vivid and unusual sensory experiences combined with euphoric sensations. Hallucinations, delusions, and panic can occur; this is known as a 'bad trip' and can be terrifying.

Clinical uses: Psychotomimetic drugs have no clinical uses.

Tolerance, dependence, and withdrawal: Tolerance to, dependence on, and withdrawal from psychotomimetic drugs are not significant.

Adverse effects: Acute toxicity from psychotomimetic drugs causes frightening delusions or hallucinations that can lead to accidents or violence. In chronic toxicity, 'flashbacks' (a recurrence of hallucination) may occur long after the 'trip'. Other psychotic symptoms may also occur.

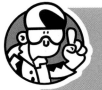
Try to use the correct chemical name when describing drugs of misuse, rather than a streetname or personal favourite—i.e. amphetamines rather than Whizz or Speed—it tends to go down better with examiners!

○ Discuss the concepts behind the misuse of drugs: positive and negative reinforcement, tolerance, dependence, and withdrawal.

○ What are the basic laws relating to the misuse of drugs, the control of drugs, supply of addicts etc., that a doctor should know about?

○ Name the different classes of drug that are subject to misuse, and for each describe:
– The mechanism of action of the drug—what does it do?
– Effects—why do people take it?
– Aspects of tolerance, dependence, and withdrawal—is it addictive, and if so, why?
– Acute and chronic toxic effects of misuse—what problems does it cause?

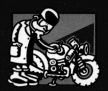

4. Cardiovascular System

THE HEART

Cardiac anatomy and physiology
The heart as a pump
The heart functions as a pump, that together with the vascular system, supplies the tissues with blood containing oxygen and nutrients as well as removing waste products.

The flow of blood around the body is as follows (Fig. 4.1):
- Deoxygenated blood from body tissues reaches the right atrium through the systemic veins (the superior and inferior venae cavae).
- Blood flows into the right ventricle, which then pumps the deoxygenated blood via the pulmonary circulation to the lungs, where the blood becomes oxygenated before reaching the left atrium.
- Blood flows from the left atrium into the left ventricle, where it is pumped into the systemic circulation, via the aorta, to supply the tissues of the body.

Cardiac rate and rhythm
The sinoatrial node (SAN), located in the roof of the right atrium near the entrance of the superior vena cava, and the atrioventricular node (AVN), located at the base of the right atrium, possess a spontaneous intrinsic rhythm.

Since the SAN discharges at a frequency higher than other regions of the heart (80 impulses/minute), it is the pacemaker for the heart, and as such determines the heart rate.

The action potential generated by the SAN spreads throughout both atria, reaching the AVN, from which it enters the interventricular septum by means of the bundle of His. The bundle of His splits into left and right branches making contact with the Purkinje fibres, which conduct the impulse throughout the ventricles, causing the ventricles to contract (Fig. 4.2)

Cardiac action potential
The shape of the action potential is characteristic of the location of its origin (i.e. whether from nodal tissue, the atria, or the ventricles) (Fig. 4.2).

Fig. 4.1 Blood flow through the heart chambers.

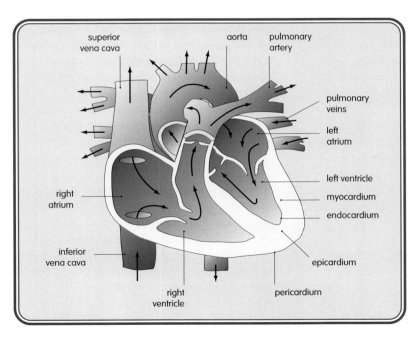

superior vena cava

aorta

pulmonary artery

pulmonary veins

left atrium

left ventricle

myocardium

endocardium

right atrium

inferior vena cava

epicardium

right ventricle

pericardium

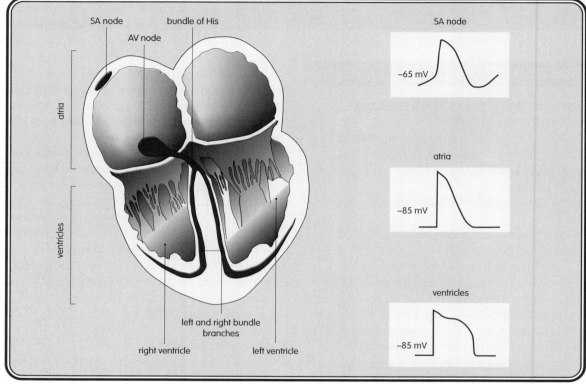

Fig. 4.2 Regional variation in cell structure and action potential configuration throughout the heart. (AV, atrioventricular; SA, sinoatrial.)

Non-nodal cells

The resting membrane potential across the ventricular cell membrane is approximately −85 mV; this is because the resting membrane is more permeable to potassium than to other ions. Four phases occurring at the ventricular cell membrane are:

- Phase 0 or depolarization. Depolarization occurs when the membrane potential reaches a critical value of −60 mV. The upstroke of the action potential is due to the transient opening of voltage-gated sodium channels, allowing sodium ions into the cell. In addition, potassium conductance falls to very low levels.
- Phase 1 or partial repolarization. Partial repolarization occurs as a result of the inactivation of the sodium current, and a transient outward potassium current.
- Phase 2 or plateau phase. The membrane remains depolarized at a plateau of approximately 0 mV. This

is due to the activation of a voltage-dependent slow inward calcium current, conducting positive charge into the cell, and a delayed rectifier potassium current conducting positive charge out of the cell.
- Phase 3 or repolarization. Repolarization is due to the inactivation of the calcium current and an increase in potassium conductance (Fig. 4.3).

Nodal cells

The resting membrane potential of nodal cells is approximately −60 mV.

In nodal cells, there is no fast sodium current. Instead, the action potential is initiated by an inward calcium current, and because calcium spikes conduct slowly, there is a delay of approximately 0.1 seconds between atrial and ventricular contraction.

Nodal cells have a phase known as phase 4 or the pacemaker potential. This phase involves a gradual depolarization that occurs during diastole and is known as the f current (I_f, funny). The f current is activated by hyperpolarization at −45 mV or more negative, and consists of sodium and calcium ions entering the cell (Fig. 4.4).

Autonomic control of the heart

Both the parasympathetic and sympathetic nervous systems influence the resting heart, but parasympathetic activity predominates and explains why the heart rate is lower than the inherent firing frequency of the SAN.

The sympathetic nervous system mediates its effects through the activation of β_1-receptors. These are linked to adenylyl cyclase and their activation causes increased levels of cyclic adenosine monophosphate (cAMP), and a subsequent increase in intracellular calcium levels.

The parasympathetic nervous system mediates its effects through the activation of M_2-receptors. These are also linked to adenylyl cyclase, but their activation causes decreased levels of cAMP, and a subsequent decrease in intracellular calcium levels.

The effects of the sympathetic and parasympathetic nervous systems on the heart are summarized in Fig. 4.5.

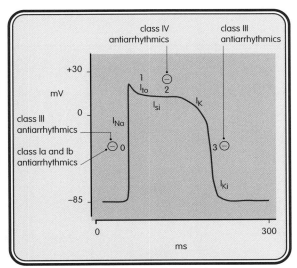

Fig. 4.3 Configuration of a typical ventricular action potential showing the ionic currents, the phases, and where Class I, III, and IV antiarrhythmic drugs act. (1, 2, and 3, phases of the action potential; I_{Na}, fast inward Na^+ current; I_{si}, slow inward Ca^{2+} current; I_{to}, transient outward K^+ current; I_K, delayed rectifier K^+ current; I_{Ki}, inward rectifier K^+ current.)

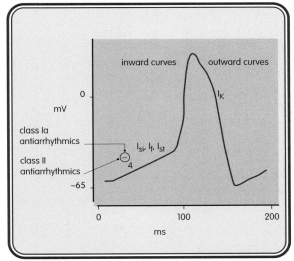

Fig. 4.4 Configuration of a typical sinoatrial node action potential showing the ionic currents, the phases, and where class Ia and II antiarrhythmic drugs act. (4, phase of the action potential; I_{si}, an inward current carried by Ca^{2+} ions; I_f, a 'funny' current carried by Na^+ and Ca^{2+} ions; I_{st}, the sustained inward Na^+ current; I_K, the delayed rectifier current which is an outward K^+ current.)

Effects of the sympathetic and parasympathetic systems on the heart		
	Sympathetic	**Parasympathetic**
heart rate	increased	decreased
force of contraction	increased	decreased
automaticity	increased	reduced
AV node conduction	facilitated	inhibited
cardiac efficiency	reduced	increased

Fig. 4.5 Effects of the sympathetic and parasympathetic system on the heart. (AV, atrioventricular.)

Cardiac contractility

Myocardial contraction is the result of calcium entry through L-type channels, giving rise to an increase in cytosolic calcium (Fig. 4.6).

The calcium is derived from two sources:
- The sarcoplasmic reticulum.
- Extracellular calcium.

Extracellular calcium enters the sarcoplasmic reticulum, causing larger amounts of calcium to be released, a process known as calcium-induced calcium release.

During contraction, the intracellular levels of calcium rise to levels 10 000 times greater than those at rest. Calcium binds to troponin C, thus modifying the position of actin and myosin filaments, and allowing contraction.

Contraction ceases only once calcium has been removed from the cytosol. This occurs through two mechanisms:
- Calcium is pumped out of the cell via the electrogenic Na^+/Ca^{2+} exchanger, which pumps one calcium ion out for every three sodium ions in.
- Calcium is re-sequestered into sarcoplasmic reticulum stores by a Ca^{2+} ATPase pump.

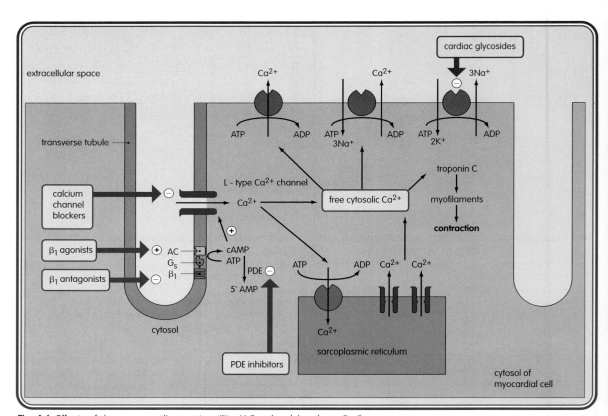

Fig. 4.6 Effects of drugs on cardiac contractility. (AC, adenylyl cyclase; β_1, β_1-adrenoceptor; G_s, stimulatory G-protein; PDE, phosphodiesterase.)

Cardiac dysfunction

Congestive heart failure

Congestive heart failure (CHF) is the combined failure of both the left and right sides of the heart.

Each year, 400 000 new cases of CHF are diagnosed in the USA alone, where it is the most common cause of hospitalization in those aged over 65 years.

CHF occurs when the cardiac output does not meet the needs of the tissues. This is thought to be due to defective excitation–contraction coupling, with progressive systolic and diastolic ventricular dysfunction.

Some of the causes and symptoms of acute and chronic heart failure are listed in Fig. 4.7.

The characteristics of left and right ventricular heart failure are listed in Fig. 4.8.

The body attempts to compensate for the effects of CHF by two processes—extrinsic and intrinsic.

Extrinsic neurohumoral reflexes: Extrinsic neurohumoral reflexes aim to maintain cardiac output and blood pressure such that hypotension → activation of baroreceptors (receptors resonding to changes in pressure)→ increased sympathetic activity → increased heart rate and vasoconstriction → increased cardiac contractility and vascular tone → increased cardiac afterload.

However, the greater resistance (afterload) against which the heart must pump, reduces the ejection fraction and thus the perfusion of the tissues.

The reduced perfusion of the kidneys activates the renin–angiotensin system (RAS), leading to renin secretion and subsequent elevated plasma angiotensin II and aldosterone levels (see Fig. 4.14).

Angiotensin II causes peripheral vasoconstriction and aldosterone increases sodium retention, leading to increased water retention, oedema, and an increased preload.

Intrinsic cardiac compensation: The increased cardiac preload leads to incomplete emptying of the ventricles and an increase in end-diastolic pressure.

The heart eventually fails, owing to the massive increase in myocardial energy requirements.

Causes and symptoms of acute and chronic heart failure			
Causes		**Symptoms**	
acute HF	**chronic HF**	**acute HF**	**chronic HF**
toxic drug exposure coronary artery disease	primary hypertension myocardial infarction myocardial ischaemia cardiac valve disease	tachycardia oedema shortness of breath reduced exercise tolerance	arrhythmias hypertension oedema cardiomegaly

Fig. 4.7 Causes and symptoms of acute and chronic heart failure (HF).

Characteristics of left and right heart failure	
Left HF: forward failure	**Right HF:** backward failure
reduced cardiac output hypotension pulmonary oedema dyspnoea fatigue	reduced cardiac output hypotension peripheral oedema hepatomegaly ascites

Fig. 4.8 Characteristics of left and right heart failure.

Arrhythmias

Sudden death as a result of arrhythmias is the most common cause of death in developed countries, and usually results from underlying cardiovascular pathology such as atherosclerosis.

Myocardial ischaemia is one of the most important causes of arrhythmias, and occurs when a coronary artery becomes occluded, such as in atherosclerosis, thus preventing sufficient blood from reaching the myocardium. Accumulation of endogenous biological mediators, including potassium, cAMP, thromboxane A_2 and free radicals, are believed to initiate arrhythmias.

Reperfusion after coronary occlusion is necessary for tissue recovery and prevention of infarction, but spontaneous resumption of coronary flow is often itself a cause of arrrhythmias.

Arrhythmias have been defined according to their appearance on the electrocardiogram (ECG) by the Lambeth Conventions. These include:

- Ventricular premature beats, tachycardia, fibrillation, and torsades de pointes.
- Atrial premature beats, tachycardia, flutter, and fibrillation.

The two main mechanisms by which cardiac rhythm becomes dysfunctional are:

- Abnormal impulse generation (automatic or triggered).
- Abnormal impulse conduction.

Abnormal impulse generation

Automatic: Automatic abnormal impulse generation automaticity is likely to cause sinus and atrial tachycardia, and ventricular premature beats. It can be:

- Enhanced: pathological conditions such as ischaemia may effect nodal and conducting tissue so that inherent pacemaker frequency is less than that of the SAN under normal conditions. Ischaemia causes partial depolarization of tissues (owing to a decrease in the activity of the electrogenic sodium pump) and catecholamine release, thus enhancing the automaticity of the slow pacemakers (AVN, Purkinje fibres, bundle of His) and often giving rise to an ectopic focus triggering the development of a premature beat.
- Abnormal: a premature beat may also develop in atrial or ventricular tissue, which are not normally automatic.

Triggered: Forms of triggered abnormal impulse generation are:

- Early after-depolarizations (EADs), which are likely to cause torsades de pointes and reperfusion-induced arrhythmias. EADs are triggered during repolarization, i.e. phase 2 or 3, by the previously normal impulse. They may result from a decrease in the delayed rectifier K^+ current and are associated with abnormally long action potentials. They are therefore more likely to occur during bradycardia and class III antiarrhythmic drug treatment.
- Delayed after-depolarizations (DADs) are triggered once the action potential has ended, i.e. during phase 4, by the previously normal impulse. DADs usually result from cellular calcium overload, associated with ischaemia, reperfusion, and cardiac glycoside intoxication.

Abnormal impulse conduction

Heart block: Heart block is likely to cause ventricular premature beats and results from damage to nodal tissue (most commonly the AVN) caused by conditions such as infarction. AV block may be first, second, or third degree, manifesting itself from slowed conduction to complete block of conduction, where the atria and ventricles beat independently.

Re-entry: Re-entry is likely to cause ventricular and atrial tachycardia and fibrillation, atrial flutter, and Wolff–Parkinson–White syndrome. Re-entry is of two types, circus movement (Fig. 4.9) and reflection.

In circus movement, an impulse re-excites an area of the myocardium, recently excited, after the refractory period has ended. This usually occurs in a ring of tissue in which a unidirectional block is present, preventing anterograde conduction of the impulse, but allowing retrograde conduction of the same impulse. This results in its continuous circulation, termed circus movement. The time taken for the impulse to propagate around the ring must exceed the refractory period; thus, administration of drugs that prolong the refractory period will interrupt the circuit and terminate re-entry.

Reflection occurs in non-branching bundles within which electrical dissociation has taken place. Owing to this electrical dissociation, an impulse can return over the same bundle.

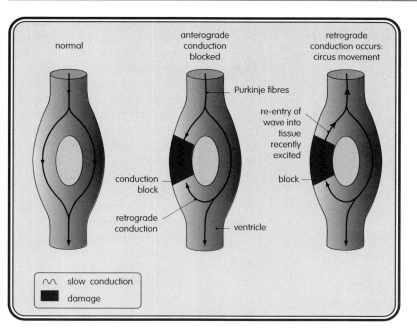

Fig. 4.9 Mechanism of re-entry due to damaged myocardium leading to circus movement.

Angina pectoris

Angina is associated with acute myocardial ischaemia, and results from underlying cardiovascular pathology. When coronary flow does not meet the metabolic needs of the heart, a radiating chest pain—anginal pain—results.

Stable or classical angina is due to fixed stenosis of the coronary arteries, and is brought on by exercise and stress.

Unstable angina or crescendo angina can occur suddenly at rest, and becomes progressively worse, with an increase in the number and severity of attacks. The following conditions can all cause unstable angina:

- Coronary atherosclerosis.
- Coronary artery spasm.
- Transient platelet aggregation and coronary thrombosis.
- Endothelial injury causing the accumulation of vasocontrictor substances.
- Coronary vasocontriction following adrenergic stimulation.

Variant angina or Prinzmetal's angina occurs at rest, at the same time each day, and is usually due to coronary artery spasm. It is characterized by an elevated ST segment on the ECG during chest pain, and may be accompanied by ventricular arrhythmias.

Treatment of cardiac dysfunction
Drugs used in heart failure
Cardiac glycosides

Examples of cardiac glycosides include digoxin, digitoxin, ouabain, and trophanthine.

Cardiac glycosides possess an aglycone steroid nucleus, conveying the pharmacological activity of these compounds; an unsaturated lactone ring, conveying cardiotonic activity; and sugar moieties, able to modulate potency and pharmacokinetic distribution.

Although the positive inotropic actions of cardiac glycosides shift the Frank–Starling ventricular function curve to a more favourable position (Fig. 4.10), thus improving the symptoms of CHF, there is no evidence that they have a beneficial effect on the long-term prognosis of patients with CHF.

Mechanism of action: Cardiac glycosides act by inhibiting the membrane Na^+/K^+ ATPase pump (Fig 4.6). This increases intracellular Na^+ concentration, thus reducing the sodium gradient across the membrane and decreasing the amount of calcium pumped out of the cell by the Na^+/Ca^{2+} exchanger during diastole. Consequently, the intracellular calcium concentration rises, thus increasing the force of cardiac contraction and maintaining normal blood pressure.

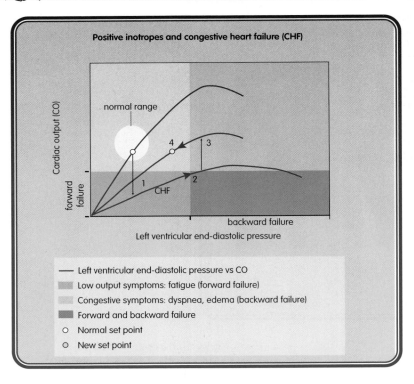

Fig. 4.10 The Frank–Starling curve, positive inotropes, and congestive heart failure (CHF). Normal cardiac output is determined by the pressure in the left ventricle at end-diastole. In CHF, the set point for cardiac output is reduced and cardiac output falls (1). Compensatory neurohumoral responses become activated which increase end-diastolic pressure and improve cardiac output; however, this can give rise to backward failure (2). Positive inotropic agents increase cardiac output. (3). The improved cardiac output reduces the drive for a high end-diastolic pressure, and decompensation occurs to a new set point (4).

In addition, cardiac glycosides alter the electrical activity of the heart, both directly and indirectly. At therapeutic doses they indirectly decrease the heart rate, slow AV conductance and shorten the atrial action potential by stimulating vagal activity. This is useful in atrial fibrillation. At toxic doses they indirectly increase the sympathetic activity of the heart, and cause arrhythmias, including heart block. The direct effects are mainly due to loss of intracellular potassium, and are most pronounced at high doses. The resting membrane potential is reduced, causing enhanced automaticity, slowed cardiac conduction, and increased AVN refractory period.

The increased cytosolic calcium concentration may reach toxic levels thereby saturating the sarcoplasmic reticulum sequestration mechanism and causing oscillations in Ca^{2+} owing to Ca^{2+}-induced Ca^{2+} release. This results in oscillatory after-potentials and subsequent arrhythmias.

In addition, cardiac glycosides have a direct effect on α-adrenoceptors, causing vasoconstriction and a consequent increase in peripheral vascular resistance, which is further enhanced by a centrally-mediated increase in sympathetic tone.

Route of administration: Cardiac glycosides are administered orally.

Indications: Cardiac glycosides are given for heart failure and supraventricular arrhythmias.

Contraindications: Cardiac glycosides should not be given to people with heart block, or hypokalaemia associated with the use of diuretics (the lack of competition from potassium potentiates the effects of cardiac glycosides on the Na^+/K^+ ATPase pump).

Adverse effects: The adverse effects of cardiac glycosides include arrhythmias, anorexia, nausea and vomiting, visual disturbances, and abdominal pain and diarrhoea.

Therapeutic notes: The cardiac glycosides have a very narrow therapeutic window, and toxicity is therefore relatively common. If this occurs, the drug should be withdrawn and, if necessary, potassium supplements and antiarrhythmic drugs (procainamide, phenytoin) administered. For severe intoxication, antibodies specific to cardiac glycosides are available.

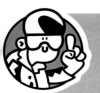

To remember the classes of drugs used in the treatment of heart failure: Norman's Aunt Promptly Collapsed And Died (Nitrovasodilators, ACE inhibitors, PDE inhibitors, Cardiac glycosides, β-Agonists, Diuretics).

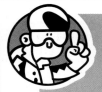

Arrhythmia means an absence of rhythm, whereas dysrhythmia means an abnormal rhythm. However, these terms are used interchangeably to mean an irregular heart beat.

Phosphodiesterase inhibitors

Examples of phosphodiesterase (PDE) inhibitors include amrinone and milrinone. These have been developed as a result of the many adverse effects and problems associated with cardiac glycosides. There is no evidence that these improve the mortality rate.

Mechanism of action: The type III PDE isoenzyme is found in myocardial and vascular smooth muscle.

Phosphodiesterase is responsible for the degradation of cAMP; thus, inhibiting this enzyme raises cAMP levels and causes an increase in myocardial contractility and vasodilatation (Fig. 4.6). Cardiac output is increased, and pulmonary wedge pressure and total peripheral resistance are reduced, without much change in heart rate or blood pressure.

Route of administration: Amrinone is short acting and is administered intravenously while milrinone is long acting and is administered orally.

Indications: PDE inhibitors are given for severe acute heart failure that is resistant to other drugs.

Adverse effects: PDE inhibitors have several adverse effects. These include nausea and vomiting, arrhythmias, liver dysfunction, abdominal pain, and hypersensitvity.

β-Adrenoceptor agonists

Examples of β-adrenoceptor agonists (p. 97) include dobutamine and dopamine. They are used intravenously in CHF emergencies (Fig. 4.6).

Diuretics

The diuretics used in CHF are:
- Thiazides.
- Loop diuretics.

Diuretics inhibit sodium and water retention by the kidneys, and so reduce oedema due to heart failure. Venous pressure and thus cardiac preload are reduced, increasing the efficiency of the heart as a pump (see Chapter 6).

Angiotensin-converting-enzyme inhibitors

For details of angiotensin converting enzyme (ACE) inhibitors see p. 94.

Nitrovasodilators

See antianginal drugs (p. 89).

Antiarrhythmic drugs

Antiarrhythmic drugs are classified according to a system devised by Vaughan Williams in 1970, and later modified by Harrison. A summary of the effects of the different classes of drug is given in Fig. 4.11.

Class I

All class I drugs block the voltage-dependent sodium channels in a use-dependent manner. Their action resembles that of local anaesthetics (see Chapter 2).

All class I drugs have the following effects:
- They prolong the effective refractory period (terminate re-entry).
- They convert unidirectional block to bidirectional block (prevent re-entry).

Class Ia

Examples of class Ia drugs include quinidine, procainamide, and disopyramide.

Class Ia drugs affect atrial muscle, ventricular muscle, the bundle of His, the Purkinje fibres, and the AVN.

Effects of antiarrhythmic drugs				
Class	Myocardial contractility	AV conduction	AP duration	Effective refractory period
Ia	↓	↓↓	↑	↑
Ib	–	–	↓	↑↑
intracellular	↓↓	↓↓	–	–
II	↓↓	–/↓	–	–
III	–	↑	↑↑↑	↑↑↑
IV	↓↓↓	↓↓	↓↓	–

Fig. 4.11 Effects of the antiarrhythmic drugs. (AP, action potential; AV, atrioventricular.) The number of arrows indicates the degree of the effect caused.

Mechanism of action: Class Ia drugs block voltage-dependent sodium channels in their open (activated) or refractory (inactivated) state (Figs 4.3 and 4.4). Their effects are to slow phase 0 (increasing the effective refractory period), slow phase 4 (reducing automaticity), and to prolong action potential duration.

Route of administration: Class Ia drugs are administered either as sustained-release tablets or intravenously.

Indications: Class Ia drugs are given to patients with ventricular and supraventricular arrhythmias.

Contraindications: Class Ia drugs should not be given to those with heart block, sinus node dysfunction, cardiogenic shock, and severe uncompensated heart failure. Procainamide should not be given to patients with systemic lupus erythematosus.

Adverse effects: Class Ia drugs have several adverse effects. These include arrhythmias, nausea and vomiting, hypersensitivity, thrombocytopenia, and agranulocytosis. Procainamide can cause a lupus-like syndrome, and disopyramide causes hypotension.

Class Ib

Examples of class Ib drugs include lignocaine, mexiletine, and phenytoin.

Mechanism of action: Class Ib drugs exert their effects in several ways (Fig. 4.3). These include:

- Blocking voltage-dependent sodium channels in their refractory (inactivated) state, i.e. when depolarized, as occurs in ischaemia.
- Binding to open channels during phase 0, and dissociating by the next beat, if the rhythm is normal, but abolishing premature beats.

- Decreasing action potential duration.
- Increasing the effective refractory period.

Route of administration: Lignocaine is administered intravenously, and mexiletine and phenytoin either orally or intravenously.

Indications: Class Ib drugs are given for ventricular arrhythmias following myocardial infarction. Phenytoin is used in epilepsy (see Chapter 3).

Contraindications: Class Ib drugs should not be given to patients with sinoatrial disorders, AV block, and porphyria.

Adverse effects: Class Ib drugs have several adverse effects. These include hypotension, bradycardia, drowsiness and confusion, convulsions, and paraesthesia (pins and needles).

Lignocaine may cause dizziness and respiratory depression; mexiletine may cause nausea and vomiting, constipation, arrhythmias, and hepatitis; and phenytoin may cause nausea and vomiting, and peripheral neuropathy.

To remember the classes of drugs used in the treatment of arrhythmias: Some Arrhythmias Can Cause Pain (Sodium blockers, β-Antagonists, Calcium antagonists, Cardiac glycosides, Potassium blockers).

Class Ic
Examples of class Ic drugs include flecainide and encainide.

These are no longer used, after the CAST (cardiac arrhythmia suppression trial) study, carried out in 1989, revealed that the mortality rate in patients taking these drugs was nearly four times as great as in those who received placebo.

Class II
Examples of class II drugs include propranolol, atenolol, and pindolol (Figs 4.4 and 4.6).

Class II drugs are β-adrenoceptor antagonists (atenolol is β_1 selective) (p. 90). They have been shown to reduce sudden death after myocardial infarction by 50% (although this is believed to be due to prevention of cardiac rupture as opposed to prevention of ventricular fibrillation).

Class III
Examples of Class III drugs include bretylium, amiodarone, sotalol, and ibutilide.

Mechanism of action: All Class III drugs used clinically are potassium channel blockers. They prolong cardiac action potential duration (increased QT interval on the ECG), and prolong the effective refractory period (Fig. 4.3).

Amiodarone also blocks sodium and calcium channels, i.e. slows phase 0 and 3, and blocks α- and β-adrenoceptors. Sotalol is a β-adrenoceptor antagonist with class III activity.

Other actions causing class III effects include α_1-adrenoceptor agonism and inhibition of sodium channel activation; the latter is thought to be responsible for the effects of a new class III drug, ibutilide, which was released for use in 1996.

Route of administration: Bretylium is administered intravenously while amiodarone and sotalol are administered orally or intravenously.

Indications: Class III drugs are given for ventricular and supraventricular arrhythmias. Amiodarone is restricted to patients resistant to other drugs while bretylium is used only in resuscitation.

Contraindications: Bretylium should not be given to patients with phaeochromocytoma while amiodarone should not be given to those with AV block, sinus bradycardia, or thyroid dysfunction.

For contraindications regarding sotalol, see under β-blockers (p. 90).

Adverse effects: Class III drugs can cause arrhythmias, especially torsades de pointes.

Bretylium may cause hypotension, nausea and vomiting while amiodarone may cause thyroid dysfunction, liver damage, pulmonary disorders, photosensitivity, and neuropathy.

For adverse effects regarding sotalol see under β blockers (p. 90).

Class IV
Examples of class IV drugs include verapamil and diltiazem (see Figs 4.3 and 4.6).

Class IV drugs are calcium antagonists, that shorten phase 2 of the action potential, thus decreasing action potential duration. They are particularly effective in nodal cells, where conduction is initiated by calcium spikes.

Details of the drugs are given in the section on antianginal drugs (p. 90).

Class V (miscellaneous)
Examples of class V drugs include the cardiac glycosides (p. 85).

Antianginal drugs
Treatment of angina
Acute attacks of angina are treated with:
- Sublingual nitrates.
- Nifedipine.

Acute anginal pain is treated with morphine (see Chapter 3).

Stable angina is treated with:
- Long-lasting nitrates.
- β-Adrenoceptor antagonists.
- Calcium antagonists.

Unstable angina is treated with:
- Aspirin (reduces platelet aggregation; p. 105).
- Dipyridamol.

Organic nitrates
The organic nitrates, glyceryltrinitrate (GTN), nitroglycerin, isosorbide mononitrate (IMN), and isosorbide dinitrate (IDN) can relieve angina within minutes.

Mechanism of action: Most nitrates are prodrugs, decomposing to form nitric oxide (NO), which activates guanylyl cyclase, thereby increasing the levels of cyclic guanosine monophosphate (cGMP). Protein kinase G is activated and contractile proteins are phosphorylated. Dilatation of the systemic veins decreases preload and thus the oxygen demand of the heart, while dilatation of the coronary arteries increases blood flow and oxygen delivery to the myocardium.

Route of administration: Organic nitrates are administered sublingually, orally (modified release), or from patches. GTN can be given by intravenous infusion.

Indications: Organic nitrates are given for the prophylaxis and treatment of angina, and in left ventricular failure.

Contraindications: Organic nitrates should not be given to patients with hypersensitivity to nitrates, or those with hypotension and hypovolaemia

Adverse effects: The side effects of organic nitrates include postural hypotension, tachycardia, headache, flushing and dizziness.

Therapeutic notes: To avoid nitrate tolerance, a drug-free period of approximately 8 hours is needed. The following routine is therefore recommended:

- During the day, a long-acting nitrate, e.g. IDN taken every 6–8 hours.
- At nighttime, a short-acting nitrate, e.g. nitroglycerin applied as a patch.

β-Blockers

Examples of β-blockers include propranolol, atenolol, and metoprolol.

Mechanism of action: β-Blockers block β_1-adrenoceptors in the heart (Fig. 4.6). This causes a decrease in heart rate (slowing of phase 4) (Fig. 4.4), in systolic blood pressure, in cardiac contractile activity, and in myocardial oxygen demand.

Route of administration: β-Blockers are administered orally (intravenously for arrhythmias and thyrotoxic crisis).

Indications: β-Blockers are used for angina, arrhythmias induced by increased sympathetic tone—such as occur after myocardial infarction, exercise or stress—hypertension, thyrotoxicosis, glaucoma, and anxiety.

Contraindications: Non-selective β-blockers (e.g. propranolol) must not be given to asthmatic patients (at high doses β_1-adrenoceptor antagonists lose their selectivity). Other contraindications for β-blockers include bradycardia, hypotension, AV block, and CHF.

Adverse effects: β-Blockers have several side effects, including bronchospasm, fatigue and insomnia, dizziness, cold extremities, bradycardia, heart block, hypotension, and decreased glucose tolerance in diabetic patients.

Calcium-channel blockers

Examples of calcium-channel blockers include verapamil, diltiazem, and nifedipine. These drugs have fewer side effects than β-blockers.

Mechanism of action: Verapamil and diltiazem block L-type calcium channels, thereby reducing calcium entry into cardiac and vascular cells (Figs. 4.3, 4.6, and 4.13). This decrease in intracellular calcium reduces cardiac contractility and causes vasodilatation, which results in several effects: reduced preload due to the reduced venous pressure; reduced afterload due to the reduced arteriolar pressure; increased coronary blood flow; reduced cardiac contractility and thus reduced myocardial oxygen consumption; and a decreased heart rate. High doses of these drugs affect AVN conduction.

Nifedipine blocks L-type calcium-channels in vascular cells. It does not affect cardiac contractility, or AVN conduction, and its beneficial effects are due to increased coronary flow and peripheral vasodilatation.

Route of administration: Calcium-channel blockers are administered orally as tablets or capsules.

Indications: Calcium-channel blockers are used for the prophylaxis and treatment of angina and hypertension. Verapamil and diltiazem are given for supraventricular arrhythmias, and nifedipine for Raynaud's syndrome.

Contraindications: Calcium-channel blockers should not be given to patients in cardiogenic shock.

Nifedipine is contraindicated in advanced aortic stenosis while verapamil and diltiazem should not be given to patients in severe heart failure (owing to their negative inotropic action), to those taking β-blockers (risk of AV block and impaired cardiac output), and those with severe bradycardia.

Adverse effects: Verapamil and diltiazem may cause hypotension, rash, bradycardia, CHF, heart block, and constipation.

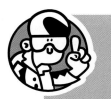

To remember the classes of drugs used in the treatment of angina: Nitrate Drugs Calm Angina (Nitrates, Dipyridamole, Calcium antagonists, β-Antagonists).

Nifedipine may cause hypotension, rash, tachycardia, peripheral oedema, and flushing and dizziness.

Dipyridamole

Mechanism of action: Dipyridamole causes inhibition of adenosine uptake, resulting in the accumulation of adenosine within the tissues. Adenosine is an endogenous vasodilator, the effect of which is most pronounced on arterioles.

Route of administration: Dipyridamole is administered orally.

Indications: Dipyridamole is used for variant angina, in which there is coronary spasm (in other forms of angina, the arterioles in ischaemic areas of the myocardium are fully dilated). It is also used in conjunction with warfarin and other oral anticoagulants in the prophylaxis of thrombosis associated with prosthetic heart valves (p. 106)

Adverse effects: The side effects of dipyridamole include hypotension, nausea, diarrhoea, and headache.

Fig. 4.12 provides a summary of the drugs used to treat angina, heart failure, and arrhythmias.

- How are the different phases of the cardiac action potential caused? Distinguish between nodal and non-nodal cells.
- Summarize the autonomic control of the heart.
- How is myocardial contraction induced?
- What are the causes and characteristics of heart failure, arrhythmias, and angina?
- Describe the classes of drugs used to treat cardiac dysfunction. For each of these list examples, their mechanism of action, route of administration, indications, and major adverse effects.

Cardiac terminology:
chronotropic: rate.
inotropic: force.
lusitropic: relaxation.
dromotropic: conduction.

Classes of drugs to treat angina, heart failure, and arrhythmias		
Angina	**Heart failure**	**Arrhythmias**
organic nitrates	cardiac glycosides	Na^+ channel blockers (Class I)
β_1-adrenoceptor antagonists	phosphodiesterase inhibitors	β_1-adrenoceptor antagonists (Class II)
Ca^{2+} antagonists	β_1-adrenoceptor agonists	K^+ channel blockers (Class III)
dipyridamole	diuretics	Ca^{2+} antagonists (Class IV)
	ACE inhibitors	cardiac glycosides
	nitrovasodilators	

Fig. 4.12 Classes of drugs used to treat angina, heart failure, and arrhythmias.

THE CIRCULATION

Control of vascular tone

α-Adrenoceptor activation

α-Adrenoceptor activation (Fig. 4.13) causes contraction of vascular smooth muscle through the activation of phospholipase C (PLC). The resulting increased levels of IP_3 cause the release of calcium from the endoplasmic reticulum, thus increasing calcium levels. Calcium then binds to calmodulin, thus activating myosin light-chain kinase (MLCK) and allowing contraction.

$β_2$-Adrenoceptor activation

$β_2$-Adrenoceptor activation (Fig. 4.13) causes relaxation of vascular smooth muscle through the activation of adenylyl cyclase. The resulting increased levels of cAMP activate protein kinase A, which phosphorylates and inactivates MLCK.

M_3-receptor activation

M_3-receptor activation causes relaxation of vascular smooth muscle through the release of endothelium-derived relaxing factor (EDRF), which is believed to be

NO (Fig. 4.13). Guanylyl cyclase is activated by NO, thus increasing the levels of cGMP and activating protein kinase G. Protein kinase G inhibits contraction by phosphorylating contractile proteins.

Renin–angiotensin system

A decrease in plasma volume results in the activation of the renin–angiotensin system (RAS), which is summarized in Fig. 4.14 (see Chapter 6).

Angiotensin-converting enzyme (ACE) catalyses the production of angiotensin II. The effects of angiotensin II are:

- Potent vasoconstriction (40 times as potent as noradrenaline).
- Release of noradrenaline.
- Secretion of aldosterone.

ACE also catalyses the inactivation of bradykinin, which is an endogenous vasodilator.

Aldosterone is a steroid that induces the synthesis of sodium channels and Na^+/K^+ ATPase pumps in the luminal membrane of the cortical collecting ducts. This results in a greater amount of sodium and

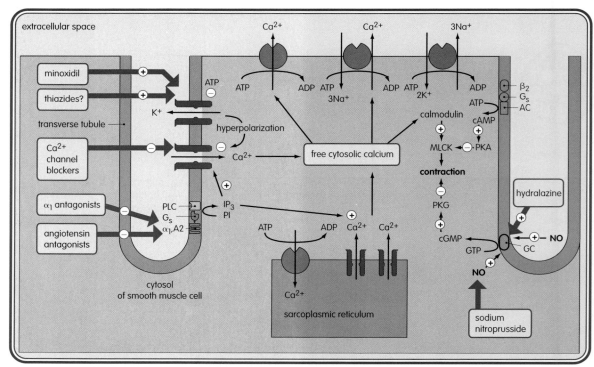

Fig. 4.13 Drugs affecting vascular tone. (A2, angiotensin II; GC, guanylyl cyclase; IP_3, inositol triphosphate; MLCK, myosin light-chain kinase; NO, nitric oxide; PLC, phospholipase C; PI, phosphatidylinositol.)

consequently water being reabsorbed, thus restoring blood volume and pressure back to normal.

Certain renal diseases and renal artery occlusion will cause activation of the RAS and result in the development of hypertension.

Treatment of hypertension
Hypertension
Normal blood pressure is 120/80 mmHg (systolic pressure /diastolic pressure). Hypertension is defined as a diastolic arterial pressure greater than 90 mmHg. The condition can be fatal if left untreated, as it greatly increases the risk of thrombosis, stroke, and renal failure.

Three factors determine blood pressure:
- Blood volume.
- Cardiac output.
- Peripheral vascular resistance.

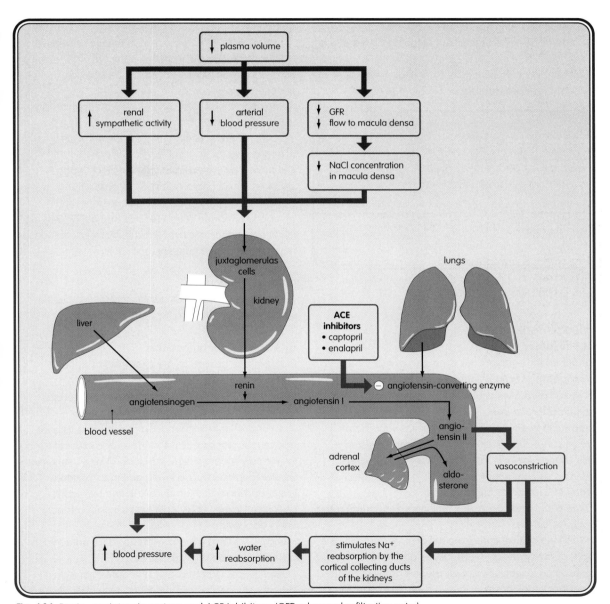

Fig. 4.14 Renin–angiotensin system and ACE inhibitors. (GFR, glomerular filtration rate.)

'Primary' or 'essential' hypertension occurs in 90–95% of patients. This has no known cause, but is associated with:
- Age (40+).
- Obesity.
- Physical inactivity.
- Smoking and alcohol consumption.
- Genetic predisposition.

'Secondary hypertension' occurs in 5–10% of patients. The cause is usually one of the following:
- Renal disease which activates the RAS.
- Endocrine disease, e.g. phaeochromocytoma, steroid-secreting tumour of the adrenal cortex, adrenaline-secreting tumour of the adrenal medulla.

The treatment of hypertension is aimed at various targets; these are summarised in Fig. 4.15.

Drugs targets in the treatment of hypertension	
Target	Control
sympathetic nerves kidneys heart arterioles endothelial cells CNS	vascular tone blood volume cardiac output peripheral vascular resistance circulating angiotensin II levels blood pressure set point systems controlling blood pressure

Fig. 4.15 Drug targets in the treatment of hypertension. (CNS, central nervous system.)

Vasodilators
ACE inhibitors
Captopril and enalapril are examples of ACE inhibitors.
Mechanism of action: Captopril and enalapril cause inhibition of ACE with consequent reduced angiotensin II and aldosterone levels (Fig. 4.14), and increased bradykinin levels. This therefore causes vasodilatation with a consequent reduction in peripheral resistance, little change in heart rate and cardiac output, and reduced sodium retention.
Many ACE inhibitors are prodrugs.
Route of administration: ACE inhibitors are administered orally as tablets.
Indications: ACE inhibitors are used for all degrees and types of hypertension, heart failure, and renal dysfunction (especially diabetic nephropathy or reduced renal functional mass).

Contraindications: ACE inhibitors should not be given in pregnancy or renovascular disease, or to those with aortic stenosis.
Adverse effects: The side effects of ACE inhibitors include a characteristic cough, hypotension, dizziness and headache, diarrhoea, and muscle cramps.
Therapeutic notes: Only a half dose should be given if used in conjunction with a diuretic in the treatment of hypertension.

Angiotensin antagonists
Losartan and EXP3174 are examples of angiotensin antagonists.
Mechanism of action: Angiotensin antagonists cause inhibition at the angiotensin II receptor (Fig. 4.13), resulting in vasodilatation with a consequent reduction in peripheral resistance.
Route of administration: Angiotensin antagonists are administered orally.
Indications: Angiotensin antagonists are used for hypertension.
Contraindications: Pregnant and breast-feeding women should not take angiotensin antagonists.
Adverse effects: The side effects of angiotensin antagonists include cough (less common than with ACE inhibitors), orthostatic hypotension, dizziness, headache and fatigue, hyperkalaemia, and rash.

Calcium antagonists
Examples of calcium antagonists include nifedipine, verapamil and diltiazem (Fig. 4.13) (p. 90).

α_1-Adrenoceptor antagonists
Prazosin and doxazocin are examples of α_1-adrenoceptor antagonists.
Mechanism of action: α_1-Adrenoceptor antagonists cause inhibition of α_1-adrenoceptor-mediated vasoconstriction—thus reducing peripheral resistance and venous pressure (Fig. 4.13). They also lower plasma low-density lipoprotein (LDL) cholesterol levels, very-low-density lipoprotein (VLDL) levels, and triacylglyceride (TGA) levels, and increase high-density lipoprotein (HDL) cholesterol levels—thus reducing the risk of coronary artery disease.
Route of administration: α_1-Adrenoceptor antagonists are administered orally as tablets.
Indications: α_1-Adrenoceptor antagonists are used in hypertension (especially in patients with CHF), prostate

hyperplasia (reduced bladder and prostate resistance), and coronary artery disease.

Contraindications: Prazocin should not be given to people with CHF due to aortic stenosis.

Adverse effects: Side effects of α_1-adrenoceptor antagonists include postural hypotension, dizziness, headache and fatigue, weakness, palpitations, and nausea.

Therapeutic notes: Gradually increase the dose from 1 mg to 2 mg daily and then 4 mg daily for doxazocin, and 500 μg 2–3 times daily to 1 mg 2–3 times daily for prazocin.

Hydralazine

Hydralazine is the second- or third-line drug for the treatment of mild to moderate hypertension.

Mechanism of action: Hydralazine acts directly by activating guanylyl cyclase and thus increasing cGMP levels (Fig. 4.13). It also relaxes smooth muscle in precapillary resistance vessels, thereby reducing peripheral resistance and blood pressure.

Route of administration: Hydralazine can be administered orally as tablets, or by intravenous injection or infusion.

Indications: Hydralazine is used for moderate to severe hypertension—with β-blockers and thiazide, in hypertensive emergencies, and in hypertensive pregnant women.

Contraindications: Hydralazine should not be given to patients with idiopathic systemic lupus erythematosus or severe tachycardia.

Adverse effects: Side effects of hydralazine include tachycardia, fluid retention, nausea and vomiting, and headache.

Minoxidil

Owing to its adverse effects, minoxidil is the drug of last resort in the long-term treatment of hypertension.

Mechanism of action: Minoxidil antagonizes the action of intracellular ATP on the ATP-sensitive K^+ channels—ATP normally functions in keeping these channels closed. This results in the activation of the ATP-sensitive potassium channels, resulting in hyperpolarization of the smooth muscle cell and consequent reduced calcium entry through L-type channels (Fig. 4.13).

Route of administration: Minoxidil is administered orally as tablets for hypertension, and as a topical cream for baldness.

Indications: Minoxidil is effective in severe hypertension (especially if accompanied by renal failure), and baldness.

Contraindications: Minoxidil should not be given to people with phaeochromocytoma or porphyria.

Adverse effects: Side effects of minoxidil include hirsutism (limits use in women), sodium and water retention. tachycardia, and cardiotoxicity.

Therapeutic notes: Minoxidil is given in combination with diuretics and α-adrenoceptor antagonists to avoid reflex fluid retention and increased cardiac output.

Sodium nitroprusside

Mechanism of action: Sodium nitroprusside is a prodrug that spontaneously decomposes into NO inside smooth muscle cells. NO activates guanylyl cyclase, thus increasing intracellular cGMP levels, and causing vasodilatation (Fig. 4.13).

Route of administration: Sodium nitroprusside is administered intravenously.

Indications: Sodium nitroprusside is given in hypertensive crisis (emergency), and for controlled hypotension in surgery, and heart failure.

Contraindications: Sodium nitroprusside should not be given to patients with severe hepatic impairment, vitamin B_{12} deficiency, or Leber's optic atrophy.

Adverse effects: Side effects of sodium nitroprusside include headache and dizziness, nausea, abdominal pain, palpitations, and retrosternal discomfort.

To remember the vasodilators used in the treatment of hypertension: Minoxidil Alleviates Hypertension, A Serious Arterial Condition (Minoxidil, ACE inhibitors, Hydralazine, Angiotensin antagonists, Sodium nitroprusside, α_1-Adrenoceptor antagonists, Calcium antagonists).

Diuretic drugs

Diuretics used in hypertension include:
- Thiazides.
- Loop diuretics.
- Potassium-sparing diuretics.

See Chapter 6 for details of each of these drugs.

Mechanism of action: The antihypertensive action of diuretic drugs does not seem to correlate with their diuretic activity: loop diuretics are powerful diuretics but only moderate antihypertensives while thiazides are moderate diuretics but powerful antihypertensives.

It has recently been suggested that the hypotensive effects of diuretics (especially the thiazides) are not necessarily due to their diuretic effect, but rather may be due to activation of ATP-regulated potassium channels in resistance arterioles, with a mechanism of action similar to that of minoxidil (p. 95). This causes hyperpolarization, and thus inhibition of calcium entry into vascular smooth muscle cells with consequent vasodilatation and reduced peripheral vascular resistance (Fig 4.13).

Centrally acting drugs

Clonidine and α-methyldopa are examples of centrally acting drugs. These drugs are second- or third-line drugs in the treatment of hypertension.

α-Methyldopa is rarely used owing to its adverse effects.

Mechanism of action: Centrally-acting drugs are α_2-adrenoceptor agonists. The activation presynaptic α_2-adrenoceptors, causes inhibition of noradrenaline release and consequent vasodilatation. The activation of postsynaptic α_2-adrenoceptors causes vasoconstriction, although presynaptic effects dominate.

Centrally acting drugs reduce the activity of the vasomotor centre in the brain, causing reduced sympathetic activity and subsequent vasodilatation. They also reduce heart rate and cardiac output.

α-Methyldopa is a prodrug that is metabolized in the CNS to α-methylnoradrenaline, which is an α_2-adrenoceptor agonist.

Route of administration: Centrally acting drugs are administered orally as tablets or capsules. α-Methyldopa is given by intravenous infusion.

Indications: Centrally acting drugs are given to hypertensive patients, especially those with renal insufficiency or cerebrovascular disease. α-Methyldopa is safe for hypertension in pregnancy, asthmatic patients and those with heart failure.

Contraindications: α-Methyldopa should not be given to people with depression, liver disease, or phaeochromocytoma.

Adverse effects: The side effects of centrally acting drugs include dry mouth, sedation, orthostatic hypotension, male sexual dysfunction, and galactorrhoea. α-Methyldopa can cause diffuse parenchymal liver injury, fever, and, rarely, haemolytic anaemia. Clonidine can cause withdrawal symptoms on stopping treatment, such as tachycardia and sweating.

Therapeutic notes: Treatment with clonidine should not be stopped abruptly, but the dose should gradually be decreased. A peripheral α_1-adrenoceptor antagonist can be given to decrease the rebound increase in blood pressure observed on withdrawal from clonidine.

Vasoconstrictors and the management of shock

Shock

Shock is a state of circulatory collapse, characterized by an arterial blood pressure unable to maintain adequate tissue perfusion. Shock is a life-threatening condition.

The body responds inappropriately to shock, releasing mediators such as histamine, prostaglandins, bradykinin, and serotonin, which cause capillary dilatation and increased capillary permeability. This further reduces blood pressure and cardiac output.

Signs of shock include:
- Very low arterial blood pressure.
- A weak, rapid pulse.
- Cold, pale, sweaty skin.
- Irregular breathing.
- Dry mouth.
- Dilated pupils.
- Reduced urine production.
- Anxiousness.

Causes of shock include:
- Haemorrhage.
- Burns.
- Dehydration.
- Severe vomiting or diarrhoea.
- Bacterial infections.
- Coronary thrombosis.
- Myocardial infarction.

- Pulmonary embolism.

Types of shock include:
- Hypovolemic, which is caused by a reduction in the circulating blood volume.
- Cardiogenic, caused by reduced activity of the heart.
- Septic, which is caused by bacterial infections.
- Anaphylactic, a severe allergic reaction, in which there is a massive generalized release of mediators such as histamine.
- Neurogenic, which is caused by emotional shock.

Management of shock

Sympathomimetic amines

Examples of sympathomimetic amines include adrenaline, noradrenaline, phenylephrine, and ephedrine.

Sympathomimetic amines raise blood pressure at the expense of vital organs such as the kidneys, and raise peripheral resistance, which is already high in patients with shock.

Mechanism of action: Adrenaline is a β/α-adrenoceptor agonist, noradrenaline an α/β-adrenoceptor agonist, and phenylephrine an α_1-adrenoceptor agonist. Ephedrine is a β-adrenoceptor agonist and causes noradrenaline release. These drugs work either by activating α-receptors which then activate PLC, causing vasoconstriction and a consequent increase in arterial blood pressure, or by activating β-receptors which then activate adenylyl cyclase, causing an increased heart rate, increased cardiac contractility, and vasodilatation.

Route of administration: Sympathomimetic amines are administered intravenously. Ephedrine can be administered intramuscularly, phenylephrine subcutaneously, and noradrenaline intracardially.

Indications: Sympathomimetic amines are used in shock, acute hypotension, and reversal of hypotension caused by spinal or epidural anaesthesia. noradrenaline is used in cardiac arrest.

Contraindications: Sympathomimetic amines should not be given to people who are pregnant or have hypertension.

Adverse effects: Side effects of sympathomimetic amines include tachycardia, anxiety, insomnia, arrhythmias, dry mouth, and cold extremities.

Therapeutic notes: Phenylephrine has a longer duration of action than noradrenaline and may cause a prolonged hypertensive response.

Dopamine and dobutamine

Mechanism of action: Dopamine is a precursor of noradrenaline. It activates dopamine receptors and α- and β-adrenoceptors. When administered by intravenous infusion, dopamine acts on:
- Dopamine receptors, causing vasodilatation in the kidneys and the mesentery.
- α_1–Adrenoceptors, causing vasoconstriction in other vasculature.
- β_1-Adrenoceptors, causing positive inotropy.

Dobutamine activates β_1-adrenoceptors.

As renal perfusion is not impaired, dobutamine and dopamine are a more appropriate means of treating shock than α-adrenoceptor agonists. This form of treatment maintains renal perfusion, and inhibits the activation of the RAS.

Dopamine and dobutamine have little effect on heart rate.

Route of administration: Both dopamine and dobutamine are administered intravenously.

Indications: Dopamine and dobutamine are given in CHF (emergencies only), cardiogenic shock, septic shock, hypovolaemic shock, cardiomyopathy, and cardiac surgery.

Contraindications: Dopamine and dobutamine should not be given to people with tachycardia; dopamine is contraindicated in people with phaeochromocytoma.

Adverse effects: Dopamine and dobutamine can cause tachycardia; dopamine causes nausea and vomiting, and hypotension.

Therapeutic notes: Although low doses of dopamine cause vasodilatation, high doses ($>5\,\mu g/kg/min$) cause vasoconstriction and may exacerbate heart failure.

Vasopressin (ADH), desmopressin, and felypressin

Vasopressin (antidiuretic hormone; ADH), desmopressin, and felypressin are examples of antidiuretic peptides.

Vasopressin and felypressin are short acting ($t_{1/2}$ = 10 minutes) while desmopressin is longer acting ($t_{1/2}$ = 75 minutes).

Mechanism of action: Antidiuretic peptides activate V_1-receptors on smooth muscle cells, which stimulate PLC, causing contraction. They also activate V_2-receptors on the tubular cells of the kidneys, which stimulate adenylyl cyclase and thereby increase the permeability of these cells to water, and reduce sodium and water excretion.

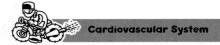

Vasopressin has a much greater affinity for V_2-receptors than V_1-receptors while desmopressin is selective for V_1-receptors.

Route of administration: Antidiuretic peptides are administered orally, by subcutaneous or intramuscular injection, intravenous infusion, or intranasally by snuff or spray.

Indications: Antidiuretic peptides are given to people in shock or with pituitary diabetes insipidus.

Contraindications: Antidiuretic peptides should not be given to people with vascular disease or chronic nephritis.

Adverse effects: The side effects of antidiuretic peptides include fluid retention, nausea, pallor, abdominal cramps and belching. They may induce anginal attacks (due to coronary vasoconstriction).

Corticosteroids

Very high doses of corticosteroids are given by intravenous injection in septic shock, although it has recently been demonstrated that these may increase mortality. They are also given by intravenous injection in the treatment of anaphylactic shock as an adjunct to adrenaline (usually 100–300 mg hydrocortisone; see Chapter 8).

Lipoprotein circulation and atherosclerosis

Lipoproteins provide a means of transporting lipids—cholesterol, triglycerides, and phospholipids—which are insoluble in the blood, around the body.

Four classes of lipoproteins exist. These differ in size, density, constituent lipids, and type of surface protein (apoprotein). These lipoproteins are:

- High-density lipoproteins (HDL).
- Low-density lipoproteins (LDL).
- Very-low-density lipoproteins (VLDL).
- Chylomicrons.

Lipid transport in the blood is via two pathways, exogenous and endogenous, which are summarized in Fig. 4.16.

In the exogenous pathway (numbers refer to those in Fig. 4.16):

1. Diet-derived lipid leads to the formation of chylomicrons.
2. Lipoprotein lipase, found in the endothelium of extrahepatic tissues, hydrolyses the triglycerides in chylomicrons to glycerol and free fatty acids (FFAs), for use by the tissues.

3. The chylomicron remnant is taken up by the liver.
4. The liver secretes cholesterol and bile acids into the gut, creating an enterohepatic circulation.

In the endogenous pathway (numbers refer to those in Fig. 4.16):

1. The liver secretes VLDLs, the components of which may be derived either endogenously or from the diet.
2. Lipoprotein lipase (LPL), found in the endothelium of extrahepatic tissues, hydrolyses triglycerides in the VLDLs to glycerol and FFAs, for use by the tissues, and leaves LDL.
3. LDL is then taken up by the liver and extrahepatic tissues.
4. HDL is secreted by the liver into the plasma, where it is modified by lecithin cholesterol acyltransferase (LCAT) and uptake of cholesterol from the tissues. LCAT transfers cholesterol esters to LDLs and VLDLs.

Hyperlipidaemias

Hyperlipidaemias are characterized by markedly elevated plasma TAG, cholesterol, and lipoprotein concentrations.

Cholesterol is deposited in various tissues:

Deposition in arterial plaques results in atherosclerosis, which leads to heart attacks, strokes, and peripheral vascular disease. Deposition in tendons and skin results in xanthomas.

Primary

Primary hyperlipidaemias are genetic. The Fredrickson/WHO classification of the primary hyperlipidaemias is summarized in Fig. 4.17.

Secondary

Secondary hyperlipidaemias are the consequences of other conditions such as:

- Diabetes.
- Liver disease.
- Nephrotic syndrome.
- Renal failure.
- Alcoholism.
- Smoking.
- Hypothyroidism.
- Oestrogen administration.

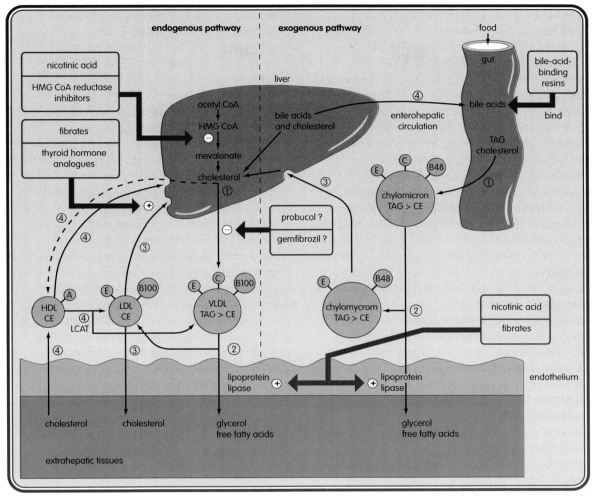

Fig. 4.16 Endogenous and exogenous pathways of lipid transport. (CE, cholesterol ester; HDL, high density lipoprotein; LCAT, lecithin cholesterol acyltransferase; TAG, triacylglycerol; VLDL, very low density lipoproteins; numbers refer to steps in pathways, see p. 98.)

Fredrickson/World Health Organisation classification of the primary hyperlipidaemias							
Type	**Occurrence**	**Plasma lipids**		**Plasma lipoproteins**			**Risk of atherosclerosis**
		Chol	TAG	LDL	VLDL	CM	
I	rare	+	+++	low	N	++	-
IIa	common	++	N	++	N	-	high
IIb	common	++	++	++	++	-	high
III	uncommon	++	++	low	+	+	moderate
IV	common	+	++	N	++	-	moderate
V	rare	+	++	low	++	++_	-

Fig. 4.17 Fredrickson/WHO classification of the primary hyperlipidaemias, (Chol, cholesterol; CM, chylomicrons; LDL, low-density lipoproteins; TAG, triacylglycerol; VLDL, very-low-density lipoproteins.)

99

Treatment (Lipid-lowering drugs)
HMG CoA reductase inhibitors
Lovastatin and simvastatin are examples of 3-hydroxy-3-methylglutaryl co-enzyme A (HMG CoA) reductase inhibitors. These drugs have been shown to reduce blood cholesterol by 33% in patients with type II hyperlipidaemia, and in combination with colestipol (see p. 100) to reduce blood cholesterol by 46% in patients with type II hyperlipidaemia. HMG CoA reductase inhibitors reduce the risk of coronary artery disease by 50–60%.

Mechanism of action: Lovastatin and simvastatin reversibly inhibit the enzyme HMG CoA reductase, which catalyses the rate-limiting step (RLS) in the synthesis of cholesterol: HMG CoA$\rightarrow$ mevalonic acid (Fig. 4.16). The decrease in cholesterol synthesis increases the number of LDL receptors, thus decreasing LDL levels.

Route of administration: Lovastatin and simvastatin are both administered orally as tablets.

Indications: Lovastatin and simvastatin are given for primary hyperlipidaemia type IIa if cholesterol is >6.5 mmol/L and resistant to dietary control.

Contraindications: Lovastatin and simvastatin should not be given to people who are pregnant or breast-feeding, or who have liver disease or porphyria.

Adverse effects: Side effects of lovastatin and simvastatin include the following: reversible myositis (rare unless also taking cyclosporin, nicotinic acid, or gemfibrozil); constipation or diarrhoea; abdominal pain and flatulence; nausea and headache; fatigue and insomnia; and rash.

Therapeutic notes: Liver function and creatine phosphokinase levels should be monitored in people taking lovastatin or simvastatin with cyclosporin, nicotinic acid, or gemfibrozil.

Fibrates
Fibrates include clofibrate, bezafibrate, and gemfibrozil. These are broad-spectrum lipid-modulating agents that are ineffective in patients with elevated cholesterol but normal triglyceride concentrations.

Mechanism of action: Fibrates work in several ways, as follows: stimulation of lipoprotein lipase (Fig. 4.16), thus reducing the triglyceride content of VLDLs and chylomicrons; stimulation of hepatic LDL clearance, by increasing hepatic LDL uptake (Fig. 4.16); reduction of plasma triglyceride, LDL, and VLDL concentrations; and increase of HDL-cholesterol concentration (except bezafibrate). Gemfibrozil decreases lipolysis and may decrease VLDL secretion.

Route of administration: Fibrates are administered orally as tablets.

Indications: Fibrates are used in type IIa, IIb, III, IV, and IV hyperlipidaemia, if patients do not respond to dietary control. In addition, gemfibrozil is indicated in the primary prevention of coronary heart disease in men aged 40–55 years with hyperlipidaemia who have not responded to diet and other measures.

Contraindications: Fibrates should not be given to patients who have gallbladder disease, severe renal or hepatic impairment, or hypoalbuminaemia, or to women who are pregnant or are breast-feeding. In addition, clofibrate should not be given to those who have not had a cholecystectomy (owing to the high risk of gall stones associated with the increase in biliary cholesterol excretion) and gemfibrozil should not be given in alcoholism.

Adverse effects: Side effects of fibrates include:
- Myositis-like syndrome (especially if renal function is impaired).
- GI disturbances.
- Dermatitis, pruritus, rash and urticaria.
- Impotence.
- Headache, dizziness, blurred vision.

Therapeutic notes: Fibrates should be taken with or after food. Gemfibrozil has been shown to reduce the incidence of coronary heart disease in men with hyperlipidaemia.

Nicotinic acid
The side effects of nicotinic acid limit its use in the treatment of hyperlipidaemias. Nicotinic acid has been shown to reduce the incidence of coronary artery disease.

Mechanism of action: Nicotinic acid has the following effects: it inhibits cholesterol synthesis (Fig. 4.16), thereby decreasing VLDL and thus LDL production; it stimulates lipoprotein lipase, thus reducing the triglyceride content of VLDLs and chylomicrons; it increases HDL-cholesterol; it increases the levels of tissue plasminogen activator (p. 104); and it decreases the levels of plasma fibrinogen (p. 103).

Route of administration: Nicotinic acid is administered orally as tablets.

Indications: Nicotinic acid is given for type IIa, IIb, III, IV and V hyperlipidaemia in patients not responding to diet and other control measures.

Contraindications: Nicotinic acid should not be given to women who are pregnant or breast-feeding.

Adverse effects: Side effects of nicotinic acid include flushing, disease, headache, palpitations, nausea and vomiting, and pruritus.

Therapeutic notes: The dose of nicotinic acid is 1–2 g three times daily.

Bile-acid-binding resins

Cholestyramine and colestipol have been shown to decrease the rate of mortality from coronary artery disease.

Mechanism of action: Basic anion exchange resins act by binding bile acids in the intestine (Fig. 4.16), thus preventing their reabsorption and promoting hepatic conversion of cholesterol into bile acids. This increases hepatic LDL receptor activity, thus increasing the breakdown of LDL-cholesterol. Plasma LDL-cholesterol is therefore lowered.

Route of administration: The bile-acid-binding resins are administered orally: cholestyramine as a powder and colestipol as granules.

Indications: Bile-acid-binding resins are especially useful when elevated cholesterol is due to a high LDL concentration. They are also used in patients in whom type IIa and IIb hyperlipidaemia is not responding to diet or other control measures, and for diarrhoea.

Cholestyramine is used in the primary prevention of coronary heart disease in men aged 35–59 years with primary hypercholesterolaemia. It also relieves pruritus associated with partial biliary obstruction and primary biliary cirrhosis.

Contraindications: Bile-acid-binding resins should not be given to patients with complete biliary obstruction.

Adverse effects: Bile-acid-binding resins are not absorbed, and therefore have very few systemic side effects. Side effects include nausea and vomiting, constipation, heartburn, abdominal pain and flatulence, and aggravation of hypertriglyceridaemia. They may interfere with the absorption of fat-soluble vitamins and certain drugs.

Therapeutic regimen: To avoid interference with their absorption, other drugs should not be taken within 1 hour before or 3–4 hours after cholestyramine or colestipol administration.

Probucol

Mechanism of action: Probucol decreases levels of plasma LDL and HDL, and may decrease VLDL secretion (Fig. 4.16). It has antioxidant properties, which may decrease the atherogenicity of LDLs. It may also inhibit the uptake of lipoproteins by macrophages.

Route of administration: Probucol is administered orally as tablets.

Indications: Probucol is used for xanthomata.

Contraindications: Probucol should not be given to women who are pregnant or breast-feeding.

Adverse effects: The side effects of probucol include nausea and vomiting, abdominal pain and flatulence, diarrhoea, and, rarely, ventricular arrhythmias.

Therapeutic regimen: As probucol is very lipophilic, its effect on plasma cholesterol does not peak until 1–3 months after administration. Probucol is taken at night.

Thyroid hormone analogues

Mechanism of action: Thyroid hormone analogues increase LDL receptor synthesis, thus stimulating LDL uptake and therefore clearance (Fig. 4.16).

Indications: Thyroid hormone analogues are given for type IIa familial hypercholesterolaemia (lack of functional LDL receptors), in which dietary treatment and other drugs have been unsuccessful. They are recommended for use in young patients in whom coronary artery disease is not yet evident.

For further details of thyroid hormone analogues, (see Chapter 8)

Fig. 4.18 provides a summary of the types of drugs used in the treatment of the hyperlipidaemias.

Drugs used in the treatment of hyperlipidaemias	
Type	Drug treatment
II	none
IIa	nicotinic acid with bile acid resin HMG-CoA reductase inhibitors probucol thyroxine? neomycin?
IIb	nicotinic acid gemfibrozil fibrates bile acid resin HMG-CoA reductase inhibitors?
III	fibrates nicotinic acid gemfibrozil
IV	nicotinic acid gemfibrozil fibrates
V	nicotinic acid gemfibrozil fibrates

Fig. 4.18 Drugs used in the treatment of the different types of hyperlipidaemias.

HAEMOSTASIS AND THROMBOSIS

Principles of haemostasis

Haemostasis is the eradication of bleeding from damaged blood vessels.

If haemostasis is defective or unable to cope with blood loss from larger vessels, blood may accumulate in the tissues. This accumulated blood is called a haematoma.

Three stages are involved in haemostasis. These are:
- Blood vessel constriction.
- Formation of a platelet plug.
- Formation of a clot.

Blood vessel constriction

The first response to a severed blood vessel is contraction of the smooth muscle of the vessel. This is mediated by the release of thromboxane A_2 and other substances from platelets.

Blood vessel constriction slows the flow of blood through the vessel, thus reducing the pressure, and pushes opposing surfaces of the vessel together. In very small vessels, this results in permanent closure of the vessel, but in most cases blood vessel constriction is insufficient for this to occur.

Platelet plug formation

Exposure to the collagen underlying the vessel endothelium, as occurs during vessel injury, allows platelets to adhere to the collagen by binding to von Willebrand factors. These factors, secreted by the platelets and endothelium, bind to the exposed collagen; platelets then bind to this complex.

- Define hypertension, distinguishing between primary and secondary types.
- Describe the classes of drugs used in the treatment of hypertension. For each of these list examples, their mechanism of action, route of administration, indications, and major adverse effects.
- Define shock, its signs and causes, and distinguish between the different types.
- Describe the classes of drugs used in the treatment of shock. For each of these list examples, their mechanism of action, route of administration, indication, and major adverse effects
- Describe the classes of drugs used in the treatment of hyperlipidaemias. For each of these list examples, their mechanism of action, route of administration, indications, and major adverse effects.

Release of ADP, serotonin, thromboxane A$_2$, and other substances, by the platelets causes the latter to aggregate, while fibrin acts to bind them together.

The synthesis and release of prostacyclin by the intact endothelium inhibits platelet aggregation and acts to limit the extent of the platelet plug.

Intact endothelial cells also produce nitric oxide (NO), a potent vasodilator and inhibitor of platelet aggregation.

Clot formation

Blood coagulation is the conversion of liquid blood into a solid gel, known as a clot. A clot:

- Consists of a meshwork of fibrin within which blood cells are trapped.
- Functions to reinforce the platelet plug.

Fibrin is formed from its precursor fibrinogen, through the action of an enzyme called thrombin.

The formation of thrombin occurs via two distinct pathways—intrinsic and extrinsic—which together are known as the coagulation cascade. Both pathways involve the conversion of inactive factors into active enzymes, which then go on to catalyse the conversion of other factors into enzymes, and so on (Fig. 4.19).

The extrinsic pathway is thus termed because the component needed for its initiation is contained outside the blood. Tissue factor binds factor VII on exposure of blood to subendothelial cells, and converts it to its active form, VIIa. This enzyme then catalyses the activation of factors X and IX.

The intrinsic pathway is thus termed because its components are contained in the blood. It merges with the extrinsic pathway at the step prior to thrombin formation.

The thrombin formed stimulates the activation of factors XI, VIII, and V, and thus acts as a form of positive feedback.

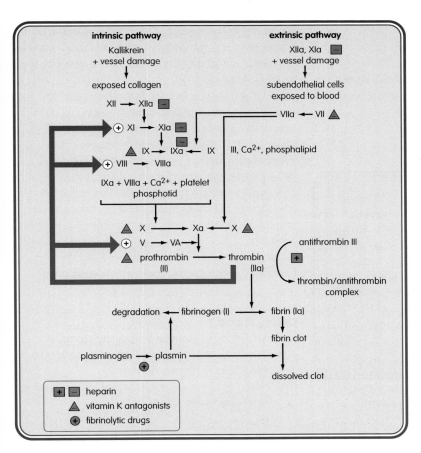

Fig. 4.19 Effects of heparin, vitamin K, and fibrinolytic drugs on the coagulation cascade. (Factor III, factor/tissue thromboplastin.)

. Three naturally occurring anticoagulants limit the extent of clot formation. These are:

- Tissue factor pathway inhibitor (TFPI), which binds to the tissue factor–VIIa complex, and inhibits its actions.
- Protein C, which is activated by thrombin, and inactivates factors VII and V.
- Antithrombin III, which is activated by heparin, and inactivates thrombin and other factors.

Fibrinolysis

The fibrinolytic or thrombolytic system functions to dissolve a clot once repair of the vessel is under way.

Plasmin digests fibrin. It is formed from plasminogen through the action of plasminogen activators, the best example of which is tissue plasminogen activator (t-PA).

Thrombosis

Thrombosis is the pathological formation of a clot known as a thrombus, which may cause occlusion within blood vessels or the heart, and result in death. Thrombosis causes:

- Arterial occlusion, which may lead to myocardial infarction, stroke, and peripheral ischaemia.
- Venous occlusion, which may lead to deep venous thrombosis and pulmonary embolism.

Arterial thrombi form because of endothelial injury, which is in turn the result of underlying arterial wall pathology, such as atherosclerosis.

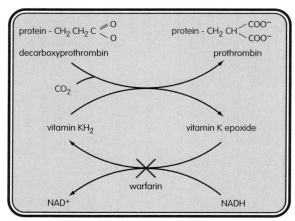

Fig. 4.20 Role of vitamin K in prothrombin formation. Warfarin inhibits the reduction of vitamin K epoxide.

Venous and atrial thrombi tend to form as a result of blood stasis, allowing the build-up of platelets and fibrin. People with hypercoagulability, due to a lack of one or more of the naturally occurring anticoagulants, are particularly susceptible.

Arterial thrombi consist mainly of platelets, whereas venous thrombi consist mainly of fibrin.

Management of disorders of haemostasis

Bleeding disorders

Hereditary bleeding disorders are rare. Haemophilia is a genetic disorder in which excessive bleeding occurs, owing to the absence of factor VIII (haemophilia A) or IX (haemophilia B). Von Willebrand's disease is characterized by abnormal bruising and mucosal bleeding.

Acquired bleeding disorders may be due to liver disease, vitamin K deficiency, or anticoagulants.

Caution should be taken when using the following drugs in patients with thromboembolic disease.

Vitamin K

Mechanism of action: Vitamin K is needed for the post-transcriptional γ-carboxylation of glutamic acid residues of prothrombin and clotting factors VII, IX, and X by the liver (Fig. 4.20).

Route of administration: Vitamin K is administered orally, intramuscularly, and intravenously.

Indications: Vitamin K is used as an antidote to the effects of oral anticoagulants, and in patients with biliary obstruction or liver disease, where Vitamin K deficiency may be a problem. It is also used after prolonged treatment with antibiotics that inhibit the formation of vitamin K_2 by intestinal bacteria, and as prophylaxis against hypoprothrombinaemia in the newborn.

Adverse effects: Side effects of vitamin K include haemolytic anaemia and hyperbilirubinaemia in the newborn.

Clotting factors

Deficient clotting factors can be replaced by the administration of fresh plasma. Factors VIII and IX are available as freeze-dried concentrates.

Mechanism of action: All clotting factors are necessary for normal blood coagulation.

Route of administration: Clotting factors are administered intravenously.

Indications: Clotting factors are used in haemophilia, and as an antidote to the effects of oral anticoagulants.

Adverse effects: The side effects of clotting factors include allergic reactions such as fevers and chills.

Desmopressin

Desmopressin or 1-deamino-(8-D-arginine)-vasopressin (dDAVP) is a synthetic analogue of vasopressin.

Mechanism of action: Desmopressin causes the release of von Willebrand factor and factor VIII.

Route of administration: Desmopressin is administered by intravenous infusion.

Indications: Desmopressin is given for mild factor VIII deficiency and von Willebrand's disease, and prophylactically before minor surgery.

Adverse effects: The side effects of desmopressin include fluid retention, hyponatraemia, and headache, nausea, and vomiting.

Anticoagulants
Vitamin K antagonists

Warfarin, nicoumalone, and phenindione are examples of vitamin K antagonists.

Mechanism of action: Vitamin K antagonists block the reduction of vitamin K epoxide, which is necessary for its action as a co-factor in the synthesis of factors II, VII, IX, and X (Fig.4.20).

Route of administration: Vitamin K antagonists are well absorbed orally.

Indications: Vitamin K antagonists are used in the prophylaxis and treatment of deep vein thrombosis and pulmonary embolism, the prophylaxis of embolization in atrial fibrillation and rheumatic disease, and in patients with prosthetic heart valves.

Contraindications: Vitamin K antagonists should not be given to patients with cerebral thrombosis, peripheral arterial occlusion, peptic ulcers, or hypertension, or to pregnant women.

Adverse effects: Haemorrhage is a side effect of vitamin K antagonists.

Therapeutic regimen: Vitamin K antagonists are given at an initial dose of 10 mg daily for 2 days, followed by maintenance dose.

Therapeutic notes: The onset of action of vitamin K antagonists takes several hours, owing to the time needed for the degradation of factors that have already been carboxylated ($t_{1/2}$: VII = 6 hours, IX = 24 hours, X = 40 hours, II = 60 hours).

Heparin

Heparin can be extracted from beef lung or hog intestinal mucosa for use clinically.

Mechanism of action: Heparin activates antithrombin III, which limits blood clotting by inactivating thrombin and other factors. Heparin must bind to both antithrombin and the factor being inactivated. It also inhibits platelet aggregation, possibly as a result of inhibiting thrombin.

Route of administration: Heparin can be administered intravenously and subcutaneously.

Indications: Heparin is used in the treatment of deep vein thrombosis and pulmonary embolism, as well as for prophylaxis against postoperative deep vein thrombosis and pulmonary embolism in high-risk patients.

Contraindications: Heparin should not be given to patients with haemophilia, thrombocytopenia, or peptic ulcers.

Adverse effects: Heparin has several side effects. These include haemorrhage (treated by stopping therapy or administering a heparin antagonist such as protamine sulphate), hypersensitivity, and osteoporosis if used long term.

Therapeutic regimen: Heparin is given intravenously (5000 units), followed by infusion of 1000–2000 units/hour or subcutaneous injection of 15 000 units every 12 hours.

Therapeutic notes: Heparin has an immediate onset and can therefore be used in emergencies.

Antiplatelet agents
Aspirin

Aspirin is acetylsalicylic acid.

Mechanism of action: Aspirin blocks the synthesis of thromboxane A_2 from arachidonic acid in platelets, by acetylating and thus inhibiting the enzyme cyclooxygenase. Thromboxane A_2 stimulates PLC, thus increasing calcium levels and causing platelet aggregation. Aspirin also blocks the synthesis of prostacyclin from endothelial cells, which inhibits platelet aggregation. However, this effect is short lived because endothelial cells, unlike platelets, can synthesize new cyclooxygenase (see Fig. 4.21).

Route of administration: Aspirin is administered orally as a tablet.

Indications: Aspirin is used prophylactically against myocardial infarction and stroke.

Contraindications: Aspirin should not be given to children under 12 years of age, to breast-feeding women, to haemophiliac people, or to patients with peptic ulcers.

Adverse effects: Side effects of aspirin include bronchospasm and gastrointestinal haemorrhage.

Therapeutic regimen: Aspirin at 150 mg daily after myocardial infarction has been shown to decrease mortality significantly. Given on alternate days, aspirin may reduce the incidence of primary myocardial infarction.

Dipyridamole

Mechanism of action: Dipyridamole causes inhibition of the phosphodiesterase enzyme that hydrolyses cAMP. Increased cAMP levels result in decreased calcium levels and inhibition of platelet aggregation.

Route of administration: Dipyridamole is administered orally.

Indications: Dipyridamole is used in conjunction with warfarin and other oral anticoagulants in the

prophylaxis against thrombosis associated with prosthetic heart valves. It is also used in angina—this has a different mechanism of action (p. 91).

Adverse effects: Dipyridamole can cause hypotension, and nausea, diarrhoea, and headache.

Therapeutic regimen: Dipyridamole is given (300–600 mg daily) in three or four divided doses before food.

Prostacyclin

Prostacyclin is synthesized from arachidonic acid through the action of cyclooxygenase.

Mechanism of action: Prostacyclin activates adenylyl cyclase in platelets, thus increasing cAMP levels, decreasing calcium levels, and inhibiting platelet aggregation.

Route of administration: Prostacyclin is administered orally.

Indications: Owing to its very short half-life, prostacyclin is limited to procedures such as cardiac bypass surgery.

Adverse effects: Prostacyclin can cause nausea, diarrhoea, and headache.

Fibrinolytic agents

Streptokinase

Mechanism of action: Streptokinase forms a complex with, and activates, plasminogen.

Route of administration: Streptokinase is administered by intravenous infusion.

Indications: Streptokinase is used in life-threatening venous thrombosis, pulmonary embolism, arterial thromboembolism, and acute myocardial infarction.

Contraindications: Streptokinase should not be given to patients with haemorrhage or bleeding disorders.

Adverse effects: Side effects of streptokinase include nausea, vomiting, and bleeding.

Therapeutic regimen: Streptokinase is given in a dose of 250 000 units over 30 minutes, then 100 000 units every hour for 24–72 hours. In myocardial infarction, 1 500 000 units are given over 1 hour, followed by aspirin.

Tissue-type plasminogen activators

Alteplase and anistreplase are examples of tPAs.

Mechanism of action: tPAs are tissue-type plasminogen activators.

Route of administration: tPAs are administered by intravenous injection.

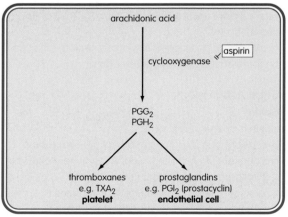

Fig. 4.21 Inhibition of cyclooxygenase by aspirin, leading to a reduction in the formation of thromboxane and prostacyclin. (PG, prostaglandin; PGI_2, prostacyclin; T_xA_2, thromboxane A_2.)

Indications: tPAs are used in acute myocardial infarction.

Contraindications: tPAs should not be given to patients with haemorrhage and bleeding disorders.

Adverse effects: Side effects of tPAs include nausea, vomiting, and bleeding.

Therapeutic regimen: Treatment should commence within 6 hours: 10 mg over 1–2 minutes, intravenous infusion of 50 mg over 1 hour, then 40 mg over 2 hours.

Antifibrinolytic agents

Tranexamic acid and aminocaproic acid

Tranexamic acid and aminocaproic acid are examples of antifibrinolytic agents.

Mechanism of action: Antifibrinolytic agents inhibit plasminogen activation; aminocaproic acid also inhibits streptokinase and urokinase.

Route of administration: Antifibrinolytic agents are administered orally and intravenously.

Indications: Antifibrinolytic agents are used for gastro-intestinal haemorrhage and conditions in which there is haemorrhage or risk of haemorhage, e.g. haemophilia, menorrhagia, and dental extraction.

Contraindications: Antifibrinolytic agents should not be given to patients with thromboembolic disease.

Adverse effects: Side effects of antifibrinolytic agents include nausea, vomiting, and diarrhoea.

Aprotinin

Mechanism of action: Aprotinin inhibits proteolytic enzymes, acting on plasmin and kallikrein.

Route of administration: Aprotinin is administered by intravenous injection or infusion.

Indications: Aprotinin is used when there is a risk of blood loss after open heart surgery, and for hyperplasminaemia.

Adverse effects: Side effects of aprotinin include allergy and localized thrombophlebitis.

Ethamsylate

Mechanism of action: Ethamsylate corrects abnormal platelet adhesion.

Route of administration: Ethamsylate is administered orally or by injection.

Indications: Ethamsylate is used to reduce capillary bleeding and periventricular haemorrhage in premature infants.

Contraindications: Ethamsylate should not be given to patients with porphyria.

Adverse effects: Side effects of ethamsylate include nausea, headache, and rashes.

The liver is important in coagulation as it is the site at which many of the clotting factors are produced.

It also produces bile salts necessary for the absorption of vitamin K, which is needed by the liver to produce prothrombin and clotting factors VII, IX, and X.

- What are the three stages of haemostasis? How are each of these mediated?
- Distinguish between the intrinsic and the extrinsic pathway of the coagulation cascade.
- Define thrombosis, its causes, implications, and consequences.
- Distinguish between arterial and venous occlusion.
- What are the classes of drugs used in the management of haemostasis? For each of these list examples, their mechanism of action, route of administration, indications, and major adverse effects.

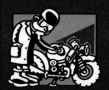
ASTHMA

Concepts of asthma

Asthma is a respiratory disease characterized by recurrent reversible obstruction to airflow in the bronchiolar airways.

Asthma may be allergic (extrinsic) or non-allergic (intrinsic).

Allergic asthma

Allergic asthma is the most common form of asthma. Allergic asthma occurs in people who are allergic to allergens—antigenic substances in inspired air. Affected individuals have high circulating levels of immunoglobulin E (IgE) and are usually atopic, i.e. prone to allergies.

Non-allergic asthma

Non-allergic asthma is an intrinsic type of asthma not attributable to any allergic reaction. It tends to develop later in life and is severe and unremitting.

Severe asthma (status asthmaticus)

Severe asthma or status asthmaticus, is a life-threatening acute deterioration of otherwise stable asthma. It is a potentially fatal condition that must be dealt with as an emergency, and requires hospital admission.

Pathogenesis of asthma

Asthma is characterized by episodes of wheezing and breathlessness caused by bronchospasm, mucosal oedema, and mucus formation. In asthma, smooth muscle that surrounds the bronchi is hyperresponsive to stimuli, and underlying inflammatory changes are present in the airways. Asthmatic stimuli include inhaled allergens (e.g. pollen, animal dander), occupational allergens, and drugs or non-specific stimuli such as cold air, exercise, stress, and pollution.

Stimuli cause asthmatic changes through several complex pathways. The possible mechanisms of these pathways include the following:

- Immune reactions (type 1 hypersensitivity) and release of inflammatory mediators: The cross-linking of IgE by allergens causes mast cell degranulation, and release of histamine and powerful eosinophil and neutrophil chemotactic factors. The eosinophils, neutrophils, and other inflammatory cells, release powerful inflammatory mediators *in situ* that cause a bronchial inflammatory reaction, tissue damage, and an increase in bronchial hyperresponsiveness. Bronchial inflammatory mediators include leucotrienes, prostaglandins, and thromboxane; platelet-activating factor, and eosinophilic major basic protein.
- An imbalance in airway smooth muscle tone involving the parasympathetic nerves (vagus), non-adrenergic non-cholinergic (NANC) nerves, and circulating noradrenaline that act under normal circumstances to control airway diameter.
- Abnormal calcium flux across cell membranes, increasing smooth muscle contraction and mast cell degranulation.
- Leaky tight junctions between bronchial epithelial cells allowing allergen access.

In many patients the asthmatic attack consists of two phases—an immediate-phase response and a late-phase response.

Immediate-phase response

An immediate-phase response occurs on exposure to the eliciting stimulus. The response consists mainly of broncho-spasm. Bronchodilators are effective in this early phase.

Late-phase response

Several hours later, the late-phase response occurs. This consists of bronchospasm, vasodilatation, oedema, and mucus secretion caused by inflammatory mediators released from eosinophils, platelets, and other cells, and neuropeptides released by axon reflexes. Anti-inflammatory drug action is necessary for the prevention and/or treatment of this phase (Fig. 5.1).

Management of asthma

Anti-asthmatic drugs include symptomatic bronchodilators (these are most effective in the immediate-phase response), and prophylactic or anti-inflammatory agents, which prevent and/or resolve the late phase response. Some drugs have more than one action (Fig. 5.2).

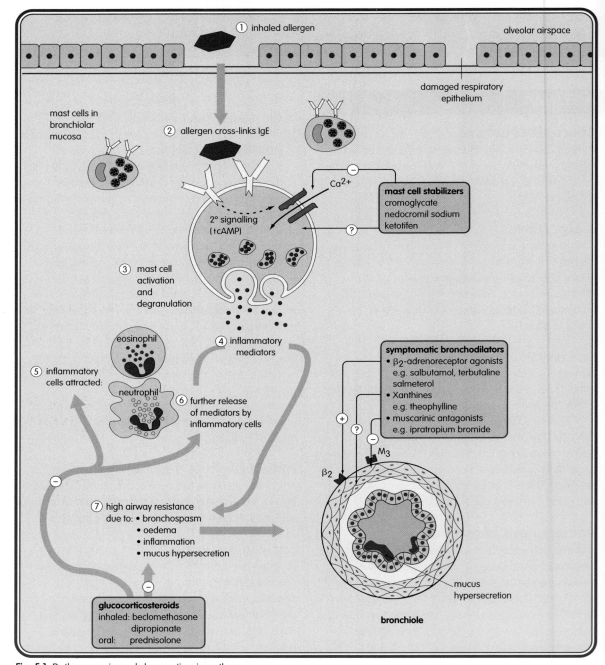

Fig. 5.1 Pathogenesis and drug action in asthma.

Bronchodilators

β₂-Adrenoceptor agonists

Examples of β_2-adrenoceptor agonists include salbutamol; terbutaline, and salmeterol.

Mechanism of action: Airway smooth muscle does not have a sympathetic nervous supply, but does contain β_2-adrenoceptors that respond to circulating adrenaline. The stimulation of β_2-adrenoceptors leads to a rise in intracellular cAMP levels and subsequent bronchial smooth muscle relaxation.

β_2-Adrenoceptor agonists may also help prevent the activation of mast cells, as a minor effect.

Modern selective β_2-adrenoceptor agonists are potent bronchodilators and have very few β_1-stimulating properties (i.e. they do not affect the heart).

Route of administration: β_2-Adrenoceptor agonists are usually delivered via a metered dose inhaler; the effects start immediately. Oral administration is reserved for children and people unable to use inhalers, and intravenous administration for status asthmaticus.

Indications: β_2-Adrenoceptor agonists are used to relieve bronchospasm. They may be used alone in mild, occasional asthma, but are more commonly used in conjunction with other drugs, e.g. corticosteroids.

Contraindications: β_2-Adrenoceptor agonists have no contraindications.

Adverse effects: Side effects of β_2-adrenoceptor agonists include fine tremor, tachycardia, and hypokalaemia after high doses.

Therapeutic notes: β_2-Adrenoceptor agonists act as 'physiological antagonists', by treating the symptoms of asthma but not the underlying disease process.

Salmeterol is a long-acting drug that can be administered twice daily. It is not suitable for relief of an acute attack.

Anticholinergics

Ipratropium bromide is an example of an anticholinergic drug.

Mechanism of action: Parasympathetic vagal fibres provide a bronchoconstrictor tone to the smooth muscle of the airways. They re activated by reflex on stimulation of sensory (irritant) receptors in the airway walls.

Anticholinergic muscarinic antagonists act by blocking muscarinic receptors, especially the M_3 subtype, which responds to this parasympathetic bronchoconstrictor tone.

Route of administration: Metered dose inhaler.

Indications: Anticholinergics are used as adjuncts to β_2-adrenoceptor agonists in the treatment of asthma.

Contraindications: Anticholinergics should not be given to patients with glaucoma or prostatic hypertrophy, or to pregnant women.

Adverse effects: When inhaled, there are virtually none of the usual side effects from anticholinergics. Dry mouth may occur.

Therapeutic notes: Anticholinergics have a synergistic effect when administered with β_2-adrenoreceptor agonists in asthma.

Xanthines

Theophylline is an example of a xanthine.

Mechanism of action: It is unclear how xanthines cause bronchodilatation in asthma. They may increase cAMP levels in the bronchial smooth muscle cells by inhibiting phosphodiesterase, an enzyme which catalyses the hydrolysis of cAMP to AMP.

Route of administration: Oral.

Indications: Xanthines are used in asthmatic children unable to use inhalers, and adults with predominantly nocturnal symptoms. They are administered intravenously in status asthmaticus.

Contraindications: Unacceptable adverse effects.

Adverse effects: Side effects of xanthines include nausea, vomiting, tremor, insomnia, and tachycardia.

Therapeutic notes: Oral xanthines are formulated as

Classification of anti-asthma drugs	
Symptomatic bronchodilators	**Examples**
β_2-adrenoreceptor agonists	short acting: salbutamol, terbutaline long acting: salmeterol
anticholinergics	Ipratopium bromide
xanthines	Theophylline
Prophylactic (prevent inflammation)	
mast cell stabilization	sodium cromoglycate, nedocromil, ketotifen
xanthines	theophylline
glucocorticosteroids	beclomethasone
Anti-inflammatory (resolve inflammation)	
glucocorticosteroids	beclomethasone

Fig. 5.2 Classification of anti-asthma drugs.

sustained-release preparations. Xanthines often cause adverse effects—the 'narrow therapeutic window'—but are useful as oral drugs, effective in preventing attacks for up to 12 hours.

Prophylactic and anti-inflammatory drugs

Mast-cell stabilizers

Cromoglycate, nedocromil sodium, and ketotifen are examples of mast-cell stabilizers.

Mechanism of action: The exact modes of action of mast-cell stabilizers are unclear. These drugs appear to stabilize antigen-sensitized mast cells by reducing calcium influx and subsequent release of inflammatory mediators.

Ketotifen also has antihistamine (H_1-receptor antagonist) actions.

Route of administration: Cromoglycate and nedocromil sodium: metered dose inhaler; ketotifen: oral.

Indications: Mast-cell stabilizers are useful in young patients (<20 years old) with marked allergic disease and moderate asthma.

Adverse effects: One side effect of mast-cell stabilizers is their foul taste.

Therapeutic notes: Mast-cell stabilizers have a prophylactic action; they must be taken regularly for several weeks before any beneficial effects are noted. These drugs are therefore of no use in acute asthma attacks.

Anti-inflammatory glucocorticoids

Anti-inflammatory glucocorticoids include beclomethasone, dipropionate, and prednisolone.

Mechanism of action: Corticosteroids depress the inflammatory response in bronchial mucosa and so diminish bronchial hyperresponsiveness. The specific effects include:

- Reduced mucosal oedema and mucus production.
- Decreased local generation of prostaglandins and leucotrienes, with less inflammatory-cell activation.
- Adrenoceptor upregulation.
- Long-term reduced T-cell cytokine production, and reduced eosinophil and mast-cell infiltration of bronchial mucosa.

For the intracellular events involved in corticosteroid action see Chapter 8.

Route of administration: Corticosteroids are usually delivered by metered dose inhaler. Oral and intravenous administration is reserved for severe asthma and status asthmaticus.

Indications: Corticosteroids are used in patients with more than minimal symptoms—often in combination with β_2-agonists or drugs that block allergies.

Contraindications: Unacceptable adverse effects.

Adverse effects: Inhaled corticosteroids may cause dysphonia, oral thrush, and systemic penetration in high dosage. If given orally, cushingoid effects may occur (see Chapter 8).

Therapeutic notes: The initial treatment of severe or refractory asthma may require oral corticosteroids. If possible, maintenance should be achieved with inhaled corticosteroids via a metered dose, to minimize side effects. Inhaled corticosteroids are usually effective in 3–7 days, but must be taken regularly.

Use of inhalers, nebulizers, and oxygen

In the treatment of asthma, inhalers and nebulizers are used to deliver drug directly to the airways. This allows higher drug concentrations to be achieved *in situ* while minimizing systemic effects. Whatever device is used, less than 15% of the dose is deposited on the bronchial mucosa.

Inhalers

There are several types of inhaler—metered dose, breath-activated spray, and breath-activated powder. They vary in cost, delivery efficiency, and ease of use.

Spacer devices, used in conjunction with inhalers, improve drug delivery and are easy to use. However, they are bulky to carry.

Nebulizers

Nebulizers convert a solution of drug into an aerosol for inhalation. They are more efficient than inhalers and are used to deliver higher doses of drug. They are useful in status asthmaticus and for the acute hospital treatment of severe asthma.

The long-term use of nebulizers is limited by cost, convenience, and the danger of patient overreliance.

Oxygen

High-concentration oxygen therapy (35–50%) is prescribed if arterial carbon dioxide levels start rising in hypoxaemic patients with severe asthma.

Oxygen increases alveolar oxygen tension and decreases the work of breathing necessary to maintain arterial oxygen tension. However, inappropriate oxygen therapy can have serious or even fatal consequences; it is not suitable as a chronic treatment for asthma.

A good understanding of the pathology involved in asthma is imperative to understanding the mechanism of action of the drugs used to treat this common condition.

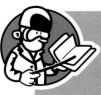

○ **What is the definition of asthma? Describe the different types that exist.**

○ **Discuss the pathological processes that occur at a cellular level in an asthmatic reaction, and how these produce the symptoms and signs of asthma, distinguishing between the immediate- and late-phase responses.**

○ **Describe the broad categories of drug that are used to counter these pathological processes: bronchodilators; prophylactic drugs that prevent inflammation; and anti-inflammatory corticosteroids that can prevent and resolve inflammation.**

○ **For each drug category, give examples and describe the different classes of drug, mechanisms of action, when they are used, how they are given, and any major side effects.**

○ **What is the role and use of inhalers, nebulizers, and oxygen therapy in asthma?**

RESPIRATORY STIMULANTS, ANTITUSSIVES, AND MUCOLYTICS

Respiratory stimulants

Respiratory stimulants, or analeptic drugs, have a very limited place in the treatment of ventilatory failure in patients with chronic obstructive airways disease. They have largely been replaced by the use of ventilatory support.

Doxapram, nikethamide, and ethmivan are examples of respiratory stimulants.

Mechanism of action: Respiratory stimulants are used to improve both rate and depth of breathing.

Doxapram is a central stimulant drug that acts on both carotid chemoreceptors and the respiratory centre in the brainstem to increase respiration. Nikethamide and ethmivan stimulate only the brainstem respiratory centre.

Route of administration: Respiratory stimulants are administered intravenously only.

Indications: Ventilatory failure in people with chronic obstructive airways disease in which ventilatory support is contraindicated.

Adverse effects: The therapeutic index of respiratory stimulants is small, although that of doxapram is larger than that of nikethamide and ethmivan. In excess, the stimulant action of these drugs on the CNS can result in restlessness, tremulousness, vomiting, and convulsions. In addition, their duration of action is very brief.

Therapeutic notes: Nikethamide and ethmivan are no longer used, owing to their narrow therapeutic window.

Antitussives

Antitussives are drugs that inhibit the cough reflex.

Cough is usually a valuable protective reflex mechanism for clearing foreign material and secretions from the airways. However, in some conditions, such as inflammation or neoplasia, the cough reflex may become inappropriately stimulated and in such cases antitussive drugs may be used.

Antitussives either reduce sensory receptor activation or work by an ill-defined mechanism, depressing a 'cough centre' in the brainstem.

Drugs that reduce receptor activation
Menthol vapour and topical local anaesthetics
Benzocaine is an example of a topical local anesthetic.

Mechanism of action: Menthol vapour and topical local anaesthetics reduce the sensitivity of peripheral sensory

'cough receptors' in the pharynx and larynx to irritation.
Route of administration: Menthol and local anaesthetics are administered topically as a spray, lozenge, or vapour.
Indications: Menthol vapour and topical local anaesthetics are used for unwanted cough.

Drugs that reduce the sensitivity of the 'cough centre'
Opioids
Opioids reduce the sensitivity of the 'cough centre'. Examples of these drugs include codeine and dextromethorphan.
Mechanism of action: Although not clearly understood, opioids seem to work via agonist action on opiate receptors, depressing a 'cough centre' in the brainstem.
Route of administration: Opioids are usually administered orally in proprietary cough preparations.
Indications: Opioids are used for inappropriate coughing.
Adverse effects: There are generally few side effects of opioids at antitussive doses. Unlike dextromethorphan, codeine can cause constipation, and inhibition of mucociliary clearance.

Mucolytics
Mucolytics are drugs that reduce the viscosity of bronchial secretions. They are sometimes used when excess bronchial secretions need to be cleared.

Acetylcysteine and bromohexine
Mechanism of action: Acetylcysteine and bromohexine reduce the viscosity of bronchial secretions by cleaving disulphide bonds cross-linking mucus glycoprotein molecules.
Route of administration: Bromohexine is administered orally, and acetylcysteine orally or by inhalation.
Indications: Acetylcysteine and bromohexine may be of benefit in chronic obstructive airways disease, although their efficacy is doubtful.

o **Describe the use of the following classes of drug, in relation to their effect on the respiratory system: respiratory stimulants, antitussives, and mucolytics.**
o **For each class of drug give an example, and describe the mechanism of action (as far as it might be known), indications, route of administration, and any major adverse effects.**

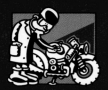

6. Kidneys

Principles of renal function

Despite making up only 1% of total body weight, the kidneys receive approximately 25% of the cardiac output.

The volume of plasma filtered by the kidneys is termed the glomerular filtration rate (GFR) and is equal to approximately 180 L/day for a person weighing 70 kg. This means that the entire plasma volume is filtered about 60 times a day.

Functions of the kidney

The kidney has several functions. These include:
- Regulation of body water content.
- Regulation of body mineral content and composition.
- Regulation of body pH.
- Excretion of metabolic waste products, e.g. urea, uric acid, and creatinine.
- Excretion of foreign material, e.g. drugs.
- Secretion of renin, erythropoietin, and 1,25-dihydroxyvitamin D_3.
- Gluconeogenesis.

The nephron

Each kidney is made up of approximately one million functional units, known as 'nephrons' (Fig. 6.1).

Each nephron consists of:
- A renal corpuscle which comprises a glomerulus and a Bowman's capsule.
- A tubule which comprises a proximal tubule, loop of Henle, distal convoluted tubule, and collecting duct system.

The renal corpuscle lies within the cortex of the kidney while the tubule extends down into the medulla.

Nephrons originating near the cortex–medulla junction are known as juxtaglomerular nephrons.

The renal process
Blood supply

Blood reaches each kidney via the renal artery, which divides into numerous branches before forming the afferent arterioles. These afferent arterioles enter the glomerular capillaries (the glomeruli) and leave as the efferent arterioles.

The efferent arteriole leaving most nephrons immediately branches into a set of capillaries known as the 'peritubular capillaries'. These branch extensively and form a network of capillaries surrounding the tubules in the cortex into which reabsorption from the tubule occurs, and from which various substances are secreted into the tubule.

In contrast, the efferent arteriole from juxtaglomerular nephrons branches into a set of capillaries termed the vasa recta, which supply medullary tubules.

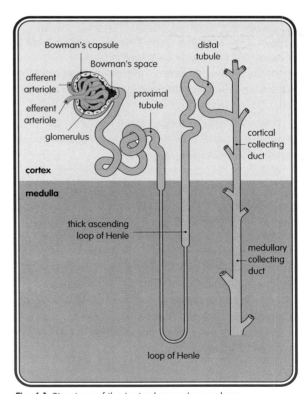

Fig. 6.1 Structure of the juxtaglomerular nephron.

115

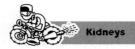

Glomerular filtration

During glomerular filtration, blood in the glomerulus is forced through the capillary endothelium, a basement membrane, and the epithelium of the Bowman's capsule, to enter a fluid-filled space known as the 'Bowman's space'.

Appoximately 20% of the plasma entering the glomerulus is filtered. The filtered fluid is known as the glomerular filtrate and consists of protein-free plasma.

Tubular function

The tubules are involved in reabsorption and secretion.

Important components of plasma tend to be reabsorbed more or less completely: e.g. sodium and glucose are 99–100% reabsorbed. Waste products are only partially reabsorbed: e.g. approximately 45% of urea is reabsorbed.

The tubules secrete hydrogen and potassium ions, as well as organic ions such as creatinine, and drugs such as penicillin.

Sodium and water reabsorption

Approximately 99% of filtered water and sodium is reabsorbed, but none is filtered.

Sodium is reabsorbed via Na^+/K^+ ATPase pumps located in the basolateral membranes of all four tubular sections. These pumps create low sodium concentrations within tubular cells and thus promote the movement of sodium from the lumen into the cells.

The mechanism of sodium movement from the lumen of the tubule into the cells varies according to the section of the tubule (Fig. 6.2–6.5).

Water is reabsorbed by passive diffusion, following the movement of sodium ions.

For water reabsorption to occur, the tubular lumen must be permeable to water; this permeability varies according to the section of the tubule.

Proximal tubule

The Bowman's capsule extends into the proximal tubule, which is made up of an initial convoluted section and a straight section. The proximal tubule is:
- The site into which many drugs are secreted.
- Permeable to water and ions.

Approximately two-thirds of the filtrate volume is reabsorbed back into the blood in the proximal tubule,

and since sodium and water are reabsorbed in equal proportions, there is practically no change in osmolarity.

Sodium movement into the cell is coupled with that of glucose and amino acids, whereas chloride movement is by passive diffusion (Fig. 6.5).

Reabsorption of bicarbonate also takes place in the proximal tubule. Carbonic acid (H_2CO_3) is formed from the action of carbonic anhydrase on carbon dioxide and water. H_2CO_3 immediately dissociates into bicarbonate (HCO_3^-), which moves down its concentration gradient across the basolateral membrane, and H^+, which is secreted into the lumen in exchange for Na^+. H^+ combines with filtered HCO_3^- to form H_2CO_3 and, subsequently, carbon dioxide and water, which are able to diffuse back into the cell.

Loop of Henle

The loop of Henle is shaped like a hairpin and consists of a descending limb, a thin ascending limb, and a thick ascending limb.

Twenty-five per cent of filtered sodium is reabsorbed in the thick ascending limb (Fig. 6.2), but this portion of the tubule is impermeable to water. This enables urine to be concentrated by generation of a hyperosmotic medullary interstitium via the countercurrent multiplier system. High medullary osmotic pressure is necessary for the reabsorption of water from the collecting tubules.

The macula densa is a collection of cells located near the afferent and efferent arterioles on the thick ascending limb. These juxtaglomerular cells secrete the hormone renin, which controls aldosterone secretion from the adrenal gland by activating angiotensin. This system, known as the aldosterone and renin–angiotensin system (RAS), controls sodium reabsorption from the cortical collecting duct and is thus able to control body plasma volume.

Distal convoluted tubule and collecting tubule

The distal tubule is continuous with the collecting duct, which is made up of a connecting tubule, a cortical collecting duct, and a medullary collecting duct.

The collecting duct is the site at which the tubules of many nephrons merge before draining into the renal pelvis. The renal pelvis is continuous with the ureter, which joins the kidney to the bladder.

The late distal tubule and collecting duct contain two cell types (Fig 6.4):

- Principal cells, which incorporate sodium and potassium channels
- Intercalated cells, which incorporate H+ATPases that secrete hydrogen ions.

Sodium movement into the principal cells exceeds potassium movement out, so that a negative potential difference is established. Sodium is transported across the basolateral membrane by Na+/K+ ATPase and potassium is moved into the cell before being forced out by the negative potential.

This part of the tubule is the major site for potassium secretion.

The H+ ATPase is involved in the reabsorption of filtered HCO_3^-.

The late distal tubule and collecting duct also contain mineralocorticoid receptors. When aldosterone binds to these, it produces an increase in the synthesis of Na+ and K+ channels, Na+/K+ ATPase, and ATP, so that Na+ reabsorption is increased, and K+ and H+ secretion are also increased.

DIURETICS

Diuretics are drugs that work on the kidneys to increase urine volume by reducing salt and water reabsorption from the tubules. They are prescribed in the treatment of oedema, where there is an increase in interstitial fluid volume leading to tissue swelling.

Underlying causes of oedema

Oedema occurs when the rate of fluid formation exceeds that of fluid reabsorption from the interstitial fluid into the capillaries.

Congestive heart failure

The decrease in cardiac output that occurs in congestive heart failure (CHF) results in underperfusion of the kidneys and a consequent reduced GFR. This leads to the activation of the RAS and subsequent sodium and water retention (see Chapter 4).

The increased pulmonary venous pressure causes pulmonary oedema, which can be fatal because of impaired respiration, while the elevated central venous pressure causes peripheral tissue swelling.

Liver disease

The decrease in protein synthesis (e.g. albumin) that occurs in liver diseases such as cirrhosis leads to a decrease in hydrostatic pressure within the blood, favouring water flow into the tissues, and thus causing oedema.

The flow of fluid into the interstitium decreases the effective circulating blood volume and results in the activation of the RAS, causing further oedema, and so the cycle continues.

Oedema is most pronounced in the peritoneal cavity. This is termed ascites.

Nephrotic syndrome

In nephrotic syndrome, the increase in the permeability of the glomerular basement membrane to proteins such as albumin leads to proteinuria (protein in the urine).

As in liver disease, reduced plasma protein levels increase hydrostatic pressure and cause water to flow into the tissues. Again, the RAS is activated.

Osmotic diuretics

Mannitol and isosorbide are examples of osmotic diuretics. These are pharmacologically inert.

Site of action: Osmotic diuretics exert their effects in tubular segments that are water permeable, such as the proximal tubule, the descending loop of Henle, and the collecting ducts.

Mechanism of action: Osmotic diuretics are freely filtered at the glomerulus, but only partially, if at all, reabsorbed. They work by increasing the tubular osmotic pressure, thereby lowering water reabsorption and subsequently decreasing sodium concentration within the lumen. This leads to a reduction in sodium reabsorption.

Loss of water from intracellular compartments increases extracellular volume, thus inhibiting renin release, which further prevents oedema.

Route of administration: Mannitol is administered intravenously and isosorbide orally.

Indications: Osmotic diuretics are used for polyuria in which there is an increase in fluid intake (polydipsia) with excessive production of dilute urine. The underlying cause is usually diabetes mellitus or diabetes insipidus. Osmotic diuretics are also used for raised intracranial or intraocular pressure (glaucoma) and prophylaxis

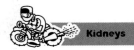

against acute renal failure, e.g. that caused by drug poisoning. Since the increase in sodium excretion is relatively small in comparison with the increase in water excretion, these drugs are not of use in treating conditions associated with sodium retention.

Contraindications: Osmotic diuretics should not be given to patients with heart failure as pulmonary oedema may occur, owing to water extraction from intracellular compartments and expansion of the extracellular volume.

Adverse effects: Side effects of osmotic diuretics include hyponatraemia (decreased plasma sodium) and possible headache, nausea, and vomiting.

Loop diuretics

Frusemide, bumetanide, torasemide, and ethacrynic acid are examples of loop diuretics.

Loop diuretics cause the excretion of 15–25% of filtered sodium as opposed to the normal 1% or less, and consequently can result in the production of up to 4 litres of urine per day.

Site of action: Loop diuretics act at the loop of Henle, in particular the thick ascending limb. Because they are bound to plasma proteins, loop diuretics are not filtered, but rather are secreted into the proximal convoluted tubule.

Mechanism of action: Loop diuretics inhibit the $Na^+/K^+/2Cl^-$ co-transporter in the luminal membrane (Fig. 6.2). This increases the amount of sodium reaching the collecting duct and thereby increases K^+ and H^+ secretion. Calcium and magnesium reabsorption is also inhibited, owing to the decrease in potential difference across the cell normally generated from the recycling of potassium.

Loop diuretics can also cause venodilatation by bringing about the release of a renal factor, believed to be prostaglandins.

Route of administration: Loop diuretics are orally active but are given intravenously in emergencies. Administered orally, they have an onset of less than an hour and last for 4–6 hours. Administered intravenously, their effect peaks within 30 minutes.

Indications: Loop diuretics are given for acute pulmonary oedema (emergency situation), oliguria due to acute renal failure, and oedema due to CHF, liver disease, or nephrotic syndrome—if no longer responsive to thiazides. They are also used for

hypertension in patients not responding to other diuretics or antihypertensives, and in hypercalcaemia or hyperkalaemia.

Contraindications: Loop diuretics should not be given to those with severe renal impairment. They should be given only with extreme caution to patients receiving (a) cardiac glycosides (as the hypokalaemia caused by loop diuretics potentiates the action of cardiac glycosides and consequently increases the risk of cardiac glycoside-

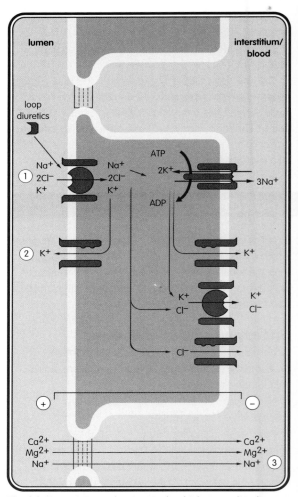

Fig. 6.2 Transport mechanism in the thick ascending loop of Henle. Loop diuretics block the $Na^+/K^+/2Cl^-$ cotransporter (1) thereby increasing the excretion of Na^+ and Cl^-. These drugs also decrease the potential difference across the tubule cell, which arises from the recycling of K^+ (2), and this leads to increased excretion of Ca^{2+} and Mg^{2+} by inhibiting paracellular diffusion (3).

Loop diuretics are termed high ceiling diuretics, owing to their strong potency.

induced arrhythmias), and (b) aminoglycoside antibiotics, as these interact with loop diuretics and increase the risk of ototoxicity and potential hearing loss.

Adverse effects: Side effects of loop diuretics include potassium loss with consequent hypokalaemia (low plasma potassium). Other side effects include hypotension and hypovolaemia, hyponatraemia, and hyperuricaemia (increased plasma uric acid) as a result of competition between uric acid and loop diuretics for tubular secretion—this may precipitate gout. Metabolic alkalosis may occur due to increased hydrogen secretion and thus excretion. Calcium and magnesium deficiency is also possible.

Thiazide diuretics

Hydrochlorothiazide, polythiazide, indapamide, chlorthalidone and metolazone are examples of thiazide diuretics.

Thiazides produce moderately potent diuresis, causing the excretion of 5–10% of filtered sodium and resulting in the production of 1–2 L urine per day.

Site of action: Thiazide diuretics act on the early distal tubule. They reach their site of action by glomerular filtration and tubular secretion.

Mechanism of action: Thiazide diuretics inhibit the Na^+/Cl^- symporter in the luminal membrane (Fig. 6.3). Like loop diuretics, they increase the secretion of K^+ and H^+ into the collecting ducts but, in contrast, they decrease Ca^{2+} excretion by a mechanism possibly involving the stimulation of a Na^+/Ca^{2+} exchange across the basolateral membrane; this is due to reduced tubular cell sodium concentration.

Route of administration: Thiazide diuretics are effective orally and have an onset time of 1–2 hours, peak effect at 4–6 hours, and duration of action of 8–12 hours; (except for chlorthalidone which lasts for 48–72 hours).

Indications: Thiazide diuretics are used for hypertension; for oedema due to CHF, liver disease, or nephrotic syndrome; and for calcium oxalate stones in the urinary tract.

Contraindications: Thiazide diuretics should not be given to patients with hypokalaemia, hyponatraemia or hypercalcaemia, those taking cardiac glycosides (p. 118), or those with diabetics mellitus (thiazides may cause hyperglycaemia).

Adverse effects: Side effects of thiazide diuretics include potassium loss with consequent hypokalaemia, metabolic alkalosis due to increased hydrogen secretion and thus excretion, hyperuricaemia, hyponatraemia, and hypermagnesaemia and hypercalcaemia.

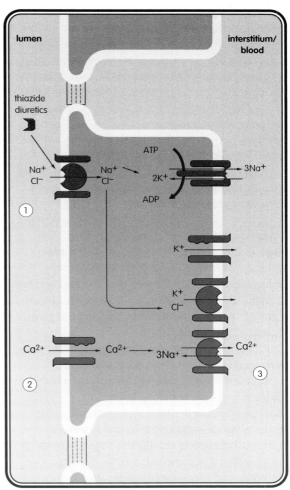

Fig. 6.3 Transport mechanisms in the early distal tubule. Thiazide diuretics increase the excretion of Na^+ and Cl^- by inhibiting the Na^+/Cl^- cotransporter (1). The reabsorption of Ca^{2+} (2) is increased by these drugs by a mechanism that may involve stimulation of Na^+/Ca^{2+} countertransport (3) due to an increase in the concentration gradient for Na^+ across the basolateral membrane.

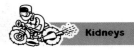

Potassium-sparing diuretics

Potassium-sparing diuretics produce mild diuresis and cause the excretion of 2–3% of filtered sodium.

Site of action: Potassium-sparing diuretics work at the late distal tubule and collecting duct.

Mechanism of action: There are two classes of potassium-sparing diuretics (Fig. 6.4), (a) sodium-channel blockers, e.g. amiloride and triamterene—these drugs block sodium reabsorption by the principal cells, thus reducing the potential difference across the cell and reducing K^+ secretion. H^+ secretion from the intercalated cells is also decreased by the reduction in potential difference across the cell, and (b) aldosterone antagonists, e.g. spironolactone. Spironolactone is a competitive antagonist at aldosterone receptors, and thus reduces Na^+ reabsorption and K^+ and H^+ secretion. The degree of diuresis depends on aldosterone levels.

Route of administration: Potassium-sparing diuretics are administered orally as tablets, capsules, or solutions.

Indications: Potassium-sparing diuretics are used in conjunction with potassium-losing diuretics (thiazides, loop diuretics) to maintain normal potassium levels. They are used for hypertension.

Aldosterone antagonists are used in the treatment of hyperaldosteronism, which can be primary (Conn's syndrome) or secondary (as a result of CHF, liver disease, or nephrotic syndrome). Aldosterone antagonists potentiate the effects of thiazides and loop diuretics, since these cause activation of the RAS which increases aldosterone secretion, thus opposing the diuretic action of these drugs.

Contraindications: Potassium-sparing diuretics interact with angiotensin-converting enzyme inhibitors, increasing the risk of hyperkalaemia. They should not be given to people with renal failure.

Adverse effects: Side effects of potassium-sparing diuretics include hyperkalaemia and metabolic acidosis. Aldosterone antagonists have a wide range of adverse effects, e.g. gynaecomastia, menstrual disorders, and male sexual dysfunction.

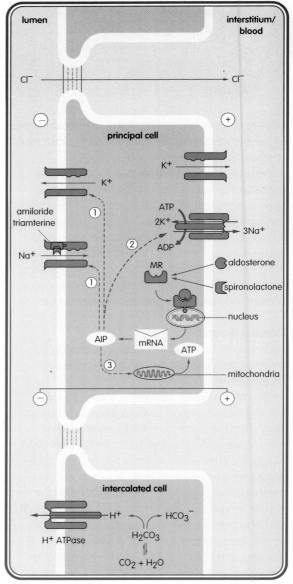

Fig. 6.4 Transport mechanisms in the late distal tubule and collecting duct. Amiloride and triamterene block the luminal Na+ channels, which reduces the lumen-negative potential difference across the principal cell and decreases the driving force for K^+ secretion from the principal cell and H^+ secretion from the intercalated cell. The net effect is increased Na^+ excretion and decreased K^+ and H^+ excretion. Aldosterone binds to a cytoplasmic mineralocorticosteroid receptor (MR) stimulating the production of aldosterone-induced proteins (AIP), which (1) activate and increase the synthesis of Na^+ and K^+ channels; (2) increase the synthesis of Na^+/K^+ ATPase, and (3) increase mitochondrial production of adenosine triphosphate (ATP). The effect of aldosterone is to decrease Na^+ excretion and increase K^+ and H^+ excretion in urine, whereas spironolactone, an aldosterone antagonist, has the opposite effects.

Carbonic anhydrase inhibitors

Amiloride and methazolamide are examples of carbonic anhydrase inhibitors. These drugs are no longer used as diuretics.

Site of action: Carbonic anhydrase inhibitors work at the proximal tubule.

Mechanism of action: Carbonic anhydrase inhibitors work by inhibiting the enzyme carbonic anhydrase, thus preventing the formation of carbonic acid from carbon dioxide and water (Fig. 6.5). This increases bicarbonate excretion and consequently reduces sodium reabsorption. The increase in sodium reaching the distal tubule and collecting duct results in increased potassium secretion, potentiated by the lack of competition from H+ ion secretion.

Route of administration: Carbonic anhydrase inhibitors are administered orally or intravenously.

Indications: Carbonic anhydrase inhibitors are used for reduction of intraocular pressure in the treatment of glaucoma, certain forms of epilepsy, and acute mountain sickness (>3000 m).

Contraindications: Carbonic anhydrase inhibitors should not be given to people taking cardiac glycosides (p. 118), or to those with severe renal impairment.

Adverse effects: Side effects of carbonic anhydrase inhibitors include metabolic acidosis and hypokalaemia.

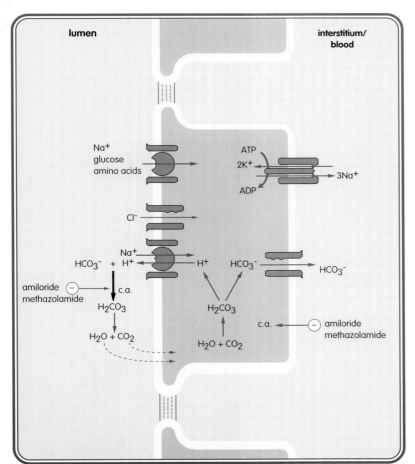

Fig. 6.5 The proximal tubule is one of the sites of bicarbonate (HCO_3^-) reabsorption. Carbonic acid (H_2CO_3) is formed from the action of carbonic anhydrase (c.a.) on carbon dioxide (CO_2) and water. H_2CO_3 immediately dissociates into HCO_3^-, which moves down its concentration gradient across the basolateral membrane, and H+ which is secreted into the lumen in exchange for Na+. In the lumen, H+ combines with filtered HCO_3^- to form H_2CO_3 and subsequently CO_2 and water which are able to diffuse back into the cell. Amiloride and methazolamide inhibit carbonic anhydrase and thus reduce sodium reabsorption by inhibiting H+ production.

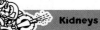

- Summarize glomerular filtration, tubular secretion, and tubular reabsorption in relation to the different sections of the kidney.
- List the main causes of oedema.
- What are the different classes of diuretics? For each of these list examples, their site of action, mechanism of action, route of administration, indications, contraindications, and major adverse effects.
- Distinguish between the potency of the various diuretics.

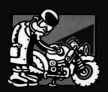

THE STOMACH

Peptic ulceration

The gastric epithelium secretes several substances—hydrochloric acid (HCl) from the parietal cells, digestive enzymes from the peptic cells, and mucus from the mucus-secreting cells. The acid and enzymes convert food into a thick semi-liquid paste called chyme, while mucus protects the stomach from its own corrosive secretions.

Peptic ulceration results from a breach in the mucosa lining the alimentary tract caused by acid and enzyme attack (Fig. 7.1). Unprotected mucosa rapidly undergoes autodigestion leading to a range of damage—inflammation or gastritis, necrosis, haemorrhage, and even perforation as the erosion deepens.

Gastric and duodenal ulcers differ in their location, epidemiology, incidence, and aetiology but are treated on similar principles. Peptic ulcer disease is chronic, recurrent, and common, affecting at least 10% of the population in developed countries. *Helicobacter pylori* plays a role in the pathogenesis of a significant proportion of peptic ulcer disease.

Protective factors

The mucosal defences against acid/enzyme attack consist of:
- The mucus barrier (approximately 500 μm thick), a mucus matrix into which bicarbonate ions are secreted, producing a buffering gradient.
- The surface epithelium, which constitutes a second line of defence; its proper functioning (mucus/bicarbonate production etc.) requires prostaglandins E_2 and I_2, synthesized by the gastric mucosa. These are thought to exert a cytoprotective action by increasing mucosal blood flow.

Weakened mucosal defence	Normal	Increased attack
weakened defences vulnerable to being breached by normal acid/enzyme levels	acid/enzyme attack is adequately balanced by mucosal and other defences	increased attack breaks down the defences that would normally be adequate
e.g. • *Helicobacter pylori* infection. • loss of normal mucosal defences, e.g. NSAIDs. (see chapter 10)	e.g. • healthy state	e.g. • hyperacidity (Zollinger-Ellison syndrome)

Fig. 7.1 Peptic ulceration. (Adapted from Underwood, J, *General and Systematic Pathology*, 2nd edition, Churchill Livingstone, Edinburgh, 1996.)

Sir Francis Avery–Jones said: 'An ulcer represents the adverse outcome of a conflict between the aggressive forces in the stomach or duodenum (acid/enzymes) and the defence mechanisms (mucus–bicarbonate barrier/surface epithelium)'. This concept can be used as a way to rationalize your thinking of the causes and thus appropriate treatment of peptic ulcers.

Acid secretion

The regulation of acid secretion by parietal cells is especially important in peptic ulceration and constitutes a major target for drug action (Fig. 7.2). Acid is secreted from gastric parietal cells by a unique proton pump that catalyses the exchange of intracellular H^+ for extracellular K^+. The secretion of HCl is controlled by the activation of three main receptors on the basolateral membrane of the parietal cell. These are:

- Gastrin receptors, which respond to gastrin secreted by the G cells of the stomach antrum.
- Histamine (H_2) receptors, which respond to histamine secreted from the enterochromaffin-like paracrine cells that are adjacent to the parietal cell.
- Muscarinic (M_1, M_3) receptors on the parietal cell, which respond to acetylcholine (ACh) released from neurons innervating the parietal cell.

Although the parietal cells possess muscarinic and gastrin receptors, both ACh and gastrin mainly exert their acid secretory effect indirectly, by stimulating nearby enterochromaffin-like cells to release histamine. Histamine then acts locally on the parietal cells where activation of the H_2 receptor results in the stimulation of adenylyl cyclase and the secretion of acid.

Prevention and treatment of peptic ulceration

Drugs that are effective in the treatment of peptic ulcers either reduce/neutralize gastric acid secretion or increase mucosal resistance to acid–pepsin attack (Fig. 7.3). Peptic ulcers thus treated will heal rapidly, but recurrence is common unless *H. pylori* is eliminated.

Reduction of acid secretion
Proton pump inhibitors
Omeprazole and lansoprazole are examples of proton pump inhibitors.
Mechanism of action: Proton pump inhibitors cause irreversible inhibition of H^+/K^+ ATPase that is responsible for H^+ secretion from parietal cells (Fig. 7.2). They are inactive prodrugs and are converted at acid pH to sulphonamide, which combines covalently and thus irreversibly with -SH groups on H^+/K^+ ATPase. This inhibition is highly specific and localized.
Route of administration: Proton pump inhibitors are administered orally.
Indications: Proton pump inhibitors are particularly useful for people with severe gastric hyperacidity—Zollinger–Ellison syndrome—and patients with stricturing or ulcerating reflux oesophagitis.
Contraindications: No important contraindications are reported with proton pump inhibitors.
Adverse effects: Side effects of proton pump inhibitors include gastrointestinal upset, nausea, and headaches. There might be a risk of gastric atrophy with long-term treatment.

Omeprazole inhibits the P_{450} enzyme system, reducing the metabolism of drugs such as warfarin, phenytoin, theophylline, and MDMA ('ecstasy').
Therapeutic notes: Acid production is drastically reduced by >90% with proton pump inhibitors. They have a long duration of action (cf. H_2 antagonists, antacids) and are given once daily.

Histamine H_2 receptor antagonists
Examples of H_2 receptor antagonists include cimetidine and ranitidine
Mechanism of action: H_2 receptor antagonists competitively block the action of histamine on the parietal cell by their antagonism of H_2 receptors (Fig. 7.2).
Route of administration: H_2 receptor antagonists are administered orally.
Indications: H_2 receptor antagonists are the first-line treatment of peptic ulcer disease.
Contraindications: Cimetidine should be avoided by patients stabilized on warfarin, phenytoin, and theophylline.

Adverse effects: H_2 receptor antagonists are generally well tolerated and side effects are uncommon. Dizziness, fatigue, gynaecomastia, and rash have occasionally been reported with all of them.

Cimetidine inhibits the P_{450} enzyme system, reducing the metabolism of drugs such as warfarin, phenytoin, theophylline and MDMA ('ecstasy').

Therapeutic notes: H_2 receptor antagonists do not reduce acid production to the same extent as proton pump inhibitors, but do relieve the pain of ulcer and promote healing. The drugs are administered at night-time when acid buffering by food is at its lowest. The usual regime is twice daily for 4–8 weeks.

Muscarinic antagonists

Pirenzepine is an example of a muscarinic antagonist.

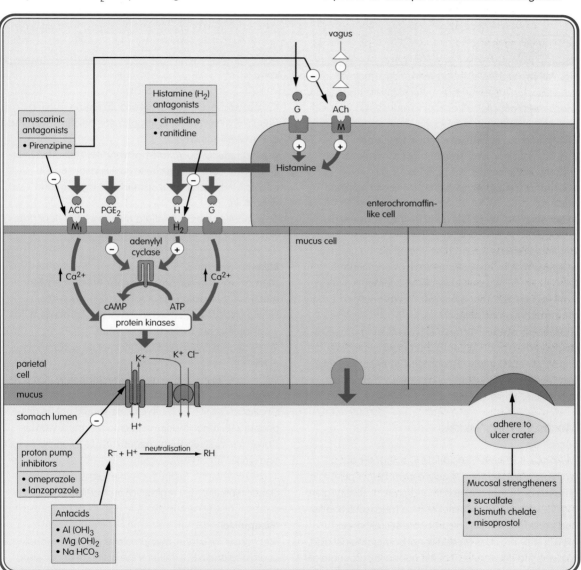

Fig. 7.2 Acid secretion from parietal cells is reduced by muscarinic antagonists, histamine (H_2) antagonists and the proton pump inhibitors. Gastrin (G) and acetylcholine (Ach) stimulate the parietal cell directly to increase acid secretion and also stimulate enterochromaffin-like cells to secrete histamine, which then acts upon the H_2 receptors of the parietal cell. Antacids raise the luminal pH by neutralising hydrogen ions. Mucosal strengthners adhere to and protect ulcer craters and may kill *H. pylori*.

Drugs used in the prevention and treatment of peptic ulceration			
Reduction of acid secretion	**Mucosal strengtheners**	**Antacids**	***Helicobacter pylori* eradication regimens**
proton pump inhibitors *omeprazole, lanzoprazole* histamine H_2 receptor antagonists *cimetidine, ranitidine* muscarinic antagonists *pirenzipine*	*sucralfate* *bismuth chelate* *misoprostol*	*aluminium hydroxide, magnesium hydroxide, sodium bicarbonate*	'classic' triple therapy *bismuth, metronidazole and tetracycline or metronidazole* dual therapy *omeprazole and amoxicillin or clarithromycin*

Fig. 7.3 Drugs used in the prevention and treatment of peptic ulceration.

Mechanism of action: Pirenzepine reduces gastric acid and pepsin secretion by blocking M_1 receptors in the enteric nervous system, and those on the parietal cell (Fig. 7.2). It is not clear what type of muscarinic receptor is present on the enterochromaffin-like cell.
Route of administration: Pirenzepine is administered orally.
Indications: Pirenzepine is used for the treatment of peptic ulcer disease.
Contraindications: Pirenzepine should not be given to people with prostatic enlargement, pyloric stenosis, paralytic ileus, and closed-angle glaucoma.
Adverse effects: Pirenzepine may occasionally cause dry mouth and blurring of vision.
Therapeutic notes: Pirenzepine is as effective as the H_2 antagonists in treating peptic ulcers, but is relatively unpopular and largely discontinued as it must be taken four times a day and there is a relatively high incidence of anticholinergic side effects.

Mucosal strengtheners
Sucralfate
Mechanism of action: Sucralfate is a polymer of aluminium and sucrose. It polymerizes below pH 4 to a gel substance that adheres to and protects ulcer craters (Fig. 7.2). It has favourable effects on mucosal blood flow, and prostaglandin and bicarbonate secretion, and presumably provides an additional barrier against acid, allowing the development of the normal bicarbonate pH gradient. Sucralfate also reduces the number of *H. pylori* and the adherence of *H. pylori* to the gastric mucosa, possibly explaining the lower recurrance rate with its use.
Route of administration: Sucralfate is administered orally.
Indications: Sucralfate is used for peptic ulcer disease.

Contraindications: Sucralfate should not be given to people with severe renal impairment, as aluminium may accumulate in the body.
Adverse effects: Sucralfate has very few side effects. Its aluminium content can cause constipation, and it interacts with tetracycline, cimetidine, digoxin, and phenytoin.
Therapeutic notes: Sucralfate must be taken four times a day.

Bismuth chelate
Mechanism of action: Bismuth chelate has a similar mechanism of action to sucralfate (Fig. 7.2). It has a strong affinity for exposed mucosal glycoproteins; it has weak antibacterial effects on *H. pylori*.
Route of administration: Bismuth chelate is administered orally.
Indications: Bismuth chelate is given for peptic ulcers with co-infection by *H.pylori*.
Contraindications: Bismuth chelate should not be given to people with renal impairment, or to pregnant women.
Adverse effects: Bismuth chelate may blacken the mouth and stools.
Therapeutic notes: Bismuth chelate forms part of the classic triple-therapy regime for eradication of *H. pylori.*.

Misoprostol
Mechanism of action: Misoprostol is a synthetic analogue of prostaglandin E. It imitates the action of endogenous prostaglandins (PGE_2 and PGI_2) in maintaining the integrity of the gastroduodenal mucosal barrier, and promotes healing (Fig. 7.2).
Route of administration: Misoprostol is administered orally.

Indications: Misoprostol is used for the prevention and cure of non-steroidal anti-inflammatory drug (NSAID)-associated ulcers.

Contraindications: Misoprostol should not be given to people with hypotension, or to women who are pregnant or breast-feeding.

Adverse effects: Misoprostol may cause diarrhoea, which can be severe.

Therapeutic notes: Misoprostol is most effective at correcting the deficit caused by NSAIDs that inhibit cyclooxygenase-1 and reduce prostaglandin synthesis. Misoprostol can prevent NSAID-associated ulcers, and therefore is particularly useful in the elderly from whom NSAIDs cannot be withdrawn.

Antacids

Examples of antacids include aluminium hydroxide, magnesium hydroxide, and sodium bicarbonate.

Mechanism of action: Antacids consist of alkaline Al^{3+}, Mg^{2+}, and Na^+ salts that are used to raise the luminal pH of the stomach. They neutralize acid and, as a result, may reduce the damaging effects of pepsin, which is pH dependent (Fig. 7.2). Additionally, Al^{3+} and Mg^{2+} salts bind and inactivate pepsin.

Route of administration: Antacids are administered orally as tablets, powders, or liquids.

Indications: Antacids are used for symptomatic relief of ulcers, non-ulcer dyspepsia, and gastro-oesophageal reflux.

Contraindications: Aluminium hydroxide and magnesium hydroxide should not be given to people with hypophosphataemia. Sodium bicarbonate should be avoided in patients on a salt-restricted diet (in heart failure and in hepatic and renal impairment).

Adverse effects: Aluminium salts can cause constipation, while magnesium salts can cause diarrhoea.

Both can bind drugs, including a variety of antibiotics and phenytoin.

Therapeutic notes: Antacids are still useful for the relief of symptoms of ulceration; frequent high dosing can promote ulcer healing but this is rarely practical.

Helicobacter pylori eradication regimes

H. pylori plays a significant role in the pathogenesis of peptic ulcer disease. It does not cause ulcers in everyone it infects (50–80% of the population) but, of those who develop ulcers, 90% can be found to have an *H. pylori* infection in their antrum.

Treatment of peptic ulcer disease should include eradication of *H. pylori*. The rate of recurrence of duodenal ulcer after healing can be as high as 80% within 1 year when *H. pylori* eradication is not part of the treatment, but less than 5% when *H. pylori* is eradicated.

The ideal treatment for *H. pylori* eradication is not yet clear. Current regimes under evaluation include:

- The 'classic' triple therapy: 1 or 2 weeks' treatment with omeprazole, metronidazole and amoxicillin or clarithromycin. This eliminates *H. pylori* in 90% of patients but adverse effects, compliance, and resistance can be problematic.
- Dual therapy. Omeprazole is given in combination with a single antibiotic, usually either amoxicillin or clarithromycin.

- Describe how the pathophysiology of peptic ulceration involves disturbance of the balance between the aggressive forces (acid/enzymes) and the defence mechanisms (mucus–bicarbonate barrier/surface epithelium) of the stomach or duodenum.
- Describe the factors that control acid production and maintain mucosal defences.
- Relate these first two points to the principles by which the pharmacological treatments work.
- Name examples of each of the different classes of drug.
- Discuss the significant role *H. pylori* plays in the pathogenesis of peptic ulcer disease, and the approaches used to eradicate it.

INTESTINES, MOTILITY, AND SECRETIONS

Intestinal motility, constipation, and diarrhoea

Normal motility, or peristalsis, of the intestinal tract acts to mix bowel contents thoroughly and to propel them in a caudal direction. Regulation of normal intestinal motility is under neuronal and hormonal control.

Neuronal control

Two principal intramural plexi form the enteric nervous system. These are:

- The myenteric plexus (Auerbach's plexus), located between the outer longitudinal and middle circular muscle layers.
- The submucous (Meissner's) plexus, on the luminal side of the circular muscle layer.

Together, these autonomic ganglionated plexi control the functioning of the gastrointestinal tract through complex local reflex connections between sensory neurons, smooth muscle, mucosa, and blood vessels.

Extrinsic parasympathetic fibres from the vagus are excitatory while extrinsic sympathetic fibres are inhibitory.

The enteric autonomic nervous system is a major target in the pharmacological therapy of gastro-intestinal disorders.

Hormonal control

The activity of the gastrointestinal tract is influenced both by endocrine (e.g. gastrin) and paracrine (e.g. histamine, secretin, cholecystokinin, vasoactive intestinal peptide) secretions. Other than in the context of local control of acid secretion in the stomach (pp. 123–127), an understanding of these other hormones is not of immediate relevance to an understanding of the pharmacological therapy of gastrointestinal disorders.

Drugs that affect intestinal motility

Four classes of drug are used clinically for their effects on gastrointestinal motility (Fig. 7.4). These are:

- Motility stimulants.
- Antispasmodics.
- Laxatives.
- Antidiarrhoeals.

Motility stimulants

Agents that increase the motility of the gastro-intestinal tract without a laxative effect are used for motility disorders such as gastro-oesophageal reflux disease (GORD) and gastric stasis (slow stomach emptying), or for diagnostic techniques such as duodenal intubation.

The main drugs used are:

- Cisapride.
- Domperidone.
- Metoclopramide.

Cisapride

Mechanism of action: Cisapride facilitates the release of ACh in the gut wall enteric plexi. It might also stimulate 5-hydroxytryptamine (5-HT$_3$; serotonin) receptors.
Route of administration: Cisapride is administered orally.
Indications: Cisapride is used for the treatment of GORD and gastric stasis.
Contraindications: Cisapride should not be given when gastrointestinal stimulation could be dangerous, e.g. blockage.
Adverse effects: Side effects of cisapride include abdominal cramps and diarrhoea.
Therapeutic notes: Cisapride should be taken before meals and before bedtime for maximum benefit.

Dopamine antagonists

Domperidone and metoclopramide are examples of dopamine antagonists.
Mechanism of action: The prokinetic actions of the dopamine agonists are blocked by atropine, suggesting that they result from the facilitation of ACh release in the enteric plexi rather than from antagonism of dopamine receptors. An agonist action on 5-HT interneurons in the enteric plexi appears to be the mechanism by which ACh release is facilitated.

Domperidone may also enhance motility by blocking α_1-adrenoceptors.

The antinausea/antiemetic effect of dopamine antagonists is caused by blockade of central dopamine (D$_2$) receptors in the chemoreceptor trigger zone.
Route of administration: Domperidone and metoclopramide can be administered orally, intravenously, or intramuscularly.
Indications: Both domperidone and metoclopramide are used for antinausea/antiemesis. Metoclopramide is used for diagnostic techniques such as duodenal intubation, or for speeding the transit of barium during intestinal

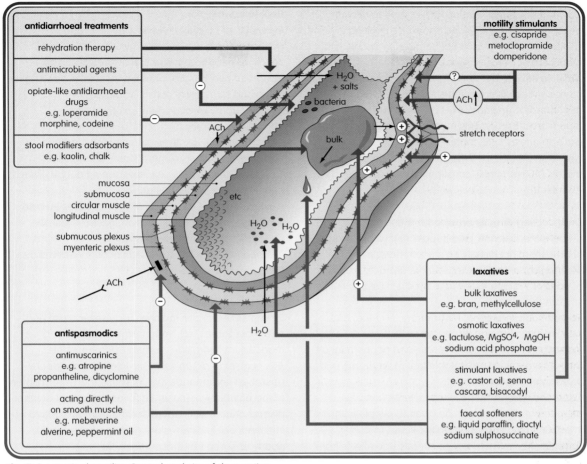

Fig. 7.4 Intestinal motility: Control and site of drug action.

investigation, and as an accessory treatment for GORD, while domperidone is used for disorders of gastric emptying and GORD.

Adverse effects: Domperidone and metoclopramide may induce an acute dystonic reaction, particularly in young women and children (see Chapter 3, Parkinsonism).

Therapeutic notes: Domperidone and metoclopramide stimulate gastric emptying and small intestinal transit, and enhance the strength of oesophageal sphincter contraction; these effects are reflected in their clinical use.

Antispasmodics

The smooth muscle relaxant properties of antispasmodic drugs may be useful as adjunctive treatment in non-ulcer dyspepsia, irritable bowel syndrome, and diverticular disease.

There are two classes of antispasmodic drug. These are:
- Antimuscarinics.
- Drugs acting directly on smooth muscle.

Antimuscarinics

Examples of antimuscarinics include atropine, propantheline, and dicyclomine.

Mechanism of action: Antimuscarinics act by antagonism at muscarinic ACh receptors in the enteric plexi causing relaxation of gastrointestinal smooth muscle.

Route of administration: Antimuscarinics are administered orally.

Indications: Antimuscarinics are used for non-ulcer dyspepsia, irritable bowel syndrome, and diverticular disease.

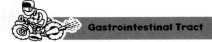

Contraindications: Antimuscarinics tend to relax the oesophageal sphincter and should be avoided in GORD. Also, they should not be given to people with glaucoma or paralytic ileus.

Adverse effects: The quaternary ammonium compounds (e.g. propantheline) are less lipid soluble than atropine and so are less likely to cross the blood–brain barrier. This means that central atropine-like side effects (e.g. confusion, amnesia) are reduced. However, peripheral atropine-like side effects (e.g. dry mouth, blurred vision, constipation) remain (see Chapter 2).

Drugs acting directly on smooth muscle

Mebeverine, alverine, and peppermint oil are examples of drugs that act directly on smooth muscle.

Mechanism of action: Mebeverine, alverine, and peppermint oil are believed to be direct relaxants of smooth muscle.

Route of administration: Mebeverine, alverine, and peppermint oil are administered orally.

Indications: Mebeverine, alverine, and peppermint oil may relieve pain in the irritable bowel syndrome and diverticular disease

Contraindications: Mebeverine, alverine, and peppermint oil should not be given to people with intestinal obstruction, or paralytic ileus.

Adverse effects: There are no serious side effects from mebeverine, alverine, and peppermint oil. Nausea, headache, and heartburn are occasional problems.

Laxatives

Laxatives are drugs used to increase the motility of the gut and encourage defecation. Laxatives are used to relieve constipation (an infrequent or difficult passage of stool) and to clear the bowel prior to medical and surgical procedures.

It should be remembered that individual bowel habit can vary considerably—the passage of stools twice a day to once every 3 days is normal. Laxatives are commonly overused by the public, owing to health misconceptions.

The frequency and volume of stool are best regulated by diet, but drugs may be necessary. The passage of food through the intestine can be hastened by:

- Bulk laxatives.
- Osmotic laxatives.
- Stimulant laxatives.
- Faecal softeners.

Bulk laxatives

Examples of bulk laxatives include bran and methylcellulose.

Mechanism of action: Bulk laxatives increase the volume of non-absorbable solid residue, distending the colon and stimulating peristaltic activity.

Route of administration: Bulk laxatives are administered orally.

Indications: Bulk laxatives are used for constipation, particularly when small hard stools are present.

Contraindications: Bulk laxatives should not be given to people with intestinal obstruction.

Adverse effects: Side effects of bulk laxatives include flatulence, abdominal distension, gastro-intestinal obstruction, and hypersensitivity.

Therapeutic notes: The full effects of bulk laxatives may take a few days to develop.

Osmotic laxatives

Examples of osmotic laxatives include lactulose and saline purgatives, e.g. magnesium sulphate, magnesium hydroxide, sodium acid phosphate.

Mechanism of action: Osmotic laxatives are poorly absorbed compounds that increase the water content of the bowel by osmosis. Lactulose is a semi-synthetic disaccharide that is not absorbed from the gastro-intestinal tract. Magnesium and sodium salts are poorly absorbed and osmotically active.

Route of administration: Osmotic laxatives are administered orally.

Indications: Osmotic laxatives are used for constipation.

Contraindications: Osmotic laxatives should not be given to people with intestinal obstruction, or acute gastrointestinal conditions.

Adverse effects: Side effects of osmotic laxatives include flatulence, cramps, and abdominal discomfort.

Therapeutic notes: Magnesium salts are useful for rapid bowel evacuation. Sodium salts should be avoided if possible as they can lead to sodium and water retention in susceptible individuals.

Stimulant laxatives

Castor oil, senna, cascara, bisacodyl, and sodium picosulphate are examples of stimulant laxatives.

Mechanism of action: Stimulant laxatives increase gastrointestinal peristalsis by stimulating the mucosa of the gut (probably by irritating local reflexes), the signal arising in the mucosa and being transmitted through the intramural plexi to the smooth muscle of the intestine.

Anthraquinones are compounds released from senna and cascara that stimulate the myenteric plexus.
Route of administration: Stimulant laxatives are administered orally.
Indications: Stimulant laxatives are used for constipation.
Contraindications: Stimulant laxatives should not be given to children, or people with intestinal obstruction.
Adverse effects: In the short term, side effects of stimulant laxatives include intestinal cramp. Prolonged use can lead to damage to the nerve plexi resulting in the deterioration of intestinal function and atonic colon.
Therapeutic notes: Stimulant laxatives should be given for short periods only.

Faecal softeners

Liquid paraffin and dioctyl sodium sulphosuccinate are examples of faecal softeners.
Mechanism of action: Faecal softeners promote defaecation by softening (e.g. dioctyl sodium sulphosuccinate) and/or lubricating (e.g. liquid paraffin) faeces to aid their passage through the gastrointestinal tract.
Route of administration: Faecal softeners are administered orally. Dioctyl sodium sulphosuccinate can also be admininstered rectally as suppositories or enemas.
Indications: Faecal softeners are used for constipation, faecal impaction, and haemorrhoids.
Contraindications: Faecal softeners should not be given to children less than 3 years old.
Adverse effects: The prolonged use of liquid paraffin may impair the absorption of fat-soluble vitamins A and D and cause 'paraffinomas'.
Therapeutic notes: The prolonged use of faecal softeners is not recommended.

Antidiarrhoeal drugs

Diarrhoea is the too-frequent passage of stools that are liquid. Causes of diarrhoea include infectious agents, toxins, drugs, chronic disease, and anxiety.

Acute secretory diarrhoea usually results from an infection, is extremely common, and causes much preventable mortality, especially in children under 2 years of age in developing countries. The vigour with which diarrhoea should be treated depends very much on the cause and the clinical evaluation of patient risk.

There are four approaches to the treatment of severe acute diarrhoea. These are:

- Maintenance of fluid and electrolyte balance through oral rehydration therapy (ORT).
- Use of antimicrobial drugs.
- Use of opiate-like antimotility drugs.
- Use of stool modifiers/adsorbents.

Maintenance of fluid and electrolyte balance through ORT

ORT should be the first priority in the treatment of acute diarrhoea of all causes, and can be lifesaving.

ORT solutions are isotonic or slightly hypotonic; they vary in their composition but a standard formula would contain NaCl, KCl, sodium citrate, and glucose in appropriate concentrations.

Intravenous rehydration therapy is needed if there are severe electrolyte imbalances.

Use of antimicrobial drugs

Antibiotic treatment of diarrhoea is useful only in certain infections and should be undertaken sparingly.

Acute infectious diarrhoea is usually self-limiting and antibiotic therapy has the risks of :

- Spreading antibiotic resistance among enteropathogenic bacteria.
- Destroying normal commensal gut flora, allowing overgrowth of the bacterium *Clostridium difficile*, a serious condition called pseudomembranous colitis.

Antibiotic treatment is indicated in:

- Severe cholera or *Salmonella typhimurium* infection—tetracycline.
- *Shigella* species infections—ampicillin.
- *Campylobacter jejuni*—erythromycin or ciprofloxacin.

Antibiotics are discussed in detail in Chapter 12.

Use of opiate-like antimotility drugs

Examples of opiate-like antimotility drugs include loperamide, morphine, and codeine.
Mechanism of action: Opiate-like antimotility drugs act on μ-opiate receptors in the myenteric plexus, and possibly on 5-HT receptors, to cause hyperpolarization of the neurons, thus inhibiting ACh release. The overall effect is a reduction in peristaltic activity, while enhancing gut segmental activity and tone.
Route of administration: Opiate-like antimotility drugs are administered orally.

Indications: Opiate-like antimotility drugs have a limited role as an adjunct to fluid and electrolyte replacement in acute diarrhoea. They are also used as adjunctive therapy in some chronic diarrhoeal conditions.

Contraindications: Opiate-like antimotility drugs should not be given to people with diarrhoeal conditions such as acute ulcerative colitis or antibiotic-associated colitis. They are not recommended for children.

Adverse effects: Side effects of opiate-like antimotility drugs may include nausea, vomiting, abdominal cramps, and drowsiness. Loperamide does not easily penetrate the blood–brain barrier and hence has much fewer central actions.

Therapeutic notes: Loperamide is the most appropriate opioid for local effects on the gut.

Use of stool modifiers/adsorbents

Examples of stool modifiers/adsorbents include kaolin, chalk, charcoal, and methylcellulose.

Mechanism of action: It has been suggested that stool modifiers/adsorbents act by absorbing toxins or by coating and protecting the intestinal mucosa, although the evidence for this is largely anecdotal.

Route of administration: Stool modifier/adsorbents are administered orally.

Indications: There is little evidence to recommend adsorbents at all.

Adverse effects: Stool modifiers/adsorbents may reduce the absorbtion of other drugs.

Therapeutic notes: Adsorbents are popular remedies for the treatment of diarrhoea, although there is little evidence of their benefits.

Inflammatory bowel disease

Crohn's disease and ulcerative colitis are both chronic inflammatory conditions of unknown aetiology. They are characterized by episodes of remission and relapse. The inflammatory bowel diseases fall into two categories that share a number of features in their pathology. These are:
- Crohn's disease, which can affect the entire gut.
- Ulcerative colitis, which affects only the large bowel.

Treatment of these conditions is not only pharmacological but also depends on psychological support, correction of nutritional deficiencies, and possibly surgery.

Drug treatment is aimed at controlling inflammation and bringing about remission. Two classes of drugs are used:
- Glucocorticoids.
- Aminosalicylates.

Glucocorticoids

Examples of glucocorticoids include prednisolone, budesonide, and hydrocortisone (Fig. 7.5)

Mechanism of action: Glucocorticoids have an anti-inflammatory effect (see Chapter 8).

Route of administration: In localized disease, glucocorticoids may be administered rectally as enemas, suppositories, or foams. In extensive disease, oral or intravenous therapy is required.

Indications: Glucocorticoids are given for inflammatory bowel conditions.

Contraindications: Glucocorticoids should not be given to people with obstruction or perforation of the bowel.

Adverse effects: Cushingoid side effects may occur with glucocorticoids (iatrogenic Cushing's syndrome) (see Chapter 8).

Therapeutic notes: Glucocorticoids are the first-line drugs used for acute attacks, but their serious side effects make them unsuitable for long-term maintenance treatment.

Drugs used in the treatment of gastrointestinal disorders		
Inflammortory bowel disease	**Pancreatic insufficiency**	**Gallstones**
glucocorticorteroids *prednisolone,* *budesonide,* *hydrocortisone* aminosalicylates *sulfasalazine,* *mesalazine,* *olsalazine*	pancreatin	bile salts *chenodeoxycholic acid* *(chenodiol)* *ursodeoxycholic acid* *(ursodiol)*

Fig. 7.5 Drugs used in the treatment of gastro-intestinal disorders.

Budesonide is a newly-developed corticosteroid that is locally acting and poorly absorbed.

Aminosalicylates

Sulphasalazine, mesalazine, and olsalazine are examples of aminosalicylates (see Fig. 7.5).
Mechanism of action: Sulphasalazine is broken down in the gut to the active component 5-aminosalicylate (5-ASA) and sulphapyridine.

Mesalazine is 5-ASA and olsalazine is two molecules of 5-ASA linked by a diazo bond. The mechanism of action of the active molecule 5-ASA is unknown.
Route of administration: Aminosalicylates are administered orally or rectally.
Indications: Aminosalicylates are used for inflammatory bowel conditions.
Contraindications: Aminosaclicylates should not be given to people with salicylate hypersensitivity and renal impairment.
Adverse effects: Side effects of aminosalicylates are mainly due to sulphapyridine; nausea, vomiting, headache, and rashes are common. Rarely, blood disorders and oligospermia are reported.
Therapeutic notes: Aminosalicylates are used in the treatment of inflammatory bowel disease to maintain remission; they are of limited value in acute relapses.

Pancreatic supplements

Pancreatic exocrine secretions contain important enzymes that break down proteins (trypsin, chymotrypsin), starch (amylase), and fats (lipase), and are essential for efficient digestion.

Pancreatin is an extract of pancreas containing protease, lipase, and amylase, that is given by mouth to compensate for reduced or absent exocrine secretions in cystic fibrosis, and following pancreatectomy, total gastrectomy, or chronic pancreatitis. Pancreatin is inactivated by gastric acid and so precautions must be taken to optimize delivery of the pancreatin to the duodenum (see Fig. 7.5).

Pancreatin preparations are best taken with food; histamine H_2 antagonists (e.g. cimetidine) may be taken an hour before to ingestion of the pancreatin in order to reduce gastric acid secretion.

Acid-resistant formulations that deliver the pancreatin to the duodenum prior to release are available.

Gall stones

Bile is secreted by the liver and is stored in the gall bladder. Bile contains cholesterol, phospholipids, and bile salts. Bile salts are important for keeping cholesterol in solution. The formation of 'stones' in the bile is relatively common (cholelithiasis), and this is frequently accompanied by inflammation of the gall bladder (cholecystitis). Stones can be formed from a variety of chemical compositions; only small stones that are formed when cholesterol precipitates out of solution are amenable to being dissolved by drug therapy. Surgery is necessary for other symptomatic stones.

The dissolution of small cholesterol stones is carried out by prolonged oral administration of the bile acids, chenodeoxycholic acid and ursodeoxycholic acid (Fig. 7.5).

Chenodeoxycholic acid

The bile salt chenodexoycholic acid (or chenodiol) commonly causes diarrhoea, and liver abnormalities may occur.

Ursodeoxycholic acid

The bile salt ursodeoxycholic acid (or ursodiol) has largely superseded chenodiol as it has a lower incidence of side effects.

Both these bile acids work by :
- Decreasing secretion of cholesterol into the bile.
- Decreasing cholesterol absorption from the intestine.

The net effect is a reduced cholesterol concentration in the bile and a tendency for the dissolution of existing stones.

All the drugs listed in this chapter are taken by the oral (or occasionally rectal) route of administration. (Note that antiemetics and glucocorticoids may also be given by injection under certain limited circumstances.)

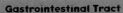

- Describe how the motility of the gastro-intestinal tract is controlled and co-ordinated in health, and the conditions that can result when this goes wrong.
- Name the four classes of drug that are used to affect the motility of the gastrointestinal tract and state why and when they are indicated for use.
- Describe the different mechanism of actions by which these drugs work and give examples from each class.
- Discuss the drugs used in the pharmacological treatment of the gastrointestinal conditions: Inflammatory bowel disease, pancreatic insufficiency, and gall stones. Describe their mechanism of action.

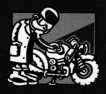

8. Endocrine and Reproductive Systems

THE THYROID GLAND

Principles of thyroid function
Production of thyroid hormones

The thyroid gland secretes two hormones: an active hormone, triiodothyronine (T_3), and its precursor, thyroxine (T_4).

The principal effects of the thyroid hormones are determination of basal metabolic rate, and influence of growth through stimulation of growth hormone synthesis and action. Other effects are summarized in Fig. 8.1.

The follicular cells of the thyroid gland synthesize and glycosylate thyroglobulin before secreting it into their lumen. Iodination of the tyrosine residues of this molecule (organification) is catalysed by thyroid peroxidase and results in the formation of monoiodotyrosine (MIT) or

diiodotyrosine (DIT), according to the position on the ring at which this occurs. The coupling of MIT with DIT

Physiological effects of thyroid hormone
• fetal development (physical and cognitive)
• metabolic rate
• body temperature
• cardiac rate and contractility
• peripheral vasodilatation
• red cell mass and circulatory volume
• respiratory drive
• peripheral nerves (reflexes)
• hepatic metabolic enzymes
• bone turnover
• skin and soft tissue effects

Fig. 8.1 Physiological effects of thyroid hormones.

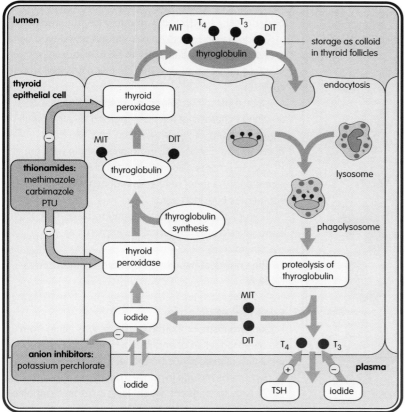

Fig. 8.2 Synthesis of thyroid hormones. (DIT, diiodotyrosine; MIT, monoiodotyrosine; PTU, propylthiouracil; T_3, triiodothyronine; T_4, thyroxine; TSH, thyroid-stimulating hormone.)

135

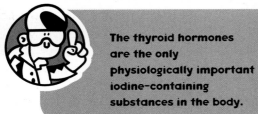

The thyroid hormones are the only physiologically important iodine-containing substances in the body.

produces T$_3$, and the coupling of two DIT molecules produces T$_4$. Coupling is also catalysed by thyroid peroxidase.

The thyroglobulin, now known as colloid, is endocytosed into the follicular cells, where it is broken down to release T$_3$, T$_4$, MIT and DIT. T$_3$ and T$_4$ are secreted into the plasma; MIT and DIT are metabolized within the cells and their iodide is re-used (Fig. 8.2).

The iodine required for the synthesis of T$_3$ and T$_4$ comes mainly from the diet in the form of iodide. Through the action of a thyrotrophin-dependent pump, iodide is concentrated in the follicular cells, where it is converted into iodine by thyroid peroxidase.

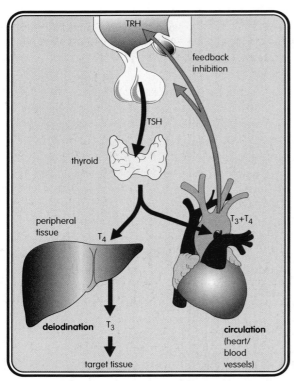

Fig. 8.3 Control of thyroid hormone synthesis. (T$_3$, triiodothyronine; T$_4$, thyroxine; TSH, thyroid-stimulating hormone; TRH, thyrotrophin-releasing hormone.)

Control of thyroid hormone secretion

The production of thyroid hormones is slow but constant, and control of their plasma levels is determined by influencing their secretion (Fig. 8.3).

The hypothalamus contains thyroid hormone receptors that are able to detect and respond to decreased levels of T$_3$ and T$_4$ by causing the release of thyrotrophin-releasing hormone (TRH) from the hypothalamus.

TRH reaches the anterior pituitary via the portal circulation and stimulates TRH receptors on the thyrotroph cells of the pituitary which in turn secrete thyroid-stimulating hormone (TSH).

TSH reaches the thyroid gland through the systemic circulation where it stimulates the secretion of T$_3$ and T$_4$. T$_3$ is the active form of the hormone that influences target tissues, and T$_4$ must be deiodinated to T$_3$ in the liver.

T$_3$ and T$_4$ are able to exert negative feedback on the hypothalamus and pituitary.

Thyroid dysfunction
Hypothyroidism

Hypothyroidism, a decrease in the activity of the thyroid gland, is relatively common in adults and associated with tiredness and lethargy, weight gain, intolerance to cold, dry skin, bradycardia, and mental impairment.

Children with hypothyroidism manifest delayed bone growth, whereas a deficiency *in utero* also results in mentally retarded infants; this condition is known as cretinism.

Hashimoto's thyroiditis is an autoimmune disease resulting in fibrosis of the thyroid gland. It is the most common cause of hypothyroidism and, like most autoimmune diseases, is more prevalent in women.

Myxoedema is also immunological in origin, and represents the most severe form of hypothyroidism—sometimes causing coma.

Thyroid hormone resistance and reduced TSH secretion will also produce the symptoms of hypothyroidism.

The causes of hypothyroidism are summarized in Fig. 8.4.

Hyperthyroidism

Hyperthyroidism, or thyrotoxicosis, results either from the overproduction of endogenous hormone or ingestion of exogenous hormone.

Symptoms include increased basal metabolic rate (BMR) with consequent weight loss, increased appetite, increased body temperature, and sweating, as well as nervousness, tremor, tachycardia, and retracted eyelids.

Graves' disease (diffuse toxic goitre) is the most common cause of hyperthyroidism. It is an autoimmune disease caused by the activation of TSH receptors by antibodies. This results in an enlargement of the gland and therefore excess hormone production. Because the extraocular muscles are attacked by the antibodies, protruding eyes are characteristic of the condition.

Toxic nodular goitre is the second most common cause of hyperthyroidism. It is due to either a single adenoma (hyperfunctioning adenoma) or multiple adenomas (multinodular goitre).

The causes of hyperthyroidism are summarized in Fig. 8.5.

Management of thyroid dysfunction
Hyperthyroidism and antithyroid drugs
Thionamides
Carbimazole, methimazole, and propylthiouracil (PTU) are examples of thionamides. The thionamides are the first-line drugs for treatment of hyperthyroidism.

Carbimazole is converted to methimazole in the body.
Mechanism of action: The thionamides cause inhibition of thyroid peroxidase with a consequent reduction in thyroid hormone production and storage (see Fig. 8.2). The effects of PTU may take weeks to show because of the stores of T_3 and T_4. PTU also inhibits the deiodination of T_4 to T_3.
Route of administration: The thionamides are administered orally as tablets.
Indications: The thionamides are used for hyperthyroidism. Patients sensitive to carbimazole are given PTU.
Contraindications: The thionamides should not be given to people with a large goitre. PTU should be given at a reduced dose in patients with renal impairment.
Adverse effects: Side effects of the thionamides include nausea and headache; allergic reactions, including rashes; hypothyroidism; and, rarely hepatotoxicosis, bone marrow suppression, and alopecia.
Therapeutic regime: Carbimazole is given at 20–60 mg daily until the patient is euthyroid (4–8 weeks later), then the dose is progressively reduced to a maintenance level of 5–15 mg daily. Treatment is usually given for 18 months. PTU is given at 300–600 mg daily until the patient is euthyroid, then the dose is progressively reduced to a maintenance level of 50–150 mg daily.

Anion inhibitors
Iodine, iodide, and potassium perchlorate are examples of anion inhibitors.

Potassium perchlorate inhibits the uptake of iodine by the thyroid (Fig. 8.2), but is no longer used, owing to the risk of aplastic anaemia.

Iodide is the most rapidly acting treatment against thyrotoxicosis and is given in thyrotoxic crisis ('thyroid storm').
Mechanism of action: Iodine and iodide cause inhibition of conversion of T_4 to T_3, of organification, and of hormone secretion. They also reduce the size and vascularity of the gland, which is evident after 10–14 days.
Route of administration: Iodine and iodide are administered orally as Lugol's solution.
Indications: Iodine and iodide are given for thyrotoxicosis, preoperatively.
Contraindications: Iodine and iodide should not be given to breast-feeding women as they cause goitre in infants.

Causes of hypothyroidism		
primary		chronic lymphocytic thyroiditis (Hashimoto's disease)
		subacute thyroiditis
		painless thyroiditis (postpartum thyroiditis)
		radioactive iodine ingestion
		iodine deficiency or excess
		inborn errors of thyroid hormone synthesis
secondary		pituitary disease
target tissues		thyroid hormone resistance

Fig. 8.4 Causes of hypothyroidism.

Causes of hyperthyroidism
• thyroid hormone ingestion
• diffuse toxic goitre (Graves' disease)
• hyperfunctioning adenoma (toxic nodule)
• toxic multinodular goitre
• painless thyroiditis
• subacute thyroiditis
• thyroid stimulating hormone (TSH)-secreting adenoma
• human chorionic gonadotrophin (hCG)-secreting tumours

Fig. 8.5 Causes of hyperthyroidism.

Adverse effects: Iodine and iodide can cause hypersensitivity reactions including rashes, headache, lacrimation, conjunctivitis, laryngitis, and bronchitis. With long-term treatment, depression, insomnia, and impotence can occur.

Therapeutic regime: Iodine and iodide are given 10–14 days before partial thyroidectomy, with either carbimazole or PTU. They should not be given long term as iodine becomes less effective.

β-Adrenoceptor antagonists

Propranolol and atenolol are examples of β-adrenoceptor antagonists. They are used to attenuate the symptoms of increased thyroid hormone levels, and the effect of increased numbers of adrenoceptors caused by thyroid hormone.

Mechanism of action: β-Adrenoceptor antagonists reduce tachycardia, the BMR, nervousness, and tremor.

Route of administration: β-Adrenoceptor antagonists are administered orally.

Indications: β-Adrenoceptor antagonists are used in thyrotoxic crisis.

Contraindications: β-Adrenoceptor antagonists should not be given to people with asthma.

Adverse effects: The side effects of β-adrenoceptor antagonists are given in Chapter 2.

Therapeutic regime: β-Adrenoceptor antagonists are used in conjunction with antithyroid drugs.

Hypothyroidism and thyroid replacement therapy
Levothyroxine

Thyroxine is given as thyroxine sodium in maintenance therapy. It has a half-life of 6 days and a peak onset of 9 days.

Mechanism of action: Thyroxine is converted to T_3 *in vivo.*

Route of administration: Thyroxine is administered orally as tablets.

Indications: Thyroxine is used for hypothyroidism.

Contraindications: Throxine should not be given to people with cardiovascular disorders.

Adverse effects: Side effects of thyroxine include arrhythmias, tachycardia, anginal pain, cramps, headache, restlessness, sweating, and weight loss.

Therapeutic regime: The starting dose of thyroxine should be no greater than 100 μg daily (reduce in elderly or those with cardiovascular disease) and increased by 25–50 μg every 4 weeks until a dose of 100–200 μg is reached.

Liothyronine (L-triiodothyronine sodium)

As liothyronine is bound only slightly by thyroid-binding globulin, it has a more rapid onset of effects and a shorter duration of action than levothyroxine.

Mechanism of action: Liothyronine is rapidly metabolized *in vivo* to T_3. It has a half-life of 2–5 days and a peak onset of 1–2 days.

Route of administration: Liothyronine is administered orally as tablets, or by intravenous injection in hypothyroid coma.

Indications: Liothyronine is given for severe hypothyroidism where a rapid effect is needed.

Contraindications: Liothyronine should not be given to people with cardiovascular disorders.

Adverse effects: Side effects of liothyronine include arrhythmias, tachycardia, anginal pain, cramps, headache, restlessness, sweating, and weight loss.

Therapeutic regime: The dosage of liothyronine should be gradually increased as with thyroxine (20 μg liothyronine is equivalent to 100 μg thyroxine).

- **How are thyroid hormones produced and how is this process controlled?**
- **Distinguish between hypothyroidism and hyperthyroidism.**
- **Describe the classes of drugs used to treat hyperthyroidism. For each of these list examples, their mechanism of action, route of administration, indications, and major adverse effects.**
- **Describe the classes of drugs used to treat hypothyroidism. For each of these list examples, their mechanism of action, route of administration, indications, and major adverse effects.**

THE ENDOCRINE PANCREAS AND DIABETES MELLITUS

Control of plasma glucose

Blood glucose levels are maintained at a concentration of 5 mmol/L, and usually do not exceed 8 mmol/L. A plasma glucose concentration of 2.2 mmol/L or less may result in hypoglycaemic coma and death due to a lack of energy reaching the brain. A plasma glucose concentration of more than 10 mmol/L exceeds the renal threshold for glucose and means that glucose will be present in the urine. Osmotic diuresis then occurs.

The islets of Langerhans, located in the pancreas, contain glucose receptors and are able to secrete the hormones glucagon and insulin. These hormones are short-term regulators of plasma glucose levels with opposite effects. In addition, their release can be influenced by gastrointestinal hormones and autonomic nerves.

Glucose receptors are also found in the ventromedial nucleus and lateral areas of the hypothalamus. These are able to regulate appetite and feeding, and also indirectly stimulate the release of a variety of hormones, including adrenaline, growth hormone, and cortisol, all of which affect glucose metabolism.

The hormones involved in blood glucose regulation target the liver, skeletal muscle, and adipose tissue.

Insulin

Insulin is a 51-amino-acid peptide made up of an α- and a β-chain linked by disulphide bonds. It has a half-life of 3–5 min and is metabolized to a large extent by the liver (40–50%), but also by the kidneys and muscles.

In response to high blood glucose levels (such as occur after a meal), as well as glucosamine, amino acids, fatty acids, ketone bodies, and sulphonylureas (see below), the β-cells of the endocrine pancreas secrete insulin along with a C-peptide.

Insulin release is mediated by ATP-dependent potassium channels, located in the membrane of the β-cells. These close in response to elevated cytoplasmic ATP and decreased cytoplasmic ADP levels, resulting in depolarization of the membrane and action potential generation. This triggers calcium entry into the cell through voltage-dependent calcium channels, and subsequent insulin release (Fig. 8.6).

Insulin release is inhibited by low blood glucose levels, growth hormone, glucagon, cortisol, and sympathetic nervous system activation.

The insulin receptor consists of two α- and two β-subunits linked by disulphide bonds. Insulin binds to the extracellular α-subunits, resulting in the internalization of the receptor and its subsequent breakdown.

The β-subunits display tyrosine kinase activity upon the binding of insulin to the receptor. Autophosphorylation of

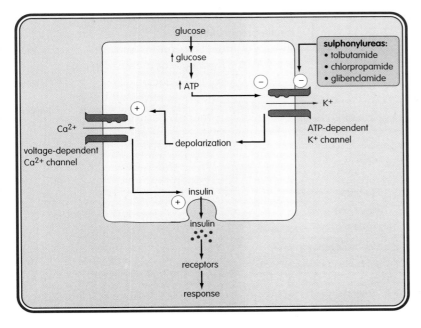

Fig. 8.6 Mechanism of insulin secretion.

the β-subunits ensues, resulting in the phosphorylation of phospholipase C with subsequent diacylglycerol (DAG) and inositol triphosphate (IP_3) generation.

The effects of insulin are summarized in Fig. 8.7.

Diabetes mellitus

Diabetes mellitus involves an inability to regulate plasma glucose within the normal range. It is characterized by an insulin deficiency, leading to hyperglycaemia, glycosuria (glucose in the urine), polyuria (production of large volumes of dilute urine) associated with cellular potassium depletion, and polydipsia (intense thirst).

Lipolysis is increased, as is the production of ketone bodies from fatty acids. This leads to ketonuria and metabolic acidosis and eventually coma and death.

Some untreated diabetic patients have a plasma glucose concentration of up to 100 mmol/L, at which level body fluids become hypertonic, resulting in cellular dehydration, hyperosmolar coma, and death.

Consequences of untreated diabetes mellitus include weight loss, muscle wasting, neuropathy, atherosclerosis, retinopathy and subsequent blindness, and ischaemic foot and leg disease leading to gangrene.

There are two forms of diabetes mellitus—type 1 and type 2. The differences between the two forms are summarized in Fig. 8.8.

Type 1: insulin-dependent diabetes mellitus

In type 1 or insulin-dependent diabetes mellitus (IDDM), pancreatic β-cells are destroyed by an autoimmune T-cell attack. This leads to a complete inability to secrete insulin and ketoacidosis is a problem.

IDDM is apparent at a young age.

Type 2: non-insulin-dependent diabetes mellitus

In type 2 or non-insulin-dependent diabetes mellitus (NIDDM), insulin is secreted but ineffective (insulin resistance). This can be due to any of the following:
- Defective glucose transporters.
- Insulin-receptor desensitization.
- Toxicity of hyperglycaemia.
- Metabolic demands of obesity.
- Pancreatitis or pancreatic cancer.
- Cushing's syndrome or acromegaly.

Management of diabetes mellitus
Insulin preparations

The aim of insulin preparations is to mimic basal levels of insulin and meal-induced increases in insulin.

Effects of insulin on fuel homeostasis	
carbohydrates	increase glucose transport increase glycogen synthesis increase glycolysis inhibit gluconeogenesis
fats	increase lipoprotein lipase activity increase fat storage in adipocytes inhibit lipolysis (hormone-sensitive lipase) increase hepatic lipoprotein synthesis inhibit fatty acid oxidation
proteins	increase protein synthesis increase amino acid transport

Fig. 8.7 Effects of insulin on fuel homeostasis.

Fig. 8.8 Features of type 1 and type 2 diabetes mellitus.

Features of type 1 and type 2 diabetes mellitus	
Type 1	**Type 2**
IDDM (insulin-dependent diabetes mellitus)	NIDDM (non-insulin-dependent diabetes mellitus)
0.5% prevalence in adults	5% prevalence in adults
juvenile onset (<30 years)	maturity onset (>30 years)
absolute lack of insulin	relative lack of, or excess, insulin
not associated with obesity	often associated with obesity
insulin therapy	oral agents (sulphonylureas) usually suffice
ketoacidosis frequent	ketoacidosis uncommon
linked to the presence of islet cell antibody and genetic markers (HLA antigens)	no known genetic or autoimmune origin

Insulin preparations are:
- Human, porcine, or bovine in origin.
- Available as short-, medium-, and long-acting preparations (Fig. 8.9).

Short-acting insulins are soluble and the presence of Zn^{2+} in the solution maintains the solubility. These preparations most resemble endogenous insulin.

Intermediate-acting insulins are not as soluble as the short-acting preparations. The solubility can be decreased by using a buffer, such as large insulin crystals, or the addition of protamine (a cationic protein). There are four types of intermediate-acting insulins. These are:
- Semilente, which is a suspension of amorphous insulin zinc.
- Lente, which is morphous insulin zinc (30%) and insulin zinc crystals (70%).
- Isophane insulin, or neutral protamine Hagedorn (NPH), which is protamine and insulin.
- Biphasic fixed mixtures, such as soluble and isophane insulin.

The long-acting insulin, ultralente, contains insulin zinc crystals.

Mechanism of action: Insulin preparations mimic endogenous insulin.

Route of administration: Insulin must always be given parenterally (intravenously, intramuscularly or subcutaneously), as it is a peptide and thus destroyed in the gastrointestinal tract. Short-acting insulin is given intravenously in emergencies, but administration of the insulin preparations in maintenance treatment is usually subcutaneous.

Indications: Insulin preparations are given for IDDM.

Adverse effects: Side effects of insulin preparations include local reactions and, in overdose,

Insulin preparations			
Insulin preparation	Action	Peak activity (h)	Duration (h)
regular	rapid	1–3	5–7
semilente	rapid	3–4	10–16
neutral protamine Hagedorn	intermediate	6–14	18–28
lente	intermediate	6–14	18–28
ultralente	prolonged	18–24	30–40

Fig. 8.9 Insulin preparations.

hypoglycaemia. Protamine can cause allergic reactions. Rarely, there may be immune resistance.

Therapeutic regime: The following regimes are recommended according to the patient:
- Short-acting insulin three times daily (before breakfast, lunch, and dinner) and intermediate-acting insulin at bedtime.
- Short-acting insulin and intermediate-acting insulin mixture twice daily before meals.
- Short-acting insulin and intermediate-acting insulin mixture before breakfast, short-acting insulin before dinner, and intermediate-acting insulin before bedtime.
- Short-acting insulin and intermediate-acting insulin mixture before breakfast is adequate for some NIDDM patients needing insulin.

Sulphonylureas
Tolbutamide, chlorpropamide, and glibenclamide are examples of sulphonylureas.

There is a failure rate of approximately 30% with sulphonylureas.

Mechanism of action: Sulphonylureas block ATP-dependent potassium channels in the membrane of the pancreatic β-cells, causing depolarization, calcium influx, and insulin release.

Route of administration: Sulphonylureas are administered orally as tablets.

Indications: Sulphonylureas are given for diabetes mellitus, in patients with some β-cell activity.

Contraindications: Sulphonylureas should not be given to breast-feeding women, or people with ketoacidosis. Long-acting sulphonylureas (chlorpropamide, glibenclamide) should be avoided in the elderly and in those with renal and hepatic insufficiency, as these drugs can induce hypoglycaemia.

Adverse effects: Side effects of sulphonylureas include weight gain; sensitivity reactions, including rashes; gastrointestinal disturbances; headache; and hypoglycaemia.

Therapeutic regime: Tolbutamide is given at 500 mg two or three times daily and lasts for 6 hours; chlorpropamide is given at 100–250 mg daily and lasts for 12 hours; and glibenclamide is given at 2.5–15 mg daily and lasts for 12 hours.

Biguanides
Metformin is an example of a biguanide.

Mechanism of action: Metformin increases the

peripheral utilization of glucose, by increasing uptake, and decreases gluconeogenesis. To work, metformin requires the presence of endogenous insulin; thus, patients must have some functioning β-cells.
Route of administration: Metformin is administered orally as tablets.
Indications: Metformin is given for NIDDM where dieting and sulphonylureas have proved ineffective.
Contraindications: Metformin should not be given to patients with hepatic or renal impairment (owing to the risk of lactic acidosis) or heart failure.
Adverse effects: Side effects of metformin include anorexia, headache, nausea and vomiting, lactic acidosis, and decreased vitamin B_{12} absorption.
Therapeutic regime: Metformin is given at 1 g two or three times daily. It can be used alone or with sulphonylureas. Metformin should be taken with or after food.

Dietary control
Dietary control is important for both type 1 and type 2 diabetes mellitus.

The diet should aim to derive its energy from the following constituents, in the following amounts:
- 50% carbohydrate (slowly absorbed forms).
- 35% fat.
- 15% protein.

This implies a reduction in total fat intake, an increase in protein intake, and an increase in the intake of high fibre foods, which slow the rate of absorption from the gut.

Simple sugars, as found in sweet drinks and cakes, should be avoided.

Meals should be small and regular, thus avoiding large swings in blood glucose levels.

Rehydration therapy
In the acute diabetic patient the fluid deficit can be as high as 7–8 L. Rehydration therapy is essential in order to regain fluid and electrolyte balance and takes precedence over the administration of insulin. At least 1.5 L/h of 0.9% saline is given over 2 hours by intravenous infusion, followed by 500 ml/h over the next 4 hours, and subsequently 500 ml/2 h.

Untreated diabetic patients suffer from hyperkalaemia due to the breakdown of cells at high glucose concentrations. However, as soon as insulin is administered , potassium follows glucose into cells, and hypokalaemia becomes the danger. The rehydration

fluid should therefore contain potassium, and plasma K^+ should be measured every hour.

Diabetic patients are also at risk of metabolic acidosis due to excessive ketone body production. If the acidosis is severe (pH < 7.1), bicarbonate can be administered intravenously.

In an acute hyperglycaemic attack, it is essential that fluids and soluble insulin are given intravenously to rehydrate the patient rapidly and decrease blood sugar levels.

- **How are plasma glucose levels controlled?**
- **Distinguish between type 1 and type 2 diabetes mellitus.**
- **What are the different insulin preparations used to treat diabetes mellitus, their mechanism of action, route of administration, indications, and major adverse effects?**
- **What are the other classes of drugs used to treat diabetes mellitus? For each of these, list examples, their mechanism of action, route of administration, indications, and major adverse effects.**

ADRENAL CORTICOSTEROIDS

Adrenal function and corticosteroids
Introduction
The adrenal cortex secretes several steroid hormones into the bloodstream. These are categorized by their actions into two main classes—mineralocorticoids and glucocorticoids.
Of the mineralocorticoids, aldosterone is the main endogenous hormone, synthesized in the zona

glomerulosa. It affects water and electrolyte balance, and possesses salt-retaining activity.

Of the glucocorticoids, hydrocortisone and cortisone are the main endogenous hormones, synthesized in the zona fasciculata and zona reticularis. They affect carbohydrate, fat, and protein metabolism, and suppress inflammatory and immune responses. They also possess some mineralocorticoid activity.

Small quantities of some sex steroids, mainly androgens, are also produced by the adrenal cortex.

Synthesis and release
Adrenal corticosteroids are not pre-formed, but are synthesized when required from cholesterol.

Glucocorticoids
The release of cortisol is controlled in a negative feedback fashion by the hypothalamo–pituitary–adrenal system (Fig. 8.10). There is a diurnal pattern of activity with an early morning peak in cortisol release.

A variety of sensorineural inputs regulate the release of corticotrophin-releasing factor (CRF) in the

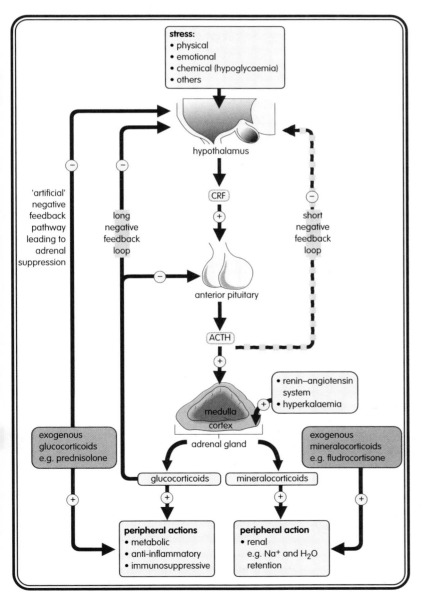

Fig. 8.10 Control of adrenal corticosteroid synthesis and secretion. (ACTH, adrenocorticotrophin hormone; CRF, corticotrophin-releasing factor.)

hypothalamus; examples include physiological and psychological 'stress', injury, and infection.

CRF, a 41-amino-acid polypeptide, reaches the anterior pituitary in the hypothalamo–hypophysial portal system where it stimulates the release of adrenocorticotrophic hormone (ACTH) or corticotrophin.

ACTH is formed from a larger molecule, pro-opiomelanocortin, and is released into the circulation where it stimulates the synthesis and release of cortisol from the zona fasciculata of the adrenal cortex.

Natural and artificial corticosteroids circulating in the blood exert a negative feedback effect on the production of both CRH and ACTH.

Mineralocorticoids

Aldosterone release is also partially controlled by ACTH, but other factors, especially the renin–angiotensin system (RAS), and plasma potassium levels, are more important.

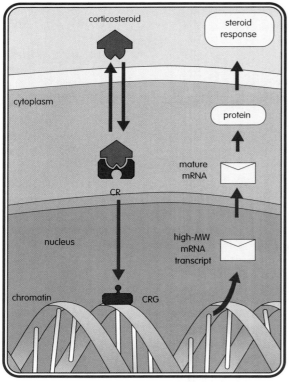

Fig. 8.11 Mechanism of action of corticosteroids at the cellular level. (CR, corticosteroid receptor; CRG, corticosteroid response gene; MW, molecular weight.)

Mechanism of action of corticosteroids

Endogenous and synthetic corticosteroids act in a similar way (Fig. 8.11). The hormone or drug circulates to peripheral tissues where it enters cells (steroids are lipid soluble) and binds to cytosolic corticosteroid receptors (CR). After hormone binding, these receptors are translocated to the nucleus where they lead to the transcription of corticosteroid-responsive genes (CRG), initially to form mRNA transcripts which are subsequently translated into protein products.

The products of these CRGs lead to diverse effects on the target tissues (Fig. 8.12). The actions of corticosteroids are divided into effects on inorganic metabolism (mineralocorticoid effects) and effects on organic metabolism (glucocorticoid effects).

Therapeutic use of corticosteroids

Corticosteroids have wide-ranging and powerful effects on human physiology. There are two main areas where these properties are taken advantage of in the therapeutic use of corticosteroids—physiological replacement therapy of corticosteroid deficiency, and anti-inflammatory therapy and immunosuppression.

Exogenous corticosteroids

Both naturally occurring and a number of synthetic corticosteroids are available for clinical use. These vary in their potency, half-life, and the balance between glucocorticoid versus mineralocorticoid activity (Fig. 8.13). *Mechanism of action:* Exogenous corticosteroids imitate endogenous corticosteroids.

Indications: The therapeutic use of corticosteroids falls into the two main categories of physiological replacement therapy, and anti-inflammatory therapy and immunosuppression.

Corticosteroid replacement therapy is necessary when endogenous hormones are deficient, as can happen in:
• Primary adrenocortical destruction (Addison's disease).
• Secondary adrenocortical failure due to deficient ACTH from the pituitary.
• Suppression of the hypothalamo–pituitary–adrenal axis due to prolonged glucocorticoid therapy.

As all the actions of natural corticosteroids are required, a glucocorticoid with mineralocorticoid activity (cortisol) or separate glucocorticoid and mineralocorticoid are given.

The anti-inflammatory and immunosuppressive effects of glucocorticoids are used to treat a wide

Fig. 8.12 Major effects of corticosteroids.

Major effects of the corticosteroids	
Glucocorticoids	
immunological	• decreased production of T and B lymphocytes and macrophages, involution of lymphoid tissue • decreased function of T and B lymphocytes, and reduced responsiveness to cytokines • inhibition of complement system
anti-inflammatory	• profound generalized inhibitory effects on inflammatory response. • reduced production of acute inflammatory mediators, especially the eicosanoids (prostaglandins, leukotrienes, etc.); owing to production of lipocortin, an enzyme that inhibits phospholipase A_2, thus blocking the formation of arachidonic acid and its metabolites—see Chapter 10 • reduced numbers and activity of circulating immunocompetent cells, neutrophils, and macrophages • decreased activity of macrophages and fibroblasts involved in the chronic stages of inflammation, leading to decreased inflammation and decreased healing
carbohydrate metabolism	• increased gluconeogenesis, decreased cellular uptake and utilization of glucose, increased storage of glycogen in the liver (hyperglycaemic actions)
fat metabolism	• redistribution of lipid from steroid-sensitive stores (limbs) to steroid-resistant stores (face, neck, trunk)
protein metabolism	• increased catabolism, decreased anabolism, leading to protein degradation
cardiovascular	• increased sensitivity of vascular system to catecholamines, reduced capillary permeability leading to raised blood pressure
central nervous system	• high levels can cause mood changes, (euphoria/depression) or psychotic states, perhaps due to electrolyte changes
anterior hypothalamus and pituitary	• negative feedback effect of CRF and ACTH with the result that endogenous secretion of glucocorticoids is reduced, and may remain so after prolonged glucocorticoid therapy ('adrenal suppression')
Mineralocorticoids	
kidney	• increases permeability of the apical membrane of cells in the distal renal tubule to sodium • stimulates the Na^+/K^+ ATPase pump leading to reabsorption of Na^+ and loss of K^+ in the urine • water is passively reabsorbed owing to sodium retention; thus extracellular fluid and blood volume are increased (raising blood pressure)

Corticosteroids used therapeutically		
Glucocorticoids		**Mineralocorticoids**
'Natural hormones'	Synthetic	Synthetic
hydrocortisone (cortisol)	prednisolone betamethasone dexamethasone beclomethasone triamcinolone	fludrocortisone deoxycortone

Fig. 8.13 Examples of corticosteroids used therapeutically.

variety of conditions (Fig. 8.14). In these cases, synthetic glucocorticoids with little mineralocorticoid activity are used.

Contraindications: Exogenous corticosteroids should not be given to people with systemic infection, unless specific antimicrobial therapy is being given.

Route of administration: Replacement therapy is given orally twice a day at physiological doses to try to mimic as closely as possible the level and rhythm of natural corticosteroid secretion.

When used to suppress inflammatory and immune responses, corticosteroids may be given orally or intravenously, but, depending on the condition, the topical administration of glucocorticoids is preferred, if feasible, as it can deliver high concentrations to the target site while minimizing systemic absorption and adverse effects (see Fig. 8.14).

At high doses, even topically administered glucocorticoids can achieve systemic penetration.

Adverse effects: Overdosage or prolonged use of corticosteroids may exaggerate some of their normal physiological actions (see earlier), leading to mineralo-corticoid and glucocorticoid side effects. Many of these effects are similar to those seen in Cushing's syndrome, a condition caused by excess secretion of endogenous corticosteroids (Fig. 8.15).

The metabolic effects of glucocorticoids include:

- Central obesity and a 'moon' face, as fat is redistributed.
- Hyperglycaemia, which may lead to clinical diabetes mellitus, due to disturbed carbohydrate metabolism.
- Osteoporosis, due to catabolism of protein matrix in bone.

- Loss of skin structure, with purple striae, and easy bruising, due to altered protein metabolism.
- Muscle weakness and wasting, due to protein catabolism.
- Suppression of growth in children.

Corticosteroid therapy suppresses endogenous secretion of adrenal hormones via negative feedback on the hypothalamo–pituitary–adrenal axis.

Adrenal atrophy can persist for years after withdrawal from prolonged corticosteroid therapy. Replacement corticosteroid therapy is needed to compensate for the lack of sufficient adrenocortical response in times of stress (e.g. illness, surgery).

Steroid therapy must be withdrawn slowly after long-term treatment, as sudden withdrawal can lead to an acute adrenal insufficiency crisis.

With glucocorticoid therapy, the modification of inflammatory and immune reactions leads to an increased susceptibility to infections. This can progress unnoticed because of the suppression of normal indicators of infection, such as inflammation.

Increased susceptibility occurs to normally pathogenic and opportunistic bacterial, viral, and fungal organisms. Re-activation of latent infections (e.g. tuberculosis, herpesviruses) can occur.

The effects are most serious when corticosteroids are being used systemically, although topical use can exacerbate superficial skin infections, and inhaled corticosteroids can encourage oropharyngeal thrush etc.

The other effects of glucocorticoids include mood changes—euphoria and, rarely, psychosis, peptic ulceration due to inhibition of gastrointestinal

Conditions in which corticosteroids are used for their anti-inflammatory and immunosuppressive effects		
Systemic uses	**Topical uses**	

acute inflammatory conditions
  e.g. anaphylaxis, status asthmaticus,
  fibrosing alveolitis, angionecrotic oedema
	asthma	aerosol

chronic inflammatory conditions
  e.g. rheumatoid arthritis, inflammatory
  bowel disease, systemic lupus
  erythematosus, glomerulonephritis
	allergic rhinitis	nasal spray

neoplastic disease
  myelomas, lymphomas, lymphatic
  leukaemias
	eczema	ointment or cream

miscellaneous
  organ transplantation
	inflammatory bowel
	  disease
		foam enema

Fig. 8.14 Examples of conditions in which corticosteroids are used for their anti-inflammatory and immunosuppressive effects.

Fig. 8.15 Effects of prolonged corticosteroid use.

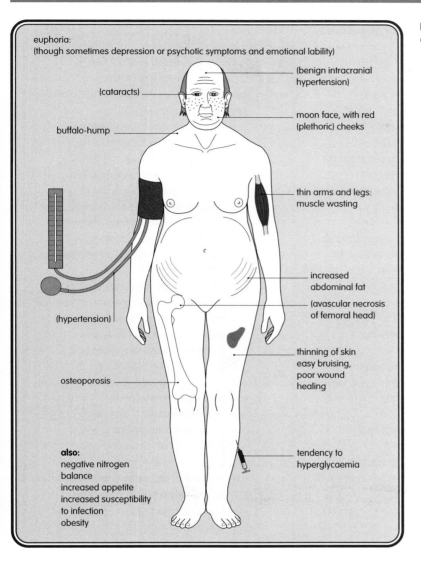

euphoria:
(though sometimes depression or psychotic symptoms and emotional lability)

(benign intracranial hypertension)

(cataracts)

moon face, with red (plethoric) cheeks

buffalo-hump

thin arms and legs: muscle wasting

(hypertension)

increased abdominal fat

(avascular necrosis of femoral head)

osteoporosis

thinning of skin easy bruising, poor wound healing

also:
negative nitrogen balance
increased appetite
increased susceptibility to infection
obesity

tendency to hyperglycaemia

---

prostaglandin synthesis, and eye problems such as cataracts and exacerbation of glaucoma.

Fluid retention, hypokalaemia, and hypertension can all be side effects of any corticosteroids that possess significant mineralocorticoid activity.

Therapeutic notes on specific steroid agents
Glucocorticoids

Hydrocortisone (cortisol):
- Is administered orally for adrenal replacement therapy, and possesses mineralocorticoid activity.
- Is administered intravenously in status asthmaticus and anaphylactic shock.

- Is applied topically for eczema, inflammatory bowel conditions, etc.

Prednisolone:
- Is predominantly glucocorticoid in activity.
- Is the oral drug most widely used in allergic and inflammatory diseases.

Betamethasone and dexamethasone:
- Have very high glucocorticoid activity with insignificant mineralocorticoid activity.
- Are very potent drugs used orally and by injection to suppress inflammatory and allergic disorders, and to

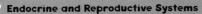
reduce cerebral oedema—they do not possess salt-
or water-retaining actions.

Beclomethasone:
- Is the dipropionate ester of betamethasone.
- Is a very potent drug with no mineralocorticoid
  activity that is useful topically, as it is poorly
  absorbed through membranes and skin.
- Is used as an aerosol in asthma, and as a cream and
  ointment in eczema to provide high local anti-
  inflammatory effects with minimal systemic penetration.

Triamcinolone:
- Is a moderately potent drug used in severe asthma.
- Is also administered by intra-articular injection for
  rheumatoid arthritis.

Mineralocorticoids
Fludrocortisone:
- Has such high mineralocorticoid activity that
  glucocorticoid activity is insignificant.
- Is administered orally, in combination with a
  glucocorticoid, in replacement therapy.

Deoxycortone:
- Has such high mineralocorticoid activity that
  glucocorticoid activity is insignificant.
- Is administered as slow-release intramuscular
  injections, used in combination with a glucocorticoid,
  in replacement therapy.

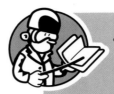

- What are the two
  different types of
  endogenous corticosteroid
  secreted by the adrenal
  glands? Describe their
  respective roles in normal
  physiology.
- Discuss the factors involved in
  controlling the release of
  endogenous corticosteroids, the
  role of negative feedback, and
  how the use of exogenous
  therapeutic corticosteroids can
  affect this.
- Describe the major physiological
  effects induced by corticosteroids
  and how these effects are
  initiated at a molecular level. List
  the major adverse effects of
  corticosteroid therapy.
- When are exogenous
  corticosteroids used
  therapeutically, how may they
  be administered, and what
  problems are involved in
  corticosteroid therapy?
- Describe the major characteristics
  of the corticosteroids used
  therapeutically.

Know the adverse effects
caused by corticosteroid
therapy as they are
numerous, common, and
a popular exam question. Some
of the adverse effects caused by
corticosteroids are logical
exaggerations of their normal
physiological actions, others are
more unexpected and must
therefore be learnt individually.

THE REPRODUCTIVE SYSTEM

Hormonal control of the reproductive system

Physiology of the female reproductive tract

The female gonads, or ovaries, are responsible for
oogenesis and the secretion of the steroid sex hormones,
namely oestrogens (mainly oestradiol) and progesterone.

The production of the female sex hormones is
controlled by the hypothalamic–pituitary–ovarian axis
(Fig. 8.16).

Gonadotrophin-releasing hormone (GnRH) is secreted
by the hypothalamus and stimulates the pulsatile
secretion of follicle-stimulating hormone (FSH) and

luteinizing hormone (LH) by the anterior pituitary. In turn, these act upon the ovaries to stimulate the release of oestradiol, progesterone, and other ovarian hormones.

The ovarian hormones are able to exert a negative feedback on the hypothalamus and/or the pituitary. Some of these are selective in their inhibition; for example, inhibin selectively inhibits FSH release from the pituitary, activin selectively stimulates FSH release from the pituitary, and gonadotrophin-surge-attenuating factor selectively inhibits LH secretion from the pituitary.

Menstrual cycle

The menstrual cycle is divided into a follicular phase (days 1–14) and a luteal phase (days 14–28).
The cycle proceeds as follows (numbers refer to Fig. 8.17):

1. Day 1 is the first day of menstruation, which involves the shedding of the uterine endometrium. Plasma oestrogen levels are low and thus little negative feedback occurs. As a result, the secretion of LH and FSH begins to increase.
2. Ten to twenty-five pre-antral follicles start to enlarge and secrete oestrogen.

3. FSH stimulates the granulosa cells to secrete oestrogen, the levels of which rise.
4. About 1 week into the cycle, one of the follicles becomes dominant, and the others undergo atresia. The dominant follicle secretes large amounts of oestrogen.
5. Plasma oestrogen levels rise significantly as a result of increased sensitivity of the granulosa cells to FSH.
6. Elevated oestrogen levels provide negative feedback, and FSH secretion decreases.
7. Plasma oestrogen levels are now so high (>200 pg/mL) that they exert a positive feedback on gonadotrophin secretion. This occurs for about 2 days, during which FSH stimulates the appearance of LH receptors on the granulosa cells.
8. An LH surge occurs. This results in a decrease in oestrogen secretion, an increase in progesterone secretion by the granulosa cells, and the resumption of meiosis in the egg.
9. Oestrogen levels decline after ovulation.
10. The first meiotic division is completed.

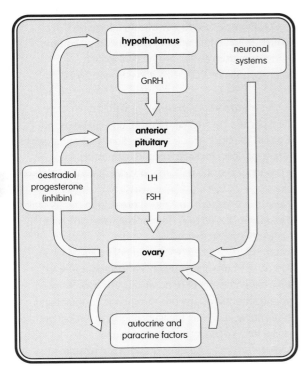

Fig. 8.16 Hypothalamic–pituitary–ovarian axis. (GnRH, gonadotrophin-releasing hormone; LH, luteinizing hormone; FSH, follicle-stimulating hormone.)

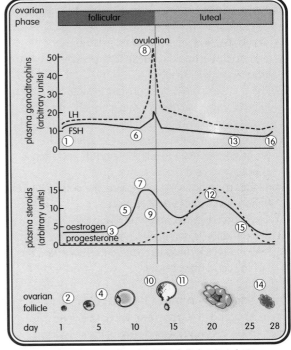

Fig. 8.17 The menstrual cycle. (FSH, follicle-stimulating hormone; LH, luteinizing hormone.)

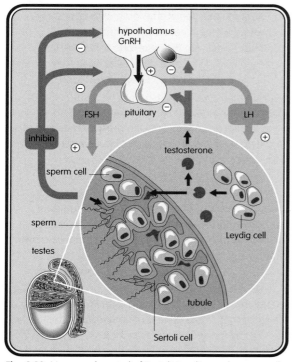

Fig. 8.18 Hormonal control of Sertoli, Leydig, and sperm cell function. (FSH, follicle-stimulating hormone; GnRH, gonadotrophin-releasing hormone; LH, luteinizing hormone.)

11. On day 14, ovulation, the release of the ovum, occurs. This is approximately 18 hours after the LH surge.
12. The granulosa cells are transformed into the corpus luteum, which secretes both oestrogen and progesterone in large quantities.
13. There is a rise in the levels of oestrogen and progesterone. As a result, FSH and LH secretion is suppressed, and the levels fall.
14. If fertilization does not take place, the corpus luteum degenerates after about 10 days.
15. Oestrogen and progesterone levels fall; menstruation is imminent.
16. FSH and LH secretion increase once more, and the 28-day cycle begins again.

Physiology of the male reproductive tract
The male gonads, or testes, are responsible for spermatogenesis and the secretion of the steroid sex hormone testosterone.

Spermatogenesis takes place in the lumen of the seminiferous tubules of the testis.

The production of the male sex hormones is controlled by the hypothalamic–pituitary axis (Fig. 8.18).

The Sertoli cells are connected to one another by tight junctions, and extend from the basement membrane of the seminiferous tubules into the lumen. Under the influence of FSH, these synthesize testosterone receptors and inhibin.

The Leydig cells are found in the connective tissue between the tubules. Under the influence of LH, these synthesize testosterone. Testosterone acts locally to increase sperm production, and also peripherally on the testosterone-sensitive tissues of the body.

Testosterone and inhibin are able to exert negative feedback control over the anterior pituitary, the former decreasing LH secretion and the latter decreasing FSH secretion. In addition, testosterone and inhibin act on the hypothalamus to decrease GnRH secretion.

Drugs that affect the reproductive system
Oral contraceptives
Combined oral contraceptive pill
The combined oral contraceptive pill (COCP) contains both an oestrogen (usually ethinyl oestradiol, 20–50 µg) and a progestogen (an analogue of progesterone).

COCPs provide a highly effective form of contraception. Their efficacy is reduced by some broad-spectrum antibiotics, which reduce enterohepatic recirculation of oestrogen by killing gut flora.

Mechanism of action: The levels of steroids mimic the luteal phase of the menstrual cycle, and suppress, via negative feedback effects, the secretion of gonadotrophins. As a result, follicular selection and maturation, the oestrogen surge, the LH surge, and thus ovulation, do not take place.

Route of administration: COCPs are administered orally.

Indications: COCPs are used for contraception and menstrual symptoms.

Contraindications: COCPs should not be given to women who are pregnant or breast-feeding, or to those with a history of heart disease or hypertension, hyperlipidaemia or any pro-thrombotic coagulation abnormality, diabetes mellitus, migraine, breast or genital tract carcinoma, or liver disease.

Adverse effects: Side effects of COCPs include nausea, vomiting and headache, weight gain, breast tenderness, impaired liver function, impaired glucose tolerance in diabetic women, 'spotting' (slight bleeding at the start of the menstrual cycle), thrombosis and hypertension, a slightly increased risk of cervical cancer, and a possibly increased risk of breast cancer.

Therapeutic regime: COCPs are taken for 21 days (starting on the first day of the menstrual cycle) at about the same time each day, with a 7-day break to induce a withdrawal bleed. If the delay in taking the pill is greater than 12 hours, the contraceptive effect may be lost.

The combined pill may be looked upon as a synthetic corpus luteum.

Progesterone-only pill (minipill)

The minipill consists of low-dose progestogen; ovulation still takes place and menstruation is normal. The minipill is not as effective as the COCP.

Mechanism of action: The minipill causes thickening of cervical mucus preventing sperm penetration. It also causes suppression of gonadotrophin secretion, and consequently ovulation, but the latter effect does not occur in the majority of women.

Route of administration: The minipill is administered orally.

Indications: The minipill is used for contraception. It is more suitable for heavy smokers and patients with hypertension or heart disease, diabetes mellitus, and migraine.

Contraindications: The minipill should not be given to pregnant women or those with arterial disease, liver disease, or breast or genital tract carcinoma.

Adverse effects: Side effects of the minipill include menstrual irregularities, nausea, vomiting and headache, weight gain, and breast tenderness.

Therapeutic regime: The minipill is taken as one tablet daily, at the same time, starting on day 1 of the menstrual cycle and then continuously. If the delay in taking the pill is greater than 3 hours, the contraceptive effect may be lost.

Other contraceptive regimes

Depot-progesterone

Examples of depot-progesterone drugs include medroxyprogesterone acetate and a levonorgestrel-releasing implant system. These provide contraception that is long term and as effective as the COCP.

Mechanism of action: Depot-progesterone causes thickening of cervical mucus. It also causes suppression of gonadotrophin secretion, and consequently ovulation, but the latter effect does not occur in the majority of women.

Route of administration: Medroxyprogesterone acetate is administered intramuscularly. The levonorgestrel-releasing implant system relies on capsules placed subdermally.

Indications: Depot-progesterone drugs are used for contraception.

Contraindications: Depot-progesterone drugs should not be given to pregnant women or to those with arterial disease, liver disease, or breast or genital tract carcinoma.

Adverse effects: Side effects of depot-progesterone drugs include menstrual irregularities, nausea, vomiting and headache, weight gain, and breast tenderness.

Therapeutic notes: Medroxyprogesterone acetate provides protection for about 12 weeks. The levonorgestrel implant system provides protection for 5 years.

Post-coital ('morning-after' pill)

The post-coital or 'morning-after' pill provides a form of emergency contraception.

Mechanism of action: High doses of oestrogen prevent implantation of the fertilized egg. This is 75% effective. Contractions of the smooth muscle are induced, and these accelerate the movement of the fertilized egg into the unprepared uterine endometrium.

Route of administration: The morning-after pill is administered orally.

Indications: The morning-after pill is used for emergency contraception after unprotected intercourse.

Contraindications: The morning-after pill should not be given to women with a history of thrombosis.

Adverse effects: Side effects of the morning-after pill include nausea, vomiting and headache, dizziness, and menstrual irregularities.

Therapeutic regime: The morning-after pill regime consists of four tablets. The first two (50 μg ethinyloestradiol) must be taken within 72 hours of coitus, followed 12 hours later by the second two tablets (250 μg levonorgestrel). If, within 3 hours of taking the tablets, vomiting occurs, two replacement tablets should be taken with an antiemetic.

Possible contraceptives for males

Possible contraceptives for males are still under trial and have not yet been released for use. Examples of these include gossypol and medroxyprogesterone.

Mechanism of action: Gossypol damages the seminiferous tubules while medroxyprogesterone inhibits gonadotrophin release, affecting spermatogenesis and androgen secretion.

Route of administration: Male contraceptives are administered intramuscularly.

Indications: Male contraceptives are used for contraception.

Adverse effects: Side effects of male contraceptives include the suppression of testosterone secretion. If this occurs, exogenous testosterone can be administered.

Oestrogens and antioestrogens

Agonists

The adverse symptoms of the menopause can be attributed to the decreased levels of oestrogen that occur at this time.

Evidence suggests that oestrogen given in low doses to menopausal women will reduce postmenopausal osteoporosis, vaginal atrophy, and the incidence of stroke and myocardial infarction.

A progestogen is co-administered with oestrogen in order to inhibit oestrogen-stimulated endometrial growth and thus reduce the risk of uterine cancer and fibroids.

Examples of oestrogen agonists include oestradiol, ethinyloestradiol, oestriol, mestranol, and stilboestrol.

Mechanism of action: Oestrogen agonists mimic pre-menopausal endogenous oestrogen levels.

Route of administration: Oestrogen agonists are administered orally, or by transdermal patches, gels, or subcutaneous implants.

Indications: Oestrogen agonists are used for hormone replacement therapy (HRT) in menopausal women, usually in conjunction with a progestogen to inhibit endometrial growth.

Contraindications: Oestrogen agonists should not be given to women with cardiovascular disease or hepatic impairment.

Adverse effects: Side effects of oestrogen agonists include an increased risk of endometrial cancer and possibly an increased risk of breast cancer after years of treatment.

Therapeutic regime: Oestrogen agonists are given for several years, starting in the perimenopausal period.

Antagonists

Examples of oestrogen antagonists include tamoxifen and clomiphene.

Mechanism of action: Antioestrogens act at oestrogen receptors in the hypothalamus, antagonizing the normal feedback of endogenous oestrogen and thereby inducing gonadrotrophin release.

Route of administration: Tamoxifen is administered orally or by intravenous or subcutaneous injection while clomiphene is administered orally.

Indications: Oestrogen antagonists are used for female infertility and breast cancer.

Contraindications: Oestrogen antagonists should not be given to women with hepatic disease, ovarian cysts, or endometrial carcinoma.

Adverse effects: Side effects of oestrogen antagonists include multiple pregnancies and hot flushes. Withdrawal causes visual disturbances and ovarian hyperstimulation.

Progestogens and anti-progestogens

Agonists

Examples of progestogen agonists include progesterone, medroxyprogesterone, norgestrel, and ethisterone.

Mechanism of action: Progestogen agonists mimic endogenous progesterone.

Route of administration: Progestogen agonists are administered orally, or by transdermal patches, gels, or subcutaneous implants.

Indications: Progestogen agonists are given for premenstrual symptoms, severe dysmenorrhea, menorrhagia, endometriosis, contraception, and HRT.

Contraindications: Progestogen agonists should not be given to pregnant women or to those with arterial disease, liver disease, or breast or genital tract carcinoma.

Adverse effects: Side effects of progestogen agonists include menstrual irregularities, nausea, vomiting and headache, weight gain, and breast tenderness.

Antagonists

Mifepristone is an example of a progestogen antagonist.

Mechanism of action: Progestogen antagonists bind to progesterone receptors but exert no effect. They sensitize the uterus to prostaglandins and can therefore be used in combination with prostaglandins in the termination of early pregnancy.

Route of administration: Progestogen antagonists are administered orally.

Indications: Progestogen antagonists are used for early abortions (alone or with prostaglandins), breast cancer, and contraception.

Contraindications: Progestogen antagonists should not be given to pregnant women (64 days' gestation or more), to women with adrenal failure or haemorrhagic disorders, or to those on anticoagulant or long-term corticosteroid treatment, or to smokers aged 35 years and over.

Adverse effects: Side effects of progestogen antagonists include vaginal bleeding, faintness, and nausea and vomiting.

Androgens and antiandrogens
Agonists
Testosterone and fluoxymesterone are examples of androgen agonists.

Mechanism of action: Androgen agonists mimic endogenous androgens.

Route of administration: Androgen agonists are administered orally, intramuscularly, or by implant.

Indications: Androgen agonists are given as androgen-replacement therapy in castrated men, for pituitary or testicular disease causing hypogonadism, and for breast cancer.

Contraindications: Androgen agonists should not be given to men with breast or prostate cancer, to people with hypercalcaemia, and to women who are pregnant or breast-feeding.

Adverse effects: Side effects of androgen agonists include sodium retention causing oedema, hypercalcaemia, suppression of spermatogenesis, virilism in women, and premature closure of epiphyses in prepubertal boys.

Therapeutic regime: Androgen agonists are administered orally (daily), intramuscularly (every 2–6 weeks depending on the disorder), or by implant (every 6 months).

Antagonists
Cyproterone is an androgen antagonist that is a progesterone derivative.

Mechanism of action: Androgen antagonists are partial agonists at androgen receptors, and act on the hypothalamus to reduce the synthesis of gonadotrophins. They inhibit spermatogenesis, causing reversible infertility, but are not contraceptives.

Route of administration: Androgen antagonists are administered orally.

Indications: Androgen antagonists are used for male hypersexuality and sexual deviation, prostate cancer, acne, female hirsutism, and precocious puberty.

Contraindications: Androgen antagonists should not be given to people with hepatic disease or severe diabetes, or to those aged 18 and under as their bones are not fully matured.

Adverse effects: Side effects of androgen antagonists include fatigue and lethargy, and hepatotoxicity.

Anabolic steroids
Nandrolone, ethyloestrenol, oxymetholone, and stanozolol are examples of anabolic steroids.

Mechanism of action: Anabolic steroids are androgenic; stimulate protein synthesis and promote wound and fracture healing.

Route of administration: Nandrolone is administered by deep intramuscular injection, and oxymetholone and stanozolol orally.

Indications: Anabolic steroids can be used for osteoporosis in post-menopausal women, aplastic anaemias, and chronic biliary obstruction.

Contraindications: Anabolic steroids should not be given to people with hepatic impairment, to men with prostate or breast cancer, or to pregnant women.

Adverse effects: Side effects of anabolic steroids include acne, sodium retention causing oedema, virilization in women, amenorrhoea, inhibition of spermatogenesis, and liver tumours.

GnRH agonists and antagonists
Agonists
Leuprolide and buserelin are examples of GnRH agonists.

Mechanism of action: GnRH agonists are given intermittently, and mimic endogenous GnRH. Continuous use desensitizes the GnRH receptors on the gonadotrophs and inhibits gonadotrophin synthesis.

Route of administration: GnRH agonists can be administered by a small battery-operated syringe pump leading to an intravenous or subcutaneous cannula. Buserelin is administered intranasally while leuprolide is administered by subcutaneous injection.

Indications: GnRH agonists are used for ovulation induction in those with GnRH deficiency (pulsatile administration), endometriosis (continuous administration), precocious puberty (continuous administration), and sex-hormone-dependent cancers

and prostate cancer (continuous administration).
Adverse effects: Side effects of GnRH agonists include menopause-like symptoms, including hot flushes, palpitations, and decreased libido due to hypo-oestrogenism, and breakthrough bleeding.
Therapeutic regime: Pulsatile adminisistration of GnRH agonists is every 90 minutes for a few minutes. The treatment must not exceed 6 months, and should not be repeated.

Antagonists

Danazol is an example of a GnRH antagonist.
Mechanism of action: GnRH antagonists inhibit the release of GnRH and the gonadotrophins. They bind to the sex steroid receptors, displaying androgenic, anti-oestrogenic, and anti-progestogenic effects.
Route of administration: GnRH antagonists are administered orally.
Indications: GnRH antagonists are given for endometriosis, menstrual disorders, including menorrhagia, cystic breast disease, gynaecomastia, and possibly contraception.
Contraindications: GnRH antagonists should not be given to pregnant women, or to people with hepatic, renal, or cardiac impairment, or those with vascular disease.
Adverse effects: Side effects of GnRH antagonists include nausea and vomiting, weight gain, and androgenic effects such as acne and hirsutism.

Oxytocic drugs

The oxytocic drugs, oxytocin, ergometrine, prostaglandins E and F [e.g. gemeprost (PGE$_1$ analogue) dinoprostone (PGE$_2$), and carboprost (15-methyl PGF$_{2\alpha}$)], all cause uterine contractions.

Oxytocin is a posterior pituitary hormone that acts on uterine muscle to induce powerful contractions. It does this directly and also indirectly by stimulating the muscle to synthesize prostaglandins.

In addition, prostaglandins ripen and soften the cervix, further aiding the expulsion of a uterine mass.
Mechanism of action: Oxytocin acts on oxytocin receptors. The mechanism for ergometrine is not well understood, but may be via partial agonist action at α-adrenoceptors or 5-hydroxytryptamine receptors. The prostaglandins act at prostaglandin receptors.

Route of administration: Gemeprost and dinoprostone are administered by vaginal pessary; dinoprostone can also be administered extra-amniotically; oxytocin is administered by slow intravenous infusion and oxytocin and ergometrine are injected intramuscularly. Prostaglandins can be administered by intravenous infusion.
Indications: Prostaglandins are used to induce abortion. Oxytocin and dinoprostone are used for the induction of labour while oxytocin, ergometrine and carboprost (in those unresponsive to oxytocin and ergometrine) are used for the management of third-stage labour and prevention and treatment of postpartum haemorrhage.
Contraindications: Oxytocic drugs should not be given to women with vascular diseases; ergometrine should not be used to induce labour.
Adverse effects: Side effects of oxytocic drugs include nausea and vomiting, vaginal bleeding, and uterine pain. Oxytocin can cause hypotension and tachycardia.

- ○ **Describe the physiology of the female reproductive tract and its control, in particular the menstrual cycle.**
- ○ **Summarize the physiology of the male reproductive tract and its control.**
- ○ **What are the different drugs used as contraceptives? For each of these list the mechanism of action, route of administration, indications, contraindications, major adverse effects, and, where relevant, the therapeutic regime.**
- ○ **What are the other classes of drugs that affect reproductive function? For each of these, list the mechanism of action, route of administration, indications, and major adverse effects.**

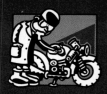

9. Eyes and Skin

THE EYES

Anatomy and physiology

The eyeball is a 25 mm sphere made up of two fluid-filled compartments (the anterior and posterior chambers), a lens, and an enclosure made up of four layers (Fig. 9.1). The four layers include:

- The cornea and sclera.
- The uveal tract comprising the iris, ciliary body, and choroid.
- The pigment epithelium.
- The retina (neural tissue containing photoreceptors).

Light entering the eye is focused by the lens onto the retina and subsequently reaches the brain via the optic nerve.

Control of pupil size
Light

Light levels affect the pupil in two ways (Fig. 9.2):

- High light levels cause pupil constriction, termed miosis.
- Low light levels cause pupil dilation, termed mydriasis.

Autonomic control

The pupils are innervated by the autonomic nervous system, such that:

- Parasympathetic stimulation causes miosis.
- Sympathetic stimulation causes mydriasis.

The dilator pupillae (radial smooth muscle of the iris) is innervated by the sympathetic system, which causes contraction when noradrenaline activates

Fig. 9.1 Anatomy of the eye.

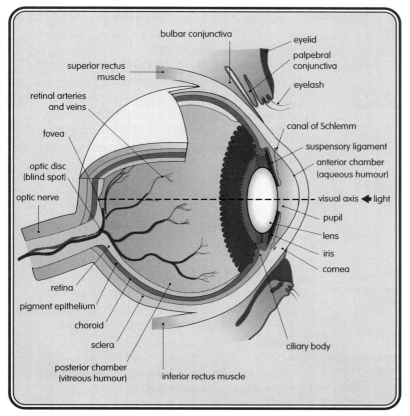

bulbar conjunctiva
eyelid
palpebral conjunctiva
superior rectus muscle
eyelash
retinal arteries and veins
canal of Schlemm
fovea
suspensory ligament
anterior chamber (aqueous humour)
optic disc (blind spot)
optic nerve
visual axis ◀ light
pupil
lens
iris
cornea
retina
pigment epithelium
choroid
sclera
ciliary body
posterior chamber (vitreous humour)
inferior rectus muscle

α_1-adrenoceptors. The constrictor pupillae (sphincter smooth muscle of the iris) is innervated by the parasympathetic system, which causes contraction when acetylcholine activates M_3 receptors.

Accommodation

Accommodation is the ability of the eye to change its refractive power. This is determined by the curvature of the lens.

Suspensory ligaments connect the lens to the ciliary muscle. When the ciliary muscle:

- Contracts (parasympathetic M_3 receptor activation), the suspensory ligaments relax, resulting in the lens becoming more spherical so that it is able to focus near objects.
- Relaxes, the opposite effect results.

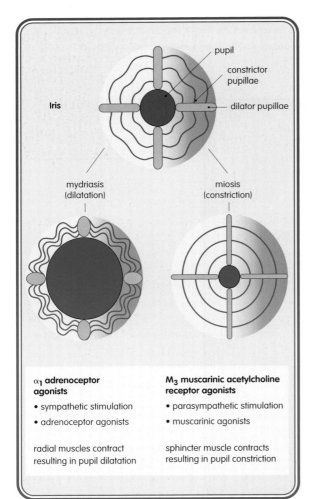

α_1 adrenoceptor agonists	M_3 muscarinic acetylcholine receptor agonists
• sympathetic stimulation • adrenoceptor agonists	• parasympathetic stimulation • muscarinic agonists
radial muscles contract resulting in pupil dilatation	sphincter muscle contracts resulting in pupil constriction

Fig. 9.2 Mechanisms involved in controlling pupil size.

Production of aqueous humour

Aqueous humour fills the anterior chamber of the eyeball. It is continuously produced at a rate of 3 ml/day by a special vascular tissue associated with the ciliary body (Fig. 9.3).

The ciliary epithelial cells contain carbonic anhydrase and ATPase which transport bicarbonate and sodium.

The aqueous humour flows through the pupil and into the anterior chamber, before draining into the episcleral veins via the trabecular meshwork and the canal of Schlemm within the surface of the sclera.

Glaucoma

Glaucoma can be defined as a disorder in which the intraocular pressure (IOP) is raised to over 21 mmHg as opposed to the normal 15 mmHg.

There may be structural changes, such as cupping of the optic disc (due to nerve fibre loss), as well as visual field changes.

If left untreated, glaucoma can cause permanent damage to the optic nerve, and blindness may occur.

There are two types of glaucoma, according to the angle that exists between the iris and cornea: open angle (chronic simple) and closed angle.

Open-angle glaucoma

Open-angle glaucoma is the most common type of glaucoma and may be congenital. It is caused by pathology of the trabecular meshwork that reduces the drainage of the aqueous humour into the canal of Schlemm. Treatment involves either reducing the amount of aqueous humour produced or increasing its drainage.

Closed-angle glaucoma

In closed-angle glaucoma, the angle between the iris and the cornea is very small and results in forward ballooning of the peripheral iris against the back of the cornea (termed 'iris bombé').

Treatment of open-angle glaucoma

Any drug that works by topical application to the eye comes in the form of eye drops. To enable these drops to penetrate the cornea, they must be lipophilic or uncharged.

The drugs that reduce aqueous humor production are:
β-Adrenoceptor antagonists
Timolol is the drug of choice.

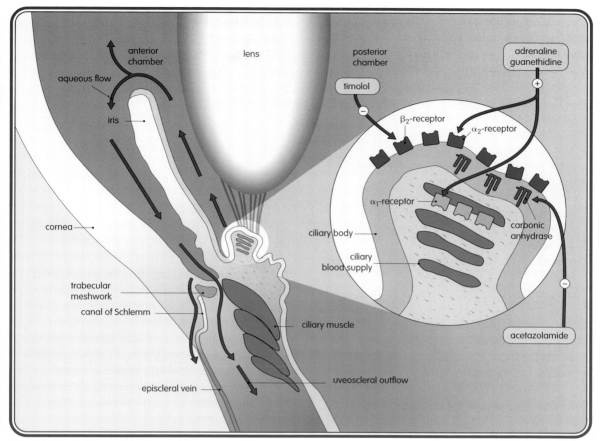

Fig. 9.3 Production and drainage of the aqueous humour.

Mechanism of action: β-Adrenoceptor antagonists block β$_2$-receptors on the ciliary body and may also block β-receptors on ciliary blood vessels, resulting in vasoconstriction (Fig. 9.3).

Route of administration: Timolol maleate is applied topically to the eye.

Indications: β-Adrenoceptor antagonists are the first-line drugs for treatment of open-angle glaucoma.

Contraindications: β-Adrenoceptor antagonists should not be given to patients with asthma, bradycardia, heart block, or heart failure.

Adverse effects: Timolol is absorbed systemically where it can provoke bronchospasm in asthmatic patients and in those with bradycardia, owing to its non-selective action on β-receptors. Other side effects include transitory dry eyes and allergic blepharoconjunctivitis.

α-Adrenoceptor agonists

Adrenaline and guanethidine are examples of α-adrenoceptor agonists.

Mechanism of action: α-Adrenoceptor agonists stimulate α$_2$-adrenoceptors on the ciliary body and α$_1$-adrenoceptors on ciliary blood vessels, resulting in vasoconstriction (Fig 9.3).

Route of administration: α-Adrenoceptor agonists are applied topically to to the eye.

Adrenaline is not very lipophilic and therefore does not penetrate the cornea effectively. This can be overcome by administering dipivefrine hydrochloride, a prodrug that crosses the cornea and is metabolized to adrenaline once inside the eye.

Indications: α-Adrenoceptor agonists are used for open-angle glaucoma.

Contraindications: α-Adrenoceptor agonists should not be used for closed-angle glaucoma, because of their mydriatic effect; it should not be given to patients with hypertension and heart disease.

Adverse effects: Side effects of α-adrenoceptor agonists include severe smarting and redness of the eye.

Carbonic anhydrase inhibitors

Acetazolamide is an example of a carbonic anhydrase inhibitor (CAI).

Mechanism of action: CAIs inhibit the enzyme carbonic anhydrase, which catalyses the conversion of carbon dioxide and water to carbonic acid. The active transport of Na^+ and bicarbonate, one of the dissociation products of carbonic acid, is necessary in the production of aqueous humour (Fig. 9.3).

Route of administration: CAIs are administered systemically; topical CAIs have recently been introduced, e.g. dorzolamide.

Indications: Topical CAIs are used synergistically with β-adrenoceptor antagonists or miotics in the treatment of open-angle glaucoma.

Contraindications: CAIs should not be given to elderly people.

Adverse effects: Side effects of CAIs are mainly due to the systemic drugs. These effects can be reduced if the drugs are administered in a slow-release form. Side effects include diuresis, and, especially in the elderly, paraesthesia, hypokalaemia, decreased appetite, and drowsiness and depression.

The drugs that increase the drainage of aqueous humour are:

Muscarinic agonists

The muscarinic agonist, pilocarpine, is often used to increase drainage of the aqueous humour.

Mechanism of action: Pilocarpine causes contraction of the ciliary muscle, resulting in stretching and separation of the trabecular meshwork.

Route of administration: Pilocarpine is a tertiary amine and is applied topically to the eye.

Indications: Pilocarpine is used for open-angle glaucoma.

Contraindications: Pilocarpine should not be given to people with asthma.

Adverse effects: Side effects of pilocarpine include permanent miosis (pupil constriction) and accommodative spasm leading to blurred vision and headache. Systemic effects include hypersalivation and bronchospasm.

Anticholinesterases

The anticholinesterase physostigmine is sometimes used in association with pilocarpine, but not usually alone.

Mechanism of action: Physostigmine causes potentiation of cholinergic transmission.

Route of administration: Physostigmine is applied topically to the eye.

Indications: Physostigmine is used for open-angle glaucoma.

Contraindications: Physostigmine should not be given to people with asthma.

Adverse effects: Side effects of physostigmine are similar to those of pilocarpine. Allergic reactions may also occur.

Treatment of closed-angle glaucoma

Drugs to treat closed-angle glaucoma are used in emergencies as a temporary measure to reduce iris bombé and lower IOP.

Mannitol and glycerol are administered systemically and reduce IOP by increasing the osmolarity of the blood. The muscarinic agonists pilocarpine and carbachol are applied topically and reduce tautening of the iris which occurs as a result of the raised IOP.

Surgery

YAG (yttrium–aluminium–garnet) laser surgery provides a permanent cure for closed-angle glaucoma. A hole is made in the iris (iridectomy) to allow increased flow of aqueous humour.

Mydriatic and cycloplegic drugs

Use of mydriatic and cycloplegic drugs

Mydriatic drugs dilate the pupil, i.e. cause mydriasis, while cycloplegic drugs cause paralysis of the ciliary muscle, i.e. cycloplegia, with consequent inhibition of accommodation for near vision and the pupillary light reflex.

Both mydriatics and cycloplegics are used in ophthalmoscopy to allow a better view of the interior of the eye.

Mydriasis and cycloplegia reduce the drainage of the aqueous humour and should therefore be avoided in patients with closed-angle glaucoma.

Muscarinic antagonists

The most effective mydriatics are the muscarinic antagonists. These block the parasympathetic control of the iris sphincter muscle and the ciliary muscle.

The type of muscarinic antagonist chosen will depend on the length of the procedure and on whether or not cycloplegia is required.

The most commonly used muscarinic antagonists, their duration of action, and their mydratic and cycloplegic effects are summarized in Fig. 9.4.

α-Adrenoceptor agonists

α-Adrenoceptor agonists can cause mydriasis, but to a lesser extent than the muscarinic antagonists, by stimulating the sympathetic control of the iris dilator muscle. However, the sympathetic system does not control the ciliary muscle and therefore these drugs do not produce cycloplegia.

The α-agonist most commonly used to produce mydriasis is phenylephrine.

Muscarinic agonists and α-antagonists

At the end of an ophthalmological examination, a muscarinic agonist such as pilocarpine, or an α-antagonist such as thymoxamine may be used to reverse mydriasis. However, this is not usually necessary.

- ○ How is pupil size controlled?
- ○ Summarize how aqueous humour is produced and drained from the eye.
- ○ What are the differences between open-angle and closed-angle glaucoma?
- ○ Describe the different classes of drugs used to treat glaucoma. For each of these classes list examples, their mechanism of action, route of administration, indications, and major adverse effects.
- ○ In which situation are mydriatic and cycloplegic drugs used?

Effects of commonly used muscarinic antagonists			
Drug	Duration (h)	Mydriatic effect	Cycloplegic effect
tropicamide	1 – 3	++	+
cyclopentolate	12 – 24	+++	+++
atropine	168 – 240	+++	+++

Fig. 9.4 Mydriatics and cycloplegics effects of the commonly used muscarinic antagonists.

Glaucoma has a prevalence of approximately 1% in people aged over 40 years.

THE SKIN

Anatomy and physiology of the skin

The skin is the largest organ in the body, making up on average 16% of the total body weight and covering an area of approximately 1.8 m^2 (Fig. 9.5).

Function of the skin

The skin has several functions. These include:

- Protection, as the skin provides a barrier against chemical, mechanical and thermal stresses, ultraviolet light, dehydration, heat loss, and microorganisms.
- Thermoregulation, as hair and subcutaneous fat provide the body with insulation, whereas sweat glands and increased dermal blood flow allow heat loss.
- Sensation, as the skin contains receptors for touch, pressure, temperature, and pain.
- Metabolism, as synthesis of vitamin D takes place in the epidermis, and adipose tissue provides a store of energy in the form of triglycerides.

Skin disorders

The most common skin diseases are eczema, acne, viral warts, urticaria, psoriasis, and skin cancer.

Eczema (dermatitis)

Eczema is an inflammatory disease of the skin, defined by the presence of epidermal intercellular oedema or spongiosis.

Eczema can be due to a number of factors, such as:
- Exogenous irritants and contact allergens.
- Infections.
- Atopy.
- Drugs.
- Certain environmental conditions such as low humidity and ultraviolet light.

Drugs used to treat eczema are summarized in Fig. 9.6.

Acne

Acne affects the pilosebaceous unit and occurs where these are numerous, such as on the face, back, and chest.

Acne is characterized by the presence of keratin plugs in the sebaceous duct opening, known as comedones. Other signs of acne include inflammatory papules, pustules, nodules, cysts, and scars.

Acne is stimulated by androgens, which is why puberty induces this disease.

The drugs used to treat acne are summarized in Fig. 9.7.

Keratolytics (see below) are first-line drugs for the treatment of acne.

The pilosebaceous follicle is colonized by *Propionibacterium acnes*. For this reason, antibiotics are sometimes used in the treatment of acne, although antibiotic resistance to this particular bacterium can be as high as 40%.

Psoriasis

Psoriasis is a genetic skin disorder that manifests under certain conditions including stress, infection, damage from ultraviolet light, or trauma.

In psoriasis, the turnover rate of skin is eight times that of normal skin (7 instead of 56 days).

Psoriasis is characterized by:
- Thickened skin plaques.
- Superficial scales.
- Dilated capilliaries in the dermis (these might act to

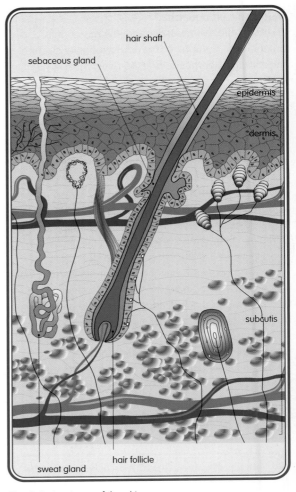

Fig. 9.5 Anatomy of the skin.

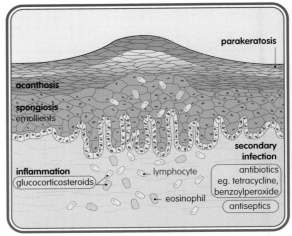

Fig. 9.6 Characteristics of eczema and its drug treatment.

initiate psoriasis or as nourishment for hyperproliferative skin).
- An infiltrate of inflammatory cells, especially lymphocytes and neutrophils, in the epidermis and dermis, respectively.

Drugs used to treat psoriasis are summarized in Fig. 9.8.

Treatment of skin disorders

Corticosteroids

Examples of corticosteroids include clobetasol propionate, betamethasone, clobetasol butyrate, and hydrocortisone.

> **Keratolytics remove keratin and are used to enhance the effect of emollients, or to reduce pore occlusion such as occurs in acne.**

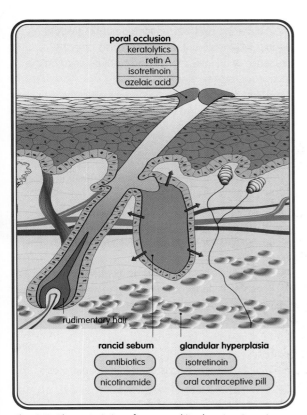

Fig. 9.7 Characteristics of acne and its drug treatment.

poral occlusion
- keratolytics
- retin A
- isotretinoin
- azelaic acid

rudimentary hair

rancid sebum
- antibiotics
- nicotinamide

glandular hyperplasia
- isotretinoin
- oral contraceptive pill

Mechanism of action: Corticosteroids suppress components of the inflammatory reaction (see Chapter 8; Fig. 9.6).

Route of administration: Corticosteroids are applied topically as creams, ointments, or lotions. In severe cases where there are local lesions, corticosteroids can be administered by intradermal injection.

Indications: Corticosteroids are used for the relief of symptoms due to inflammatory conditions of the skin other than those due to infection, e.g. in eczema.

Contraindications: Corticosteroids should not be given to people with rosacea, or ulcerative conditions, which they can exacerbate.

Adverse effects: Cessation of treatment with corticosteroids results in withdrawal, i.e. the condition rebounds. This is due to suppression of the pituitary–adrenal axis.

There are systemic side effects with potent topical corticosteroids.

Local adverse effects include thinning of the skin, spread and worsening of the untreated infection, irreversible striae atrophicae, hair growth, and perioral dermatitis.

Dithranol

Dithranol is the most potent topical drug for the treatment of psoriasis.

Mechanism of action: Dithranol modifies keratinization, but the mechanism is unclear (Fig. 9.8).

Route of administration: Dithranol is applied topically as a cream or ointment and left on the skin for 1 hour.

Indications: Dithranol is used for subacute and chronic psoriasis.

Contraindications: Dithranol should not be given to people with hypersensitivity or acute and pustular psoriasis.

Adverse effects: Side effects of dithranol include a local burning sensation and irritation, and skin and hair staining.

Vitamin D analogues

Calcipotriene is an example of a vitamin D analogue.

Vitamin D analogues are keratolytics.

Characteristics of psoriasis include an increased expression of vitamin D receptors in the basal and suprabasal layers of the epidermis and an increase in the density of vitamin D receptor positivity in intraepidermal and perivascular T cells and macrophages.

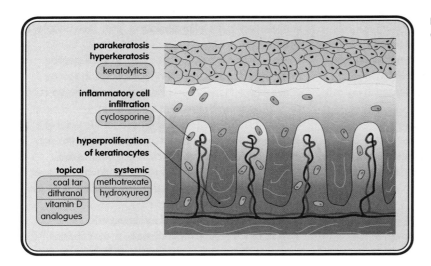

Fig. 9.8 Characteristics of psoriasis and its drug treatment.

Mechanism of action: The exact mechanism of action is still unclear, but several effects of vitamin D analogues have been observed. These include inhibition of epidermal proliferation and induction of terminal keratinocyte differentiation (Fig. 9.8).

The anti-inflammatory properties of vitamin D analogues include inhibition of T cell proliferation and of cytokine release, decreased capacity of monocytes to stimulate T cell proliferation and to stimulate lymphokine release from T cells, and inhibition of neutrophil accumulation in psoriatic skin.

Route of administration: Vitamin D analogues are applied topically as a cream, ointment, or scalp solution.

Indications: Vitamin D analogues are used for psoriasis.

Contraindications: Vitamin D analogues should not be given to people with disorders of calcium metabolism. They should not be used on the face, as irritation may occur.

Adverse effects: Side effects of vitamin D analogues include local irritation and dermatitis. High doses may affect calcium homoeostasis.

Tar preparations

Coal tar, made up of about 10 000 components, is a keratolytic that is more potent than salicylic acid. It also has anti-inflammatory and antipruritic properties.

Mechanism of action: Coal tar modifies keratinization, but the mechanism is unclear (Fig. 9.8).

Route of administration: Coal tar is applied topically.

Indications: Coal tar is used for psoriasis and sometimes for eczema.

Contraindications: Coal tar should not be given to people with acute or pustular psoriasis or in the presence of an infection. It should not be used on the face, or on broken or inflamed skin.

Adverse effects: Side effects of coal tar include skin irritation and acne-like eruptions, photosensitivity, and skin and hair staining.

Salicylates

Salicylic acid is keratolytic at a concentration of 3–6%. Approximately 95% of a single dose of salicylic acid is excreted in the urine within 24 hours.

Toxic levels (30–50 mg/dL) are usually fatal (1 g of 6% salicylic acid results in plasma concentrations of 0.5 mg/dL).

Mechanism of action: Salicylic acid causes desquamation via the solubilization of cell-surface proteins that maintain the integrity of the stratum corneum.

Route of administration: Salicylic acid is applied topically.

Indications: Salicylic acid is used for hyperkeratosis,

eczema, psoriasis (combined with coal tar or dithranol preparations), acne (concentrations up to 2%), and wart and callus eradication (concentrations up to 50%).

Contraindications: Salicylic acid should not be given to people with sensitivity to the drug, or broken or inflamed skin. High concentrations, such as those needed to treat warts, should not be given to people with diabetes mellitus or peripheral vascular disease, as ulceration may be induced.

Adverse effects: Side effects of salicylic acid include anaphylactic shock in those sensitive to the drug, skin irritation and excessive drying, and systemic effects if used long term. Concentrations above 3–6% destroy tissue.

Emollients

Emollients are used to soothe the skin. They are available as creams or ointments and require frequent applications, especially if a cream vehicle is used.

A simple preparation is aqueous cream, which is often as effective as more complex drugs.

Most creams are thin emollients, whereas a mixture of equal parts soft white paraffin and liquid paraffin is a thick emollient.

Camphor, menthol, and phenol preparations have antipruritic effects, whereas zinc- and titanium-based emollients have mild astringent effects.

Calamine and zinc oxide enhance therapeutic efficacy.

Mechanism of action: Emollients hydrate the skin and reduce transepidermal water loss.

Route of administration: Emollients are applied topically.

Indications: Emollients are used for the long-term treatment of dry scaling disorders such as ichthyosis and atopic dermatitis. They are also useful in eczema and, to a lesser extent, in psoriasis.

Contraindications: None.

Adverse effects: Some ingredients, such as lanolin or antibacterials, may induce an allergic reaction.

Preparations of drugs for use on skin

Drugs applied to the skin are delivered by a variety of vehicles such as ointments, creams, pastes, powders, aerosols, gels, lotions, and tinctures.

Factors affecting the choice of vehicle include:
- The solubility of the active drug.
- The ability of the drug to enhance penetration of the skin.
- The stability of the drug–vehicle complex.
- The ability of the vehicle to delay evaporation, this being greatest for ointments and least for tinctures.

Factors that affect the absorption of the drug include:
- Body site, in that absorption is greatest from the scrotum and vulva, high from the scalp and face, and lowest from the palms and soles.
- Skin hydration, as occlusive dressings can increase the absorption of a drug tenfold, for example.
- Skin condition, because damage caused by burns and inflammation increases absorption.
- The concentration gradient across the skin (the greater this is, the greater the rate of absorption).

- Summarize the common skin disorders (eczema, acne, psoriasis) and their treatment.
- What are the different classes of drugs used to treat skin diseases? For each of these classes list examples, their mechanism of action, route of administration, indications, and major adverse effects.
- Which factors affect the choice of vehicles for drugs used on the skin?
- Which factors affect the absorption of drugs used on the skin?

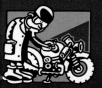

10. Immune System

INFLAMMATION AND ANTI-INFLAMMATORY DRUGS

Concepts of inflammation

Inflammation describes the changes seen in response to tissue injury or insult, as originally defined by the Latin words *dolor, rubor, calor, and tumor*, meaning pain, redness, heat, and swelling.

These changes result from alterations in local blood vessels. This leads to dilatation of the blood vessels, their increased permeability, and increased receptiveness for leucocytes, resulting in the accumulation of inflammatory cells at the site of injury. The main cells seen in an acute inflammatory response are polymorphonuclear neutrophil leucocytes and macrophages. Lymphocytes, as well as basophils and eosinophils, also accumulate, especially in certain types of inflammation.

Inflammatory responses are produced and controlled by the interaction of a wide range of inflammatory mediators, some derived from leucocytes, some from the

tissues. Examples include histamine, kinins (bradykinin), neuropeptides (substance-P, calcitonin gene-related peptide), cytokines [e.g. interleukins (ILs)] and the arachidonic acid metabolites (eicosanoids).

Arachidonic acid metabolites: the eicosanoids

Of the inflammatory mediators mentioned above, the eicosanoids are of special importance because:

- They are involved in the majority of inflammatory reactions.
- Most anti-inflammatory therapy is based on the manipulation of their biosynthesis [i.e. non-steroidal anti-inflammatory drugs (NSAIDs) and steroidal anti-inflammatory drugs (glucocorticoids)].

The eicosanoids are a family of polyunsaturated fatty acids formed from arachidonic acid. The biosynthetic pathway is shown in Fig. 10.1.

Arachidonic acid is stored mainly in the phospholipids of cell membranes, from which it is

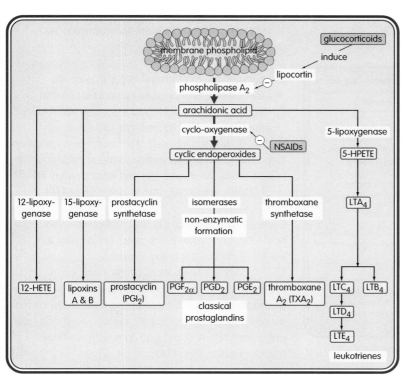

Fig. 10.1 Biosynthetic pathway of the eicosanoids. (LT, leukotrienes; HETE, hydroxyeicosatetraenoic acid; PG, prostaglandin; HPETE, hydroperoxyeicosatetraenoic acid; NSAID, non-steroidal anti-inflammatory drug.)

mobilized by the action of the enzyme phospholipase A_2 (for site of action of glucocorticoids, see later).

Arachidonic acid is then further metabolized:

- By cyclooxygenase (for site of action of NSAIDs, see later) to produce the 'classical prostaglandins', thromboxane and prostacyclin, collectively known as the prostanoids.
- By lipoxygenase to produce the leukotrienes.

The actions of eicosanoids in inflammatory reactions are listed in Fig. 10.2.

Anti-inflammatory drugs

The main drugs used for their broad-spectrum anti-inflammatory effects are:

- Non-steroidal anti-inflammatory drugs (pp . 166–168).
- Steroidal anti-inflammatory drugs (glucocorticoids) (see Chapter 8 and pp. 168–169).

Both these classes of anti-inflammatory drug exert their effect by inhibiting the formation of eicosanoids (see Fig. 10.1).

In addition, a number of other classes of drug, used clinically under certain circumstances, have more restricted anti-inflammatory actions. These are:

- Disease-modifying anti-rheumatic drugs (DMARDs) (pp. 169–170).
- Drugs used to treat gout (pp. 170–171).
- Antihistamines (pp. 172–174).

Actions of the eicosanoids in the inflammatory reaction	
Eicosanoid	**Actions in inflammation**
prostanoids	
'classical prostaglandins' e.g. PGD_2, PGE_2, PGF_2	produce increased vasodilatation, vascular permeability and oedema in an inflammatory reaction; prostaglandins also sensitize nociceptive fibres to stimulation by other inflammatory mediators
thromboxane A_2 (TXA_2)	platelet aggregation and vasoconstriction
prostacyclin (PGI_2)	inhibition of platelet aggregation and vasodilatation
leukotrienes	
e.g. LTB_4, LTC_4	increase vascular permeability, promote leucocyte chemotaxis (and cause contraction of bronchial smooth muscle)

Fig. 10.2 Actions of the eicosanoids in the inflammatory reaction.

Non-steroidal anti-inflammatory drugs

NSAIDs are a chemically diverse group of drugs that all possess the ability to inhibit the enzyme cyclooxygenase (see Fig. 10.1), an action that is responsible for their pharmacological effects (see Fig. 10.4).

The first drugs of this type were the salicylates (e.g. aspirin) extracted from the bark of the willow tree. Subsequently, many (>50 on the market) synthetic and semi-synthetic NSAIDs have been created by pharmacologists. Chemically and structurally heterogeneous, they are related through their common mechanism of action (Fig. 10.3).

Mechanism of action: The main action of all the NSAIDs is inhibition of the enzyme cyclooxygenase. This enzyme is involved in the metabolism of arachidonic acid to form the prostanoids, i.e. the 'classical prostaglandins', prostacyclin and thromboxane A_2.

Inhibition of cyclooxygenase can occur by several mechanisms:

- Irreversible inhibition—e.g. aspirin causes acetylation of the active site.
- Competitive inhibition—e.g. ibuprofen acts as a competitive substrate.
- Reversible, non-competitive inhibition—e.g. paracetamol has a free radical trapping action that interferes with the production of hydroperoxidases, which are believed to have an essential role in cyclooxygenase activity.

Cyclooxygenase exists in two enzyme isoforms:

- COX-1, which is expressed in most tissues and involved in physiological cell signalling. Most adverse effects are caused by inhibition of COX-1.
- COX-2, which is induced at sites of inflammation and produces the prostanoids involved in inflammatory responses. Analgesic and anti-inflammatory effects of NSAIDs are largely due to inhibition of COX-2.

Currently available NSAIDs are unselective, inhibiting both COX-1 and COX-2. The potential for selective inhibitors of COX-2 is being explored.

Clinical effects: NSAIDs work by the inhibition of cyclooxygenase and resulting inhibition of prostaglandin synthesis, producing three major clinical actions of potential therapeutic benefit: analgesia, an anti-inflammatory action and an antipyretic (fever reducing) action (Fig. 10.4).

Not all NSAIDs possess these three actions to exactly the same extent, an example being the lack of anti-inflammatory activity possessed by paracetamol (see Fig. 10.3).

In addition to these three main categories of effect, aspirin has a pronounced effect on inhibiting platelet aggregation, due to reduced thromboxane synthesis. This has led to its successful use after myocardial infarction to prevent vascular occlusion (see Chapter 4).

Indications: NSAIDs are widely used for a variety of complaints. They are available on prescription and 'over

the counter'. Their use includes musculoskeletal and joint diseases (strains, sprains, rheumatic problems, arthritis, gout etc.), analgesia for mild to moderate pain relief including headaches, and symptomatic relief in fever.

Contraindications: NSAIDs should not be given to people with gastrointestinal ulceration or bleeding, or a previous hypersensitivity to any NSAID.

Adverse effects: Generalized adverse effects of NSAIDs are common, especially in the elderly and in chronic users, and mostly arise from the non-selective inhibition of COX-1 and COX-2 synthesis (Fig. 10.5).

Fig. 10.3 Classes of non-steroidal anti-inflammatory drugs and comparison of their main actions.

Non-steroidal anti-inflammatory drugs				
Chemical class	Examples	Analgesic	Antipyretic	Anti-inflammatory
salicylic acids	aspirin	+	+	+
propionic acids	ibuprofen fenuprofen	+	+	+
acetic acids	indomethacin	+	+	++
oxicams	piroxicam	+	+	++
pyrazolones	phenylbutazone	+/−	+	++
fenemates	mefenamic acid	+	+	+/−
para-aminophenols	paracetemol	+	+	−

Fig. 10.4 Three major clinical actions of non-steroidal anti-inflammatory drugs (NSAIDs).

Major clinical effects of NSAIDs	
Clinical action	Mechanism of action
analgesic action	• the analgesic effect is largely a peripheral effect that is due to the inhibition of prostaglandin synthesis at the site of pain and inflammation • prostaglandins do not produce pain directly, but sensitize nociceptive fibre nerve endings to other inflammatory mediators (bradykinin, histamine, 5-HT), amplifying the basic pain message; prostaglandins of the E and F series are implicated in this sensitizing action • thus NSAIDs are most effective against pain where there is an inflammatory component • a small component of the analgesic action of NSAIDs is a consequence of a central effect in reducing prostaglandin synthesis in the CNS; paracetamol especially works in this manner
anti-inflammatory action	• prostaglandins produce increased vasodilatation, vascular permeability and oedema in an inflammatory reaction • inhibition of prostaglandin synthesis therefore reduces this part of the inflammatory reaction • NSAIDs do not inhibit the numerous other mediators involved in an inflammatory reaction; thus inflammatory cell accumulation, for example, is not inhibited
antipyretic action	• during a fever, leucocytes release inflammatory pyrogens (e.g. interleukin-1) as part of the immune response; these act on the thermoregulatory centre in the hypothalamus to cause an increase in body temperature • this effect is believed to be mediated by an increase in hypothalamic prostaglandins (PGEs), the generation of which is inhibited by NSAIDs • NSAIDs do not affect temperature under normal circumstances or in heat stroke

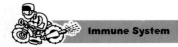

General adverse effects of NSAIDs		
System	Adverse effect	Cause
GI	dyspepsia, nausea, vomiting; ulcer formation and potential haemorrhage risk in chronic users	inhibition of the normal protective actions of prostaglandins on the gastric mucosa. PGE_2 and PGI_2 normally inhibit gastric acid secretion, increase mucosal blood flow, and have a cytoprotective action
renal	renal damage/nephrotoxicity; renal failure can occur after years of chronic abuse	inhibition of PGE_2- and PGI_2-mediated vasodilatation in the renal medulla and glomeruli
other	bronchospasm, skin rashes, other allergic-type reactions	hypersensitivity reaction/allergy to drug

Fig. 10.5 General adverse effects of non-steroidal anti-inflammatory drugs (NSAIDs). (GI, gastrointestinal.)

Less commonly, liver disorders and bone marrow depression are seen.

Other unwanted effects that are relatively specific to individual compounds are also seen (see below).

Therapeutic notes on individual NSAIDs
Salicylic acids, e.g. aspirin, which:
- Is cheap, and is still the drug of choice for many sorts of mild pain despite a relatively high incidence of gastrointestinal side effects. It is also used for antiplatelet action following myocardial infarction.
- Produces tinnitus in toxic doses.

Propionic acids, e.g. ibuprofen, which:
- Is effective and well tolerated.
- Is the drug of choice for inflammatory joint disease, owing to its low incidence of side effects.

Acetic acids, e.g. indomethacin, which:
- Is a highly potent inhibitor of COX that is effective but associated with a high incidence of side effects.
- Commonly causes neurological effects such as dizziness and confusion, as well as gastrointestinal upsets.

Oxicams, e.g. piroxicam, which:
- Is a potent drug widely used for chronic inflammatory conditions.
- Is given only once daily, but causes a relatively high incidence of gastrointestinal problems.

Pyrazolones, e.g. phenylbutazone, which:
- Is an extremely potent agent but can produce a fatal bone marrow aplasia. For this reason it is reserved for the treatment of intractable pain in ankylosing spondylitis.

Fenemates, e.g. mefenamic acid, which:
- Is a moderately potent drug.
- Commonly causes gastrointestinal upsets and occasionally skin rashes.

para-Aminophenols, e.g. paracetamol, which:
- Is used as an analgesic only and not as an anti-inflammatory drug.
- Is effective for pain, especially headaches, and fever. This is probably due to its mechanism of action in trapping free radicals and interfering with the production of hydroperoxidases, which are believed to have an essential role in cyclooxygenase activity. In areas of inflammation, phagocytic cells produce high levels of peroxide that swamp this effect.
- Causes a serious, potentially fatal hepatotoxicity in toxic doses (2–3 times therapeutic) that saturate the normal liver conjugation systems, leading to the formation of a toxic metabolite, *N*-acetyl-*p*-benzoquinone (see Chapter 1).

Steroidal anti-inflammatory drugs (glucocorticoids)
Glucocorticoids possess powerful anti-inflammatory actions that make them useful in several diseases, e.g. rheumatoid arthritis, inflammatory bowel conditions, bronchial asthma, and inflammatory conditions of the skin.

Their profound generalized inhibitory effects on inflammatory responses result from the effects of corticosteroids in altering the activity of certain corticosteroid-responsive genes. The anti-inflammatory action results from:

- Reduced production of acute inflammatory mediators, especially the eicosanoids (see Fig. 10.1). Corticosteroids prevent the formation of arachidonic acid from membrane phospholipids by inducing the synthesis of a polypeptide called lipocortin. Lipocortin inhibits phospholipase A_2, the enzyme normally responsible for mobilizing arachidonic acid from cell membrane phospholipids, and thus inhibits the subsequent formation of both prostaglandins and leukotrienes.
- Reduced numbers and activity of circulating immunocompetent cells, neutrophils, and macrophages.
- Decreased activity of macrophages and fibroblasts involved in the chronic stages of inflammation, leading to decreased inflammation and decreased healing.

Glucocorticoids are discussed in detail in Chapter 8.

Disease-modifying anti-rheumatic drugs

DMARDs are a diverse group of agents that are mainly used in the treatment of rheumatoid arthritis, a chronic, progressive, and destructive inflammatory disease of the joints (Fig. 10.6).

The mechanism of action of the DMARDs is often unclear—they appear to have a long-term depressive effect upon the inflammatory response as well as possibly modulating other aspects of the immune system.

All DMARDs have a slow onset of action, with clinical improvement not becoming apparent until 4–6 months after the initiation of treatment. DMARDs have been shown to improve symptoms and reduce disease activity. Whether they alter the long-term outcome of the disease is controversial.

DMARDs are generally indicated for use in severe, active, progressive rheumatoid arthritis when NSAIDs alone have proved inadequate. DMARDs are frequently used in combination with an NSAID and/or low dose glucocorticoids.

Disease-modifying anti-rheumatic drugs (DMARDs)	
Class	Example
gold salts	sodium aurothiomalate, auranofin
penicillamine	
antimalarials	chloroquine, hydroxyquinine
sulphasalazine	
immunosuppressants	cytotoxic drugs: methotrexate, azathioprine, cyclosporin

Fig. 10.6 Disease-modifying anti-rheumatic drugs.

Gold salts
Examples of gold salts include sodium aurothiomalate and auranofin.

Mechanism of action: The mechanism of action of gold salts is unknown—they may be taken up by, and inhibit, mononuclear macrophages, or may affect the production of free radicals.

Route of administration: Sodium aurothiomalate is given by intramuscular injection, and auranofin orally.

Adverse effects: Side effects of gold salts can be severe, including rashes, proteinuria, ulceration, diarrhoea, and bone marrow suppression.

Therapeutic notes: When administering gold salts, careful patient monitoring, including blood counts and urine analysis, is necessary. If any serious adverse effects develop, treatment must be stopped.

Penicillamine
Mechanism of action: The mechanism of action of penicillamine is unknown. It chelates metals and has immunomodulatory effects, including suppression of immunoglobulin production and effects on immune complexes.

Route of administration: Penicillamine is administered orally.

Adverse effects: Side effects of penicillamine are common and varied—many are similar to those of gold salts, such as rashes, proteinuria, ulceration, gastrointestinal upsets, fever, transient loss of taste, and bone marrow suppression.

Therapeutic notes: When administering penicillamine, careful patient monitoring, including blood counts and urine analysis, is necessary. If any serious adverse effects develop, treatment must be stopped.

Antimalarials
Examples of antimalarials include chloroquine and hydroxyquinine (see Chapter 12).

Mechanism of action: The mechanism of antimalarials is unclear. They interfere with a wide variety of leucocyte functions, including IL-1 production by macrophages, lymphoproliferative responses, and T-cell cytotoxic responses.

Route of administration: Antimalarials are administered orally.

Adverse effects: At the low doses currently recommended for antimalarials, toxicity is rare. The major adverse effect is retinal toxicity.

Therapeutic notes: People on antimalarials should have their vision monitored.

Sulphasalazine

Mechanism of action: Sulphasalazine is broken down in the gut into its two component molecules, 5-aminosalicylate (5-ASA) and sulphapyridine. It is believed that sulphapyridine is absorbed systemically and is responsible for the therapeutic effect, the mechanism being unknown.

Route of administration: Sulphasalazine is administered orally.

Adverse effects: Side effects of sulphasalazine are mainly due to sulphapyridine; they are common, but rarely serious. These include nausea, vomiting, headache, and rashes. Rarely, blood disorders and oligospermia are reported.

Therapeutic notes: People on sulphasalazine should have their blood counts monitored.

Immunosuppressants

Certain drugs with immunosuppressive actions have been shown to be effective in rheumatoid arthritis. These include azathioprine, cyclosporin A, and corticosteroids which may work by suppressing the autoimmune component of rheumatoid arthritis (pp. 175–177).

Drugs used in gout

Gout is a condition in which uric acid (monosodium urate) crystals are deposited in tissues, especially the joints, provoking an inflammatory response that manifests as an extremely painful acute arthritis. Uric acid crystallizes in the tissues when plasma urate levels are high, due to either excessive production (10%) or reduced renal excretion (90%).

There are two treatment strategies for gout—treatment of an acute attack and prophylaxis against further attacks (Fig. 10.7).

Treatment of an acute attack
Non-steroidal anti-inflammatory drugs
At the onset of an acute attack of gout, NSAIDs are used for their general anti-inflammatory and analgesic effects (pp. 166–168).

Aspirin and other salicylates are not used in gout as they antagonize uricosuric drugs.

Colchicine
Mechanism of action: Colchicine helps in gouty arthritis by inhibiting the migration of leucocytes such as neutrophils into the inflamed joint. This effect is achieved as a result of the action of colchicine binding to tubulin, the protein monomer of microtubules, resulting in their depolymerization. The end result is that cytoskeletal movements and cell motility are severely inhibited.

The inhibition of microtubular function inhibits mitotic spindle formation, giving colchicine a cytotoxic effect on dividing cells. This cytotoxic effect is responsible for side effects of colchicine.

Route of administration: Colchicine is administered orally and, rarely, intravenously.

Adverse effects: Side effects of colchicine include gastrointestinal toxicity, with nausea, vomiting, and diarrhoea, occurring in 80% of people. Rarely, bone marrow suppression and renal failure occur.

Therapeutic notes: Colchicine is rapidly effective. It is given for the first 24 hours of an attack and then no further for 7 days.

Prophylaxis against recurrent attacks
Preventative management of gout includes diet and lifestyle changes, as well as the use of drugs that reduce plasma uric acid concentration. These drugs should not be used during an acute attack, as they will initially worsen symptoms. NSAIDs or colchicine should be co-administered for the first 3 months of treatment, as initiation of treatment may precipitate an attack.

Drugs used in the treatment of gout	
Treatment of an acute attack	**Example**
NSAIDs	indomethacin
immunosuppressive	colchicine
Prophylaxis against recurrent attacks (reduction of plasma uric acid concentration)	
agents that reduce uric acid synthesis	allopurinol
agents that increase uric acid excretion (uricosurics)	sulphinpyrazone, probenecid

Fig. 10.7 Drugs used in the treatment of gout.

Agents that reduce uric acid synthesis

Allopurinol is an example of a drug that reduces uric acid synthesis.

Mechanism of action: Allopurinol inhibits the enzyme xanthine oxidase, thus reducing uric acid production.

Route of administration: Allopurinol is administered orally.

Adverse effects: Common side effects of allopurinol include headaches, dyspepsia, diarrhoea, rash, drug interactions, and acute exacerbation of gout initially. Rarely, life-threatening hypersensitivity occurs.

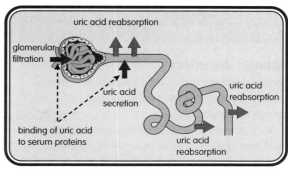

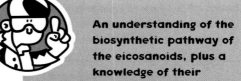

Fig. 10.8 Uric acid secretion and reabsorption in the kidney.

Agents that increase uric acid excretion

Uricosurics are drugs that increase uric acid excretion. Examples of uricosurics include sulphinpyrazone and probenecid.

Mechanism of action: Uricosurics compete with uric acid for reabsorption in the proximal tubules (see Fig. 10.8).

Route of administration: Uricosurics are administered orally.

Adverse effects: Side effects of uricosurics include gastrointestinal upset, deposition of uric acid crystals in the kidney, interference with excretion of certain drugs, and acute exacerbation of gout initially.

Therapeutic notes: Uricosurics should not be used during an acute attack of gout. NSAIDs or colchinine should be co-administered for the first 3 months of treatment, as initiation of treatment may precipitate an attack.

An understanding of the biosynthetic pathway of the eicosanoids, plus a knowledge of their inflammatory actions is central to understanding the mode of action of NSAIDs and steroidal anti-inflammatory drugs in reducing inflammation.

○ Describe the nature of inflammation, and the pathways, mediators, and cells involved. Discuss how drugs can affect this process.

○ Describe the important role of the eicosanoids in inflammation, and how NSAIDs and glucocorticoids act on this component pathway of the inflammatory process.

○ Name the various classes of NSAID and give examples of drugs from each. Describe their mechanism of action, clinical effects, indications, and adverse effects.

○ Describe the use of glucocorticoids (see Chapter 8) in inflammatory disease processes.

○ List the different classes of DMARD and when they may be of use. Describe their mechanism of action if known, clinical effects, indications, and adverse effects.

○ What are the pathological processes involved in gout, and in what way may drugs be used to affect these processes?

ALLERGIC DISORDERS AND DRUG THERAPY

Allergic disorders

Allergic reactions occur when the immune system mounts an inappropriate response to an innocuous foreign substance.

Most common allergic disorders are caused by IgE-mediated type I immediate hypersensitivity reactions that occur in a previously sensitized person re-exposed to the sensitizing antigen. Type I immediate hypersensitivity reactions are also known as atopic disorders.

Patients with atopic diseases have an inherited predisposition to develop IgE antibodies to allergens that are innocuous and non-antigenic in normal people. These specific IgE antibodies become bound to high-affinity IgE receptors (FcϵRI) on the surface of tissue mast cells and blood basophils. The cross-linking of this cell-surface-bound IgE by antigens (allergens), on subsequent exposure, induces degranulation and release of mediators such as histamine, leukotrienes,

and prostaglandins (Fig. 10.9).

The released vasoactive and inflammatory mediators produce many effects, including vasodilatation, increased vascular permeability, smooth muscle contraction, oedema, glandular hypersecretion, and inflammatory cell infiltration.

Depending on the site of this reaction and release of mediators, a variety of disorders can result (Fig. 10.10).

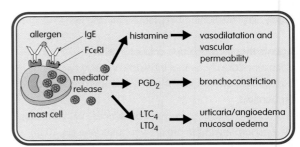

Fig. 10.9 Mechanism of type 1 hypersensitivity (allergic) reaction. (FcϵRI, cell surface IgE receptor; LT, leukotriene; PG, prostaglandin.)

Fig. 10.10 Type I hypersensitivity/allergic disorders.

Type I hypersensitivity/allergic disorders			
Disorder	**Site of reaction**	**Response**	**Common allergens**
anaphylaxis	circulation	oedema, circulatory collapse, death	venoms drugs
allergic rhinitis/ hay fever	nasal passages conjunctiva	irritation, oedema, mucosal hypersecretion	pollen dust
asthma (Chapter 5)	bronchioles	bronchoconstriction, mucosal secretion, airway inflammation	pollen dust
food allergy	GIT	vomiting, diarrhoea, urticaria (hives)	seafood milk etc.
wheal and flare	skin	vasodilatation and oedema	insect venom

Fig. 10.11 Drug therapy in allergic disorders.

Drug therapy in allergic disorders			
Disorder	**Drugs used**	**Chapter**	**Mechanism of action**
anaphylaxis	adrenaline	2 & 4	vasoconstriction (α_2) bronchodilation (β_2)
	antihistamines	5 & 11	pro-inflammatory mediator antagonism
	glucocorticoids	8 & 11	anti-inflammatory
allergic rhinitis/ hay fever	antihistamines	5 & 11	pro-inflammatory mediator antagonism
	mast-cell stabilizers	5 & 11	inhibition of mast-cell degranulation
	glucocorticoids	8 & 11	anti-inflammatory
	sympathomimetic vasoconstrictors	2, 4 & 11	decongestion of nasal mucosa
asthma	see Chapter 5	5	see Chapter 5
food allergies	antihistamines	5 & 11	pro-inflammatory mediator antagonism
wheal and flare	antihistamines	5 & 11	pro-inflammatory mediator antagonism

Drug therapy of allergic disorders

The most effective therapy in hypersensitivity reactions is avoidance of the offending antigen or environment. When this is not possible, drug therapy can be of use (Fig. 10.11).

Histamine and antihistamines

Histamine is a basic amine that is stored in mast cells (fixed in the tissues) and in circulating basophils; it is also found in the stomach and central nervous system (CNS).

The effects of histamine are mediated by three different receptor types found on target cells (Fig. 10.12).

As the major autocoid released during an allergic reaction, histamine produces a number of effects, mainly via action on H_1-receptors. Therefore H_1 antagonists (antihistamines) are of potential benefit in the treatment of allergic disorders.

H_1-Receptor antagonists: antihistamines

There are two types of antihistamines. These are:

- 'Old' sedative types, e.g. chlorpheniramine and promethazine.
- 'New' non-sedative types, e.g. terfenadine and astemizole.

Mechanism of action: Antihistamines work by antagonism of histamine H_1-receptors (Fig. 10.12). Apart from astemizole, which produces a high-affinity non-competitive block, all are competitive antagonists.

In the periphery, their action can inhibit allergic reactions where histamine is the main mediator involved.

The old-style antihistamines are able to cross the blood–brain barrier where both specific and non-specific actions in the CNS produce sedation and antiemetic effects.

Indications: The main use of antihistamines is in the treatment of seasonal allergic rhinitis ('hay fever'). They are also used for the treatment and prevention of allergic skin reactions such as urticarial rashes, pruritus, and insect bites, and in the emergency treatment of anaphylactic shock.

The old-style antihistamines can also be used as mild hypnotics (see Chapter 3), and to suppress nausea in motion sickness, owing to their actions on the CNS.

Route of administration: Antihistamines are administered orally, and applied topically as eye drops, creams, or nasal sprays. Intravenous chlorpheniramine is used in anaphylaxis.

Adverse effects: Old-style antihistamines produce quite pronounced sedation or fatigue, as well as anticholinergic effects such as dry mouth. The newer agents do not do this.

Rare hazardous arrhythmias are associated with the 'new' antihistamines (astemizole/terfenadine), especially at high plasma levels or when in combination with imidazole antifungal agents or macrolide antibiotics (Chapter 12).

Hypersensitivity reactions, especially to topically applied antihistamines, may occur.

Mast-cell stabilizers

Mast cell-stabilizers have recently been introduced for topical application and control of local inflammation in allergic rhinitis and conjunctivitis. Examples include cromoglycate and nedocromil sodium.

Fig. 10.12 Effects at histamine receptors.

Histamine receptors	
Histamine receptor	**Effect**
H_1	responsible for most of the actions of histamine in a type I hypersensitivity reaction: • capillary and venous dilatation (producing 'flare' or systemic hypotension) • increased vascular permeability (producing 'wheal' or oedema) • contraction of smooth muscle (producing bronchial and gastrointestinal contraction)
H_2	regulation of gastric acid secretion: • H_2-receptors respond to histamine secreted from the enterochromaffin-like cells that are adjacent to the parietal cell (see Chapter 7)
H_3	involved in neurotransmission: • exact physiological role not clear (presynaptic inhibition of neurotransmitter release in the CNS and autonomic nervous system? role in itch and pain perception?)

Mechanism of action: The exact modes of action of mast-cell stabilizers are unclear. These drugs appear to stabilize antigen-sensitized mast cells by reducing calcium influx and subsequent release of inflammatory mediators.

Indications: Mast-cell stabilizers are used for the prophylaxis and treatment of allergic rhinitis and conjunctivitis.

Route of administration: Mast-cell stabilizers are administered by aqueous nasal spray or eye drops.

Adverse effects: Side effects of mast-cell stabilizers include transient local irritation.

Therapeutic notes: Mast-cell stabilizers are applied topically and thus have very few adverse effects. They have a prophylactic action and thus are most effective when used regularly during the hay fever season.

Anti-inflammatory: glucocorticoids

Glucocorticoid sprays applied topically are very effective in preventing allergic rhinitis when used regularly during the hay fever season.

Glucocorticoids are administered by two routes:

- Nasally by aqueous sprays, e.g. beclomethasone dipropionate, budesonide, and fluticasone propionate.
- Intravenously, e.g. hydrocortisone. Intravenous hydrocortisone is of secondary value in the initial management of anaphylactic shock.

Mechanism of action: Corticosteroids depress the inflammatory response in the nasal mucosa and thereby reduce the rhinitis (see Chapter 8). Specific effects include:

- Reduced mucosal oedema and mucus production.
- Decreased local generation of prostaglandins and leukotrienes, with less inflammatory cell activation.
- Long-term reduced T-cell cytokine production.
- Reduced eosinophil and mast cell infiltration of nasal mucosa.

Indications: Glucocorticoids are used in the prophylaxis and treatment of allergic rhinitis, and for anaphylaxis.

Contraindications: Glucocorticoids should not be given to people with untreated nasal infection.

Adverse effects: Rarely, glucocorticoids cause dryness and irritation of the nose and throat, nosebleeds, or taste disturbances.

Therapeutic notes: Used topically, the nasally applied glucocorticoids have very few side effects. These drugs have a prophylactic action and thus are most effective

when used regularly during the hay fever season. The full effect takes 3 days to develop.

Used intravenously during anaphylaxis, hydrocortisone is useful for preventing further deterioration in severely affected people but is only of secondary value, as the onset of action is delayed for several hours.

Sympathomimetic decongestants

Examples of sympathomimetic decongestants include topical nasal sprays/drops, e.g. ephedrine, and oral decongestants, e.g. phenylephrine—contained in proprietary preparations.

Mechanism of action: Nasal congestion is caused by inflammation of the nasal mucosa (rhinitis) and hypersecretory production of mucus leading to 'streaming' of the nose (rhinorrhoea), both of which involve active vasodilatation of the nasal mucosa. Ephedrine has mixed α- and β-adrenoceptor agonist activity and also causes noradrenaline release, whereas phenylephrine is an α_1-selective adrenoceptor agonist. They cause vasoconstriction of the mucosal blood vessels, which in turn reduces the thickness of the nasal mucosa, and the rate of mucus hypersecretion (see Chapters 2 and 4).

Indications: Sympathomimetic decongestants are used for the temporary symptomatic relief of nasal congestion in allergic rhinitis and nasal infections.

Contraindications: Systemic sympathomimetics should not be given to people with cardiovascular problems or diabetes. All are contraindicated in people taking monoamine oxidase inhibitors, as they would provoke a hypertensive crisis.

Adverse effects: Topical application of sympathomimetic decongestants tends to give rise to 'rebound congestion' due to a secondary vasodilatation after the effects wear off.

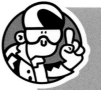

The basic mechanism of disease is the same in all atopic allergic disorders (type I immediate hypersensitivity). The variety of allergic disorders results from the differing locations where the reaction can take place.

- Describe the immunological and inflammatory processes involved in type I immediate hypersensitivity reactions.
- Name the different types of allergic disorders that can be caused by such reactions.
- Discuss the different ways in which drugs can be used therapeutically in such disorders.
- What is the importance of histamine in allergic reactions? Relate the mechanism of action of antihistamine drugs to this.
- Name the different antihistamine drugs, how they can be taken, and the major adverse effects associated with their use.
- Aside from antihistamines, what other classes of drug are used in the prophylaxis and treatment of hay fever? Name examples, give their mechanism of action, and describe how they are administered.

IMMUNOSUPPRESSANTS

Introduction

Deliberate pharmacological suppression of the immune system is used in the following three main clinical areas:

- To suppress inappropriate autoimmune responses (e.g. systemic lupus erythematosus or rheumatoid arthritis), where the host immune system is 'attacking' host tissue.
- To suppress host immune rejection responses to donor organ grafts or transplants.
- To suppress donor immune responses against host antigens (prevention of graft versus host disease after bone marrow transplant (GVHD)).

The main pharmacological agents used for immunosuppression are:

- Cyclosporin.
- Azathioprine.
- Glucocorticoids (see Chapter 8).

Immunosuppressant drugs

Cyclosporin A

Mechanism of action: Cyclosporin A is a cyclic peptide, derived from fungi, that has powerful immunosuppressive activity. It has a selective inhibitory effect on T cells by inhibiting the T-cell receptor (TCR)-mediated signal-transduction pathway. It is believed to exert its actions after entering the T cell and preventing the transcription of specific genes (Fig. 10.13).

After entry into the T cell, cyclosporin A specifically binds to its cytoplasmic binding protein, cyclophilin. This cyclosporin–cyclophilin complex then binds to a serine/threonine phosphatase called calcineurin, inhibiting its phosphatase activity. Calcineurin is normally activated when intracellular calcium ion levels rise following T-cell-receptor binding to the appropriate major histocompatibility complex:antigen complex. When calcineurin is active it dephosphorylates the cytoplasmic component of the nuclear factor of activated T cells (NF-ATc) into a form that migrates to the nucleus and induces transcription of genes such as IL-2 that are involved in T-cell activation.

Inhibition of calcineurin by the cyclosporin–cyclophilin complex therefore prevents the nuclear translocation of NF-ATc and the transcription of certain genes essential for the activation of T cells. Hence the production of IL-2 by T-helper cells, the maturation of cytotoxic T cells, and the production of some other lymphokines, such as interferon-γ, are all inhibited.

The overall action of cyclosporin A is to suppress reversibly both cell-mediated and antibody-specific adaptive immune responses.

Indications: Cyclosporin A is used for the prevention of graft and transplant rejection, and prevention of GVHD.
Route of administration: Cyclosporin A is administered orally or by intravenous infusion.
Adverse effects: Unlike most immunosuppressive agents, cyclosporin A does not cause myelosuppression. It is markedly nephrotoxic to the proximal tubule of the kidney, and renal damage

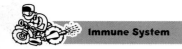

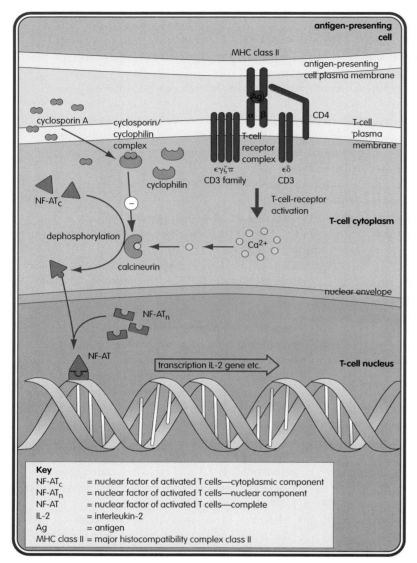

Fig. 10.13 Cyclosporin and T-cell suppression.

Key

NF-AT$_c$	= nuclear factor of activated T cells—cytoplasmic component
NF-AT$_n$	= nuclear factor of activated T cells—nuclear component
NF-AT	= nuclear factor of activated T cells—complete
IL-2	= interleukin-2
Ag	= antigen
MHC class II	= major histocompatibility complex class II

almost always occurs. This may be reversible or permanent. Hypertension occurs in 50% of people.

Less serious side effects include mild hepatotoxicity, anorexia, lethargy, gastrointestinal upsets, hirsutism, and gum hypertrophy.

Therapeutic notes: Cyclosporin A is often used as part of a post-transplantation 'triple therapy' regime with oral corticosteroids and azathioprine.

Azathioprine

Mechanism of action: Azathioprine is a prodrug that is converted into the active component 6-mercaptopurine in the liver. Mercaptopurine is a fraudulent purine nucleotide that impairs DNA synthesis, and has a cytotoxic action on dividing cells.

Indications: Azathioprine is used for the prevention of graft and transplant rejection, and autoimmune conditions when corticosteroid therapy alone is inadequate.

Route of administration: Azathioprine is administered orally or intravenously.

Adverse effects: Side effects of azathioprine include bone marrow suppression, which can lead to leucopenia, thrombocytopenia and sometimes anaemia. This is often the dose-limiting side effect.

Increased susceptibility to infections (often opportunistic pathogens), and to certain cancers (lymphomas) can occur. Common side effects include gastrointestinal disturbances, nausea, vomiting, and diarrhoea. Loss of hair (alopecia) may be partial or complete, but is usually reversible.

Drug interaction with allopurinol necessitates lowering the dose of azathioprine.

Therapeutic notes: Azathioprine is used as part of a post-transplantation 'triple therapy' regime with oral corticosteroids.

Glucocorticoids

The use of glucocorticoids as immunosuppressant agents involves both their anti-inflammatory actions and their effects on the immune system (see Chapter 8).

Immunosuppressant drugs are toxic agents, with adverse effects common, serious and frequently dose limiting. Knowledge of these adverse effects and why they occur is therefore important.

- Describe the role of therapeutic immunosuppression in transplant surgery and autoimmune conditions.
- What are the main clinically used immunosuppressant agents, their mechanism of action, indications, and major adverse effects?

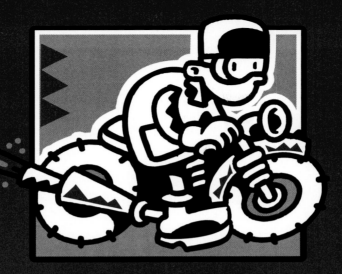

CHEMOTHERAPY

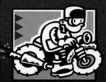

11. Cancer

Cancer

Cancers are malignant neoplastic growths ('new growths') of cells. Despite their variability, cancers share the characteristics of:

- Increased proliferation.
- Local invasiveness.
- Tendency to spread (metastasis).
- Changes in some aspects of original cell morphology/retention of other characteristics.

Cancers account for 20–25% of deaths in the western world; attempts to cure or palliate cancer employ three principal methods: surgery, radiotherapy, and chemotherapy. These methods are not mutually exclusive, often being used in combination, e.g. adjuvant chemotherapy after surgical removal of a tumour.

Chemotherapy

Chemotherapy is the use of drugs to inhibit or kill proliferating cancer cells, while leaving host cells unharmed, or at least recoverable. The techniques used include:

- Cytotoxic therapy, which is the main approach.
- Endocrine therapy.
- Immunotherapy.

Cancers differ in their sensitivity to chemotherapy, from the very sensitive (e.g. lymphomas, testicular carcinomas), where complete clinical cures can be achieved, to the resistant (generally solid tumours, e.g. colorectal, squamous cell bronchial carcinoma).

Cytotoxic chemotherapy
Mechanisms of action

Most cytotoxic drugs affect DNA synthesis. They can be classified according to their site of action on the process of DNA synthesis within the cancer cell (see Fig. 11.3). Cytotoxic drugs are therefore most active against actively cycling/proliferating cells, both normal and malignant, and least active against resting cells.

Some drugs are only effective at killing cycling cells during specific parts of the cell cycle. These are known as phase specific (Fig. 11.1). Other drugs are cytotoxic toward

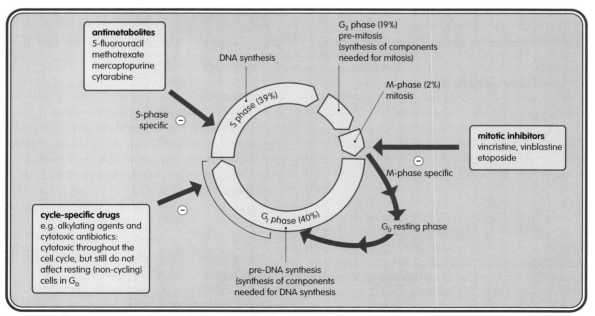

Fig. 11.1 Cell cycle and point of action of phase-specific drugs.

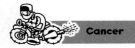

cycling cells throughout the cell cycle (e.g. alkylating agents), and are known as cycle specific.

Selectivity

Cytotoxic drugs are not specifically toxic to cancer cells, and the selectivity they show is marginal at best.

Cytotoxic drugs affect all rapidly dividing tissues, both normal and malignant, and thus are likely to have general toxic side effects (see Fig. 11.4).

Relative selectivity (a higher proportional kill of cancer cells) can occur with some cancers because:

- In malignant tumours a higher number of cells are undergoing proliferation than in normal proliferating tissues.
- Normal cells seem to recover from chemotherapeutic inhibition faster than some cancer cells.
- Synchronized cell cycling may leave discrete periods of vulnerability to cytotoxic drugs.

Knowledge of these principles and knowing that cytotoxic drugs kill a constant fraction, not a constant number, of cells, lays down the foundation for chemotherapeutic dosing schedules (Fig. 11.2).

Resistance to cytotoxic drugs

Genetic resistance to cytotoxic drugs can be inherent (*de novo*) to the cancer cell line or acquired during the course of chemotherapy, as a result of selection imposed by the chemotherapeutic agent.

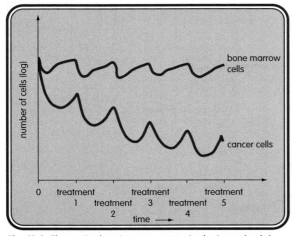

Fig. 11.2 Theoretical anticancer cytotoxic dosing schedule, allowing recovery of normal tissues.

Mechanisms of genetic resistance to cytotoxic drugs

The mechanims of genetic resistance to cytotoxic drugs include:

- Abnormal transport.
- Decreased cellular retention.
- Increased cellular inactivation (binding/metabolism).
- Altered target protein.
- Enhanced repair of DNA.
- Altered processing.

Some tumours are relatively resistant to chemotherapy because they exist in so-called 'pharmacological sanctuaries'. These occur when a tumour is in a privileged compartment, e.g. inside the blood–brain barrier, or in large solid tumours when poor blood supply and diffusion limit the penetration of the drug.

In clinical practice, cancers may be treated more successfully with combinations of cytotoxic drugs simultaneously, for example. MOPP therapy (mustine, oncovin® (vincristine), procarbazine, and prednisolone) for Hodgkin's lymphoma. The theory is that multiple attack with cytotoxic agents acting at different biochemical sites will increase efficacy while reducing the likelihood of resistance.

Cytotoxic agents

Cytotoxic agents, the major group of anticancer drugs, include the:

- Alkylating agents.
- Antimetabolites.
- Cytotoxic antibiotics.
- Mitotic inhibitors.
- Miscellaneous agents.

Alkylating agents

Examples of alkylating agents include mustine, cyclophosphamide, and chlorambucil.

Mechanism of action: Alkylating agents act via a reactive alkyl ($R\text{-}CH_2\text{-}CH_2^+$) group that reacts to form covalent bonds with nucleic acids (e.g. N7 position of guanine). There follows either cross-linking of the two strands of DNA, preventing replication, or DNA strand breakage (Fig. 11.3).

Route of administration: Mustine is administered intravenously, cyclophosphamide orally and intravenously, and chlorambucil orally.

Indications: Mustine is not used widely owing to its toxicity. Cyclophosphamide is extensively used for a variety of cancers, e.g. leukaemias, lymphomas, and solid cancers. Chlorambucil is used for leukaemias, lymphomas, and ovarian cancers.

Adverse effects: Generalized cytotoxicity is common with alkylating agents (Fig. 11.4); mustine >> cyclophosphamide >> chlorambucil.

A urinary metabolite of cyclophosphamide, acrolein, may cause serious haemorrhagic cystitis.

Damage to gametogenesis and the development of secondary acute non-lymphocytic leukaemias is a

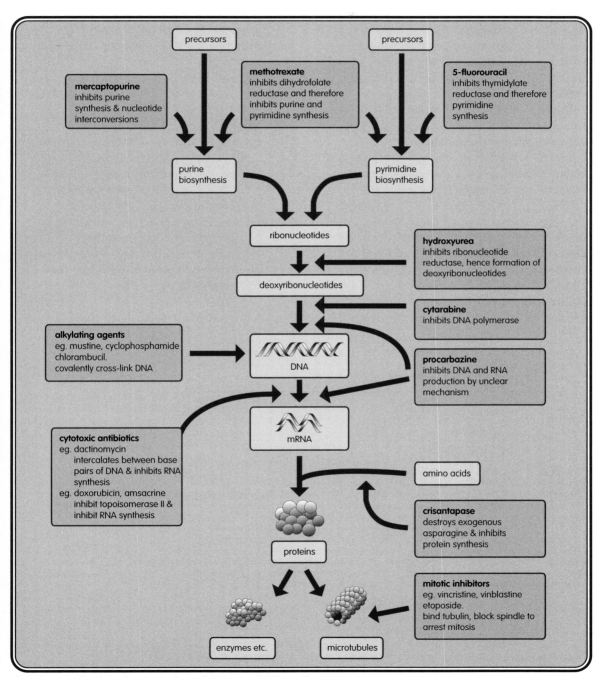

Fig. 11.3 Site of action of cytotoxic drugs that act on dividing cells.

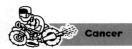
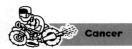

particular problem with these alkylating agents.
Therapeutic notes: Extensive clinical experience is available with aklylating agents.

Cytotoxic antibiotics

Actinomycin D (dactinomycin) and doxorubicin are examples of cytotoxic antibiotics.

Mechanism of action: Cytotoxic antibiotics contain a phenoxasone ring, which intercalates between base pairs in the DNA double helix. This process stabilizes the DNA structure and stops it being an effective template for RNA synthesis (Fig. 11.3).

Route of administration: Actinomycin D is administered intravenously and doxorubicin intravenously, or by bladder irrigation for bladder cancers.

Indications: Actinomycin is principally used in paediatric cancers. Doxorubicin is used for acute leukaemias, lymphomas, and a variety of solid tumours.

Adverse effects: A common side effect of cytotoxic antibiotics is generalized cytotoxicity (see Fig. 11.4). Doxorubicin produces dose-dependent cardiotoxicity, due to irreversible free radical damage to the myocardium.

Therapeutic notes: Simultaneous radiotherapy markedly increases the toxic adverse effects of cytotoxic antibiotics.

Mitotic inhibitors

Examples of mitotic inhibitors include the vinca alkaloids vincristine and vinblastine, and etoposide.

Mechanism of action: Mitotic inhibitors inhibit mitosis by binding tubulin and inhibiting the polymerization of microtubules necessary to form the mitotic spindle. This arrests dividing cells at metaphase (Fig. 11.3).

Route of administration: The vinca alkaloids are administered intravenously, and etoposide orally or intravenously.

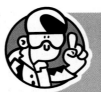

The cytotoxic drugs used in the treatment of cancer are among the most toxic agents used in modern medicine, with adverse effects almost ubiquitous and frequently dose limiting. Knowledge of these adverse effects and why they occur is therefore more important than normal in this area.

Fig. 11.4 General adverse effects of cytotoxic drugs.

General Adverse Effects of Cytotoxic Drugs	
Site	**Effect**
bone marrow	myelosuppression can lead to leucopenia, thrombocytopenia and sometimes anaemia, this is often the dose-limiting side effect; there is a high risk of haemorrhage, immunosuppression and infection as a result
gastrointestinal tract	inhibition of mucosal cell division may produce anorexia, ulceration or diarrhoea; nausea and vomiting are common, especially with alkylating agents and cisplatin
	loss of hair (alopecia) may be partial or complete but is usually reversible
wounds	impaired wound healing results from cell reproduction inhibition
reproductive system	sterility, teratogenesis, and mutagenicity are all possible
secondary cancers	many cytotoxic drugs are carcinogenic, additionally the immunosuppression resulting from myelosuppression may reduce immune surveillance of emerging dysplastic cells, leading to an increased risk of development of some cancers after chemotherapy

Indications: Mitotic inhibitors are used for acute leukaemias, lymphomas, and some solid tumours.

Adverse effects: Side effects of mitotic inhibitors result from the fact that tubulin polymerization is relatively indiscriminate, inhibiting other cellular processes that involve microtubules, as well as cell division.

Generalized cytotoxicity occurs (Fig. 11.4), except that vincristine is unusual in producing little or no bone marrow suppression.

Neurological and neuromuscular effects occur, especially with vincristine, and include peripheral neuropathy leading to paraesthesia, loss of reflexes, and weakness. Recovery from these effects occurs but is slow.

Therapeutic notes: The intrathecal administration of vinca alkaloids is contraindicated as it is usually fatal.

Antimetabolites

Examples of antimetabolites include folic acid antagonists (e.g. methotrexate), antipyrimidines (e.g. fluorouracil and cytarabine), and antipurines (e.g. mercaptopurine).

Mechanism of action: Antimetabolites are analogues of normal metabolites and act by competition, replacing the natural metabolite and then subverting cellular processes (Fig. 11.3).

Methotrexate competitively antagonizes dihydrofolate reductase and prevents the regeneration of intermediates (tetrahydrofolate) essential for the synthesis of purine and thymidylate, thus inhibiting the synthesis of DNA, RNA, and protein.

Fluorouracil is converted into a fraudulent pyrimidine nucleotide, fluorodeoxyuridylic acid, that inhibits thymidylate synthetase, impairing DNA synthesis.

Cytarabine is converted intracellularly to a triphosphate form that inhibits DNA polymerase.

Mercaptopurine is converted into a fraudulent purine nucleotide that impairs DNA synthesis.

Route of administration: Methotrexate is administered orally, intravenously, intramuscularly, and intrathecally. Fluorouracil is usually given intravenously, although it can be given orally and topically. Cytarabine is given subcutaneously, intravenously, and intrathecally, mercaptopurine is given orally.

Indications: Methotrexate is used for acute lymphoblastic leukaemia, non-Hodgkin's lymphoma, etc., fluorouracil for solid tumours and some malignant skin conditions, cytarabine for acute myeloblastic leukaemia, and mercaptopurine as maintenance therapy for acute leukaemias.

Adverse effects: Common side effects of antimetabolites are generalized cytotoxicity (Fig. 11.4).

Therapeutic notes: Methotrexate should not be given to people with significant renal impairment.

Miscellaneous agents

Several chemotherapeutic cytotoxic agents do not fall into any of the aforementioned groups.

Procarbazine

Mechanism of action: Procarbazine is a methylhydrazine derivative with monoamine oxidase inhibitor actions and cytotoxicity. It inhibits DNA and RNA synthesis by a mechanism that is unclear (Fig. 11.3).

Route of administration: Procarbazine is administered orally.

Indications: Procarbazine is the first-line drug for lymphomas such as Hodgkin's.

Adverse effects: Side effects of procarbazine include generalized cytotoxicity (Fig. 11.4). It causes an adverse reaction in combination with alcohol.

Therapeutic notes: Procarbazine forms part of MOPP therapy for Hodgkin's lymphoma.

Hydroxyurea

Mechanism of action: Hydroxyurea causes the inhibition of ribonucleotide reductase and hence the formation of deoxyribonucleotides (Fig. 11.3).

Route of administration: Hydroxyurea is administered orally.

Indications: Hydroxyurea is used for chronic myeloid leukaemia.

Adverse effects: Common side effects of hydroxyurea include generalized cytotoxicity (Fig. 11.4).

Crisantaspase

Mechanism of action: Some tumour cells lose the ability to synthesize asparagine, requiring an exogenous source of the substance to grow—normal body cells can synthesize their own. Crisantaspase is a preparation of bacterial asparaginase that breaks down any circulating asparagine, hence inhibiting the growth of some cancers, namely acute lymphoblastic leukaemia (ALL) (Fig. 11.3).

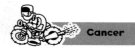

Route of administration: Crisantaspase is administered intramuscularly and subcutaneously.
Indications: Crisantaspase is used for ALL.
Adverse effects: The most serious side effects of crisantaspase include severe toxicity to the liver and pancreas. CNS depression and anaphylaxis are also risks.
Therapeutic notes: Regular testing of patients given crisantaspase is necessary to monitor organ functions.

Mitotane

Mechanism of action: Mitotane is related to the insecticide DDT. It interferes with the formation of adrenocortical steroids and has a selective cytotoxic effect on the cells of the adrenal cortex (Fig. 11.3).
Route of administration: Mitotane is administered orally.
Indications: Mitotane is used for tumours of the adrenal cortex.
Adverse effects: Side effects of mitotane include adrenosuppression.

Amsacrine

Mechanism of action: Like doxorubicin, amsacrine works by intercalation between base pairs in the DNA double helix. This stabilizes the DNA structure and stops it being an effective template for RNA synthesis.
Route of administration: Amsacrine is administered intravenously.
Indications: Amsacrine is used for acute myeloid leukaemia.
Adverse effects: Side effects of amsacrine include bone marrow suppression. Cardiotoxicity due to hypokalaemia has been reported.
Therapeutic notes: Electrolytes should be monitored in patients given amsacrine.

Endocrine therapy
Hormones and antihormones

The growth of some cancers is hormone dependent. Growth of such tumours can be inhibited by surgical removal of the gonads, adrenals, or pituitary; increasingly, however, administration of hormones or antihormones is preferred.

Endocrine therapy can cause side effects, the nature of which can normally be deduced from the physiological effects of the hormone being given or antagonized. However, endocrine therapy generally has the advantage that it carries far fewer serious adverse effects than do cytotoxic agents.

Hormones used in endocrine therapy include:
- Adrenocortical steroids (see Chapter 8), e.g. prednisolone, which inhibit the growth of cancers of the lymphoid tissues and blood. In addition they are used to treat some of the complications of the cancer (e.g. oedema).
- Oestrogen antagonists, e.g. tamoxifen, which are competitive inhibitors at oestrogen receptors. By blocking the progrowth effects of oestrogen they suppress the division of breast cancer cells. Tamoxifen is indicated for use in postmenopausal women with metastatic disease, where it has definitely been shown to increase survival times.
- Oestrogens (see Chapter 8), e.g. stilboestrol, which have an antiandrogenic effect and can be used to suppress androgen-dependent prostatic cancers.
- Progesterones (see Chapter 8), which inhibit endometrial cancer and carcinomas of the prostate and breast.
- Androgen antagonists, e.g. flutamide, which inhibit androgen-dependent prostatic cancers. Gonadotrophin-releasing hormone (GnRH) analogues have a similar effect as they inhibit GnRH release via negative feedback.

Immunotherapy

Immunotherapy of cancer is a recent advance derived from the nineteenth century observation that bacterial infections sometimes provoked the regression of cancer, i.e. indirect immunostimulation.

Approaches tried include:
- The use of tumour specific monoclonal antibodies to target drugs specifically to cancerous cells; the so called 'magic-bullet' approach.
- The use of vaccines e.g. BCG to provide non-specific immunostimulation.
- The use of specific vaccines prepared using tumour cells from similar cancers, in an attempt to raise an adaptive immune response against the cancer.
- Immunostimulation using drugs, e.g. levamisole.
- The use of cytokines to regulate the immune response so as to favourably target the cancer. Cytokines used include interferon α, interleukin-2 (IL-2), and tumour necrosis factor.
- The use of recombinant colony stimulating factors to reduce the level and duration of neutropenia after cytotoxic chemotherapy.

- Recombinant human granulocyte colony-stimulating factor (rh-G-CSF; filgrastim) and granulocyte-macrophage colony stimulating factor (GM-CSF; molgramostim) promote the development of their respective haemopoietic stem cells in the marrow.

Their use to raise white blood cell counts after cytotoxic chemotherapy is effective, although this has not been shown to alter overall survival rates.

- Describe cancer or malignant neoplastic growth, and the cellular dysfunctions it represents.
- What role does cytotoxic chemotherapy play in the treatment of human cancers?
- Summarize the broad mechanism of action of the cytotoxic drugs on cycling cells. Distinguish between phase and cycle specificity.
- Relate the broad mechanism of action of the cytotoxic drugs to their generalized adverse effects. What are these adverse effects and why do they occur?
- Name the different classes of cytotoxic drug and for each class describe the biochemical mechanism of action, indications for use, route of administration, any special adverse effects, and examples of drugs in that class.
- Describe the role of endocrine and immune therapies in the treatment of human cancer. Give examples of the agents used and, where known, how they work.

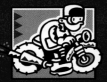

12. Infectious Disease

Concepts of antibacterial chemotherapy

Bacteria belong to the kingdom of prokaryotic organisms, some of whose species are pathogenic to humans and responsible for a number of medically important diseases.

The chemotherapy of bacterial infections aims to be selectively toxic against the invading bacteria while having the minimum of effect on the host. Antibacterial drugs therefore are chosen or designed to exploit the differences that exist between the structure and physiology of the prokaryotic bacterial cell and the host eukaryotic cell (Figs 12.1 and 12.2).

Fig. 12.1 Site of action of cytotoxic drugs that act on dividing cells.

Differences between prokaryotic and eukaryotic cells		
Site	**Exploitable difference**	**Antibacterial drugs**
peptidoglycan cell wall	peptidoglycan cell walls are a uniquely prokaryotic feature not shared by eukaryotic (mammalian) cells. Drugs that act here are therefore very selective	penicillins cephalosporins glycopeptides
cytoplasmic membrane	bacteria possess a plasma membrane within the cell wall which is a phospholipid bilayer, as in eukaryotes. However in bacteria the plasma membrane does not contain any sterols and this results in differential chemical behaviour that can be exploited	polymixins
protein synthesis	the bacterial ribosome (50S+30S subunits) is sufficiently different from the mammalian ribosome (60S+40S subunits) that sites on the bacterial ribosome are good targets for drug action	aminoglycosides tetracyclines chloramphenicol macrolides fusidic acid
nucleic acids	the bacterial genome is in the form of a single circular strand of DNA plus ancillary plasmids unenclosed by a nuclear envelope, in contrast to the eukaryotic chromosomal arrangement within the nucleus. Drugs may interfere directly or indirectly with microbial DNA and RNA metabolism, replication and transcription	antifolates quinolones rifampicin

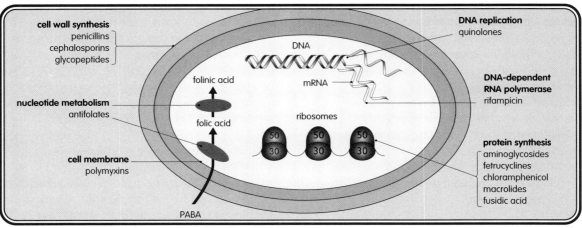

Fig. 12.2 Sites of action of different types of antibiotic agent. (PABA, *para*-aminobenzoic acid.)

Antibacterial agents can be considered as bacteriostatic (i.e. they inhibit bacterial growth but do not kill the bacteria), or bactericidal (i.e. they kill bacteria).

Note that the distinction is not clear-cut as the ability of an antibacterial agent to inhibit or kill bacteria is partially dependent on its concentration. Also, the distinction is rarely of clinical significance, the exception being immunocompromised patients in whom bactericidal agents are necessary, as the host's immune system is not capable of final elimination of the bacteria.

Antibiotics: definition

The term antibiotic strictly refers to antibacterial agents that are naturally occurring by-products of micro-organisms, e.g. penicillins from fungi. In practice, the term antibiotic has become synonymous with all antibacterial agents, whether natural or synthetic, and is used as such in this chapter.

Spectrum of activity: definition

Antibiotics have a narrow or broad spectrum of activity. Broad-spectrum antibiotics are active against many bacterial species, whereas narrow-spectrum antibiotics are active against only one or a few species.

Antibiotic resistance

When an antibiotic is ineffective against a bacterium it is said to be resistant. Resistance to antibiotics can be acquired or innate.

Innate resistance

Innate resistance is a characteristic of a particular species of bacteria. For instance, *Pseudomonas aeruginosa*, a Gram-negative bacterium that can cause serious infections of wounds, has always been resistant to treatment with several antibiotics, e.g. benzylpenicillin, vancomycin, and fusidic acid.

Acquired resistance

Acquired resistance is when bacteria that were sensitive to an antibiotic become resistant.

Biochemical mechanisms responsible for resistance to an antibiotic include:

- Production of enzymes that inactivate the drug, e.g. β-lactamases produced by many bacteria, which inactivate penicillin.

- Alteration of drug binding site, e.g. aminoglycosides and erythromycin bind to the 70S bacterial ribosome and inhibit protein synthesis. Resistant organisms have modified the sites of drug binding so that they no longer have affinity for the drugs.
- Reduction in drug uptake and accumulation, e.g. some bacteria are resistant to tetracycline because they have altered their cell membrane to make it impermeable to the drug.
- Development of altered metabolic pathways, e.g. bacteria can become resistant to trimethoprim because of acquired changes in their dihydrofolate reductase enzyme that gives it very little affinity for the drug.

The major stimulus for the development of acquired resistance is the use of antibiotics themselves. Antibiotic use exerts selective pressure on the bacteria to 'acquire' resistance to survive.

Acquired resistance to antibiotics can develop in bacterial populations in many ways, although all involve genes that code for the resistance mechanism located either on the bacterial chromosome or on plasmids.

The 'acquisition' of resistance by a bacterium can either be achived *de novo* by spontaneous mutation, or by being transferred from another bacterium.

Transferral of genes coding for the resistance mechanism can occur between bacteria of the same species and of different species. There are three main methods, which in order of importance are:

- Conjugation, which is transferral of gene during conjugation (a tube forms between bacteria) on a plasmid.
- Transduction, which is transferral of gene by a bacteriophage (a virus which infects a bacteria).
- Transformation, which is transferral of gene by bacterial uptake of DNA from its environment and subsequent incorporation.

The development of clinical antibiotic drug resistance is a major problem imposing serious constraints on the medical treatment of many bacterial infections.

Antibacterial drugs that inhibit cell wall synthesis

Examples of antibacterial drugs that inhibit bacterial cell wall synthesis include the penicillins, the cephalosporins (β-lactam antibiotics), and the glycopeptides (Fig. 12.2)

Penicillins

Examples of penicillins include benzylpenicillin, phenoxymethylpenicillin, flucloxacillin, amoxycillin, and ampicillin.

Mechanism of action: Penicillins are bactericidal. Structurally, they possess a thiazolidine ring connected to a β-lactam ring. The side chain from the β-lactam ring determines many of the pharmacological properties of the different penicillins.

Penicillins first bind to penicillin-binding proteins. They then inhibit peptidoglycan synthesis and activate autolytic enzymes. Interference with peptidoglycan synthesis is by preventing cross-linkage between the linear peptidoglycan polymer chains that make up the cell wall. The growing bacteria become unable to maintain an osmotic gradient, swell and rupture (Fig. 12.2).

Spectrum of activity: Penicillins exhibit considerable diversity in their spectrum of activity (Fig. 12.3).

Benzylpenicillin is active against aerobic Gram-positive and Gram-negative cocci and many anaerobic organisms. Many staphylococci are now resistant to benzylpenicillin. Flucloxacillin is used against penicillin resistant staphylococci as it is not inactivated by their β-lactamase. Phenoxymethylpenicillin is similar to benzylpenicillin but less active. Amoxycillin and ampicillin are broad-spectrum penicillins.

Route of administration: Benzylpenicillins must be administered intravenously as they are inactive when given orally. Phenoxymethylpenicillin, flucloxacillin, amoxycillin, and ampicillin are active orally.

Contraindications: Penicillins should not be given to people with a known hypersensitivity to penicillins or cephalosporins.

Adverse effects: Penicillins are generally very specific and safe antibiotics. Hypersensitivity reactions are the main adverse effect, including rashes (common) and anaphylaxis (rare). Neurotoxicity occurs at excessively high cerebrospinal fluid (CSF) concentrations. Diarrhoea is common, owing to disturbance of normal colonic flora.

Therapeutic notes: Resistance to penicillins is often due to production of β-lactamase, which hydrolyses the β-lactam ring. The resistance gene is located in the plasmid and is transferable. Fluocloxacillin is resistant to β-lactamase.

Cephalosporins

The cephalosporins comprise a large group of drugs. The three main groups include:

- First-generation drugs, e.g. cefadroxil (oral) and cephradine (parenteral).
- Second-generation drugs, e.g. cefuroxime (oral) and cephamandole (parenteral).
- Third-generation drugs, e.g. cefixime (oral) and cefotaxime (parenteral).

Mechanism of action: Cephalosporins are bactericidal. They are β-lactam-containing antibiotics and inhibit bacterial cell-wall synthesis in a manner similar to the penicillins. Structurally, cephalosporins possess a dihydrothiazine ring connected to the β-lactam ring that makes them more resistant to hydrolysis by β-lactamases than are the penicillins.

Spectrum of activity: The cephalosporins are broad-spectrum antibiotics that are second-choice agents for many infections (Fig. 12.3).

Route of administration: Cephalosporins are administered orally or intravenously.

Contraindications: Cephalosporins should not be given to people with a known hypersensitivity to cephalosporins or penicillins.

Adverse effects: Side effects of the cephalosporins include hypersensitivity reactions, which occur in a similar and cross-reacting fashion to the penicillins. Diarrhoea is common, owing to disturbance of normal colonic flora. Nausea and vomiting may also occur.

Therapeutic notes: The cephalosporins can be inactivated by resistant bacteria possessing β-lactamase. However, the later generations are more resistant to hydrolysis.

Glycopeptides

Vancomycin is an example of a glycopeptide.

Mechanism of action: Vancomycin is bactericidal. It inhibits peptidoglycan synthesis, with possible effects on RNA synthesis (Fig. 12.2).

Spectrum of activity: Vancomycin is active only against Gram-positive bacteria, particularly staphylococci. It is reserved for resistant staphylococcal infections and *Clostridium difficile* in antibiotic-associated pseudomembranous colitis (see Fig. 12.3).

Route of administration: Vancomycin is usually administered intravenously as it is not absorbed orally. Oral administration is reserved for when a local gastro-intestinal tract effect is required, e.g. in colitis.

Adverse effects: Side effects of vancomycin include ototoxicity and nephrotoxicity at high plasma levels, and

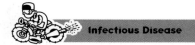
fever, rashes, and local phlebitis at the site of infection.
Therapeutic notes: Acquired resistance to vancomycin is
currently rare.

Antibacterial drugs that inhibit bacterial nucleic acids

Antibacterial drugs that inhibit bacterial nucleic acids
include (Fig. 12.2):

- The antifolates, which affect DNA metabolism.
- The quinolones, which affect DNA replication.
- Rifampicin, which affects transcription (p. 196).

Antifolates

Examples of antifolates include the sulphonamides (e.g.
sulphadimidine), trimethoprim, and co-trimoxazole.

Mechanism of action: Folates are essential co-factors in
the synthesis of purines and hence of DNA. Bacteria,
unlike mammals, must synthesize their own folate from
para-aminobenzoic acid. This pathway can be inhibited
at two points: the sulphonamides inhibit dihydrofolate
synthetase, and are bacteriostatic while trimethoprim
and co-trimoxazole inhibit dihydrofolate reductase and
are bacteriostatic.

Spectrum of activity: The sulphonamides are used for
'simple' urinary tract infections (UTIs). Trimethoprim and
co-trimoxazole are used for UTIs and respiratory tract
infections (see Fig. 12.3).

Route of administration: All the antifolates are
administered orally but may also be given intravenously.

Contraindications: Antifolates should not be given to

Drugs of choice and alternatives for selected common bacterial pathogens			
Bacterium	**Drug(s) of choice**	**Alternatives**	**Comments**
Streptococcus species	penicillin	first-generation cephalosporins erythromycin clindamycin vancomycin	a few strains are penicillin resistant, especially some *S. pneumoniae* erythromycin is only for mild infections vancomycin is only for serious infections
Enterococcus species	penicillin or ampicillin plus gentamicin	vancomycin plus gentamicin	there are some strains for which streptomycin is synergistic but gentamicin is not some strains are resistant to synergy with any aminoglycoside
Staphylococcus species	antistaphylococcal penicillin e.g. flucoxacillin	first-generation cephalosporins vancomycin	vancomycin is required for methicillin-resistant strains rifampicin is occasionally used to eradicate the nasal carriage state
Neisseria meningitidis	penicillin	chloramphenicol third-generation cephalosporins	rare strains are penicillin resistant
Neisseria gonorrhoeae	cefixime	ciprofloxacin third-generation cephalosporins	some strains are fluoroquinolone resistant (especially in Asia)
Bordetella pertussis	erythromycin	TMP–SMZ	
Haemophilus influenzae	aminopenicillin	cefuroxime third generation cephalosporins chloramphenicol	approximately 30% are aminopenicillin-resistant; aminopenicillins should not be used empirically in serious infections until susceptibility results are available rifampicin is used to eradicate the nasal carriage state
Enterobacteria in urine	TMP-SMZ	ciprofloxacin gentamicin nitrofurantoin	β lactams are less effective than TMP–SMZ or fluoroquinolones for the treatment of urinary tract infection
Enterobacteria in cerebrospinal fluid	Third-generation cephalosporin	TMP–SMZ	in neonates only, aminoglycosides are equivalent to third generation cephalosporins experience with TMP–SMZ in meningitis is limited

Fig. 12.3a Drugs of choice and alternatives for selected common bacterial pathogens. (TMP–SMZ,
Trimethoprim–sulphamethoxazole.

Drugs of choice and alternatives for selected common bacterial pathogens (continued)			
Bacterium	**Drug(s) of choice**	**Alternatives**	**Comments**
Enterobacteria elsewhere (blood, lung, etc.)	gentamicin third- generation cephalosporins ciprofloxacin	TMP–SMZ	two-drug therapy is sometimes used in serious infection monotherapy with a third-generation cephalosporin should be avoided if the pathogen is *Enterobacter cloacae, E. aerogenes, Serratia marcescens* or *Citrobacter freundii*
Pseudomonas aeruginosa	antipseudomonal penicillin plus aminoglycoside	ceftazidime ciprofloxacin	two-drug therapy recommended except for urinary tract infection
Bacteroides fragilis	metronidazole or clindamycin	imipenem penicillin β lactamase inhibitors	*B. fragilis* is usually involved in polymicrobial infections; therefore another antibiotic active against Enterobacteriaceae is often required
Mycoplasma pneumoniae	macrolides e.g. erythromycin	tetracycline	although tetracyclines are as effective as macrolides, the latter are recommended because of better activity against *Pneumococcus*, which can mimic this infection
Chlamydia trachomatis	tetracycline	azithromycin erythromycin	azithromycin is the only therapy effective in a single dose erythromycin is used in pregnancy
Rickettsial species	tetracycline	chloramphenicol	
Listeria monocytogenes	ampicillin plus gentamicin	vancomycin plus gentamicin	
Legionella species	erythromycin	tetracycline	rifampicin is occasionally used as a second agent in severe cases
Clostridium difficile	metronidazole	vancomycin (oral)	
Mycobacterium tuberculosis	isoniazid plus rifampicin plus pyrazinamide plus ethambutol	streptomycin fluoroquinolones cycloserine clarithromycin capreomycin	directly observed therapy is recommended isoniazid is used alone for preventive therapy
Mycobacterium leprae	dapsone plus rifampicin ± clofazimine	clarithromycin	thalidomide is useful for erythema nodosum leprosum

Fig. 12.3b Drugs of choice and alternatives for selected common bacterial pathogens.

pregnant women or neonates because bilirubin displacement can damage the neonatal brain (kernicterus).

Adverse effects: Antifolates can cause nausea and vomiting and hypersensitivity reactions, e.g. rashes, fever, Stevens–Johnson syndrome. The sulphonamides are relatively insoluble and can cause crystalluria, while trimethoprim and co-trimoxazole can cause myelosuppression/agranulocytosis.

Therapeutic notes: Antifolates are often used in combined preparations as they have synergistic effects. Resistance is common and is due to the production of enzymes that have reduced affinity for the drugs. Resistance can be acquired on plasmids in Gram-negative bacteria.

Quinolones

Examples of quinolones include ciprofloxacin and nalidixic acid.

Mechanism of action: Quinolones are bactericidal. They act by inhibiting the activity of DNA gyrase, the enzyme that packages bacterial DNA into supercoils and is essential for DNA replication and repair (Fig. 12.2).

Spectrum of activity: Ciprofloxacin has a broad spectrum of activity, while nalidixic acid is more narrowly active against Gram-negative organisms (see Fig. 12.3).

Route of administration: Quinolones are administered orally or intravenously.

Contraindications: Quinolones should not be given with theophylline.

Adverse effects: Side effects of quinolones include gastrointestinal disturbances. Rarely, hypersensitivity and CNS disturbances occur.

Therapeutic notes: Rarely, bacteria treated with quinolones acquire resistance due to a mutation of their DNA gyrase.

Antibacterial drugs that inhibit protein synthesis

Antibacterial drugs that inhibit protein synthesis include:

- Aminoglycosides.
- Tetracyclines.
- Chloramphenicol.
- Macrolides.
- Fusidic acid.

These drugs are summarized in Fig. 12.4.

Aminoglycosides

Examples of aminoglycosides include gentamycin, streptomycin, netilmicin, and amikacin.

Mechanism of action: Aminoglycosides are bactericidal. They bind irreversibly to the 30S portion of the bacterial ribosome. This inhibits the translation of mRNA to protein and causes more frequent misreading of the genetic code (Fig. 12.4).

Spectrum of activity: Aminoglycosides have a broad spectrum of activity but with low activity against anaerobes, streptococci, and pneumococci (see Fig. 12.3). Streptomycin is used against *Mycobacterium tuberculosis* (pp. 196–197).

Route of administration: Aminoglycosides are administered intravenously only.

Contraindications: Acute neuromuscular blockade can occur if an aminoglycoside is used in combination with anaesthesia or other neuromuscular blockers.

Adverse effects: Side effects of aminoglycosides include dose-related ototoxicity and nephrotoxicity at high plasma levels.

Therapeutic notes: Resistance to aminoglycosides is increasing and is primarily due to plasmid-borne genes encoding degradative enzymes.

Tetracyclines

Examples of tetracyclines include tetracycline, minocycline, and doxycycline.

Mechanism of action: Tetracyclines are bacteriostatic.

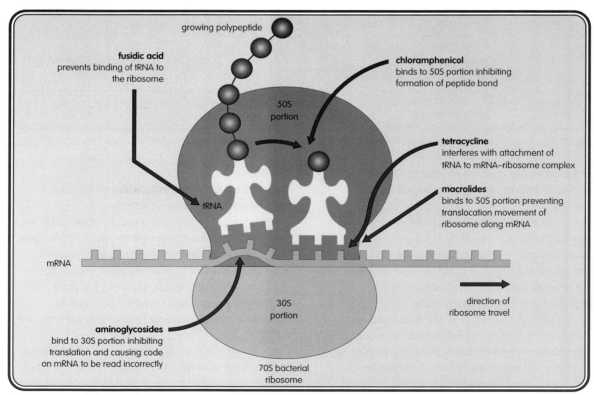

Fig. 12.4 Several classes of antibiotics inhibit bacterial protein synthesis.

They work by selective uptake into bacterial cells due to active bacterial transport systems not possessed by mammalian cells. The tetracycline then binds reversibly to the 30S subunit of the bacterial ribosome, interfering with the attachment of tRNA to the mRNA ribosome complex (Fig. 12.4).

Spectrum of activity: Tetracyclines have broad-spectrum activity against Gram-positive and Gram-negative bacteria, as well as intracellular pathogens (see Fig. 12.3).

Route of administration: Tetracyclines are administered orally or intravenously. Oral absorption is incomplete and can be impaired by calcium (e.g. milk), and magnesium or aluminium salts (e.g. antacids) (see Chapter 7).

Contraindications: Tetracyclines should not be given to children or pregnant women.

Adverse effects: Side effects of tetracyclines include gastrointestinal disturbances, which are common after oral administration. In children, tetracyclines depress bone growth, and produce permanent discoloration of teeth.

Therapeutic notes: Resistance to tetracyclines is slow to develop, but is now widespread. In the majority of cases, resistance is due to decreased uptake of the drug, and is plasmid borne.

Chloramphenicol

Mechanism of action: Chloramphenicol is bactericidal or bacteriostatic, depending on the bacterial species. It reversibly binds to the 50S subunit of the bacterial ribosome, inhibiting the formation of peptide bonds (Fig. 12.4).

Spectrum of activity: Chloramphenicol has a broad spectrum of activity against many Gram-positive cocci and Gram-negative organisms (see Fig. 12.3). Because of its toxicity, it is reserved for life-threatening infections, especially typhoid fever and meningitis.

Route of administration: Chloramphenicol is administered orally or intravenously.

Contraindications: Chloramphenicol should not be given to pregnant women or neonates.

Adverse effects: Side effects of chloramphenicol include myelosuppression and reversible anaemia. Neutropenia and thrombocytopenia may occur during chronic administration. Fatal aplastic anaemia is rare.

Neonates cannot metabolize chloramphenicol and 'grey baby syndrome' may develop including pallor, abdominal distension, vomiting, and collapse.

Therapeutic notes: Resistance to chloramphenicol is due to a plasmid-borne gene encoding an enzyme that inactivates the drug by acetylation. Blood monitoring is necessary.

Macrolides

Erythromycin is an example of a macrolide.

Mechanism of action: Erythromycin is bacteriostatic/ bactericidal. It reversibly binds to the 50S subunit of the bacterial ribosome, preventing the translocation movement of the ribosome along mRNA (Fig. 12.3).

Spectrum of activity: Erythromycin has a narrow spectrum of activity against Gram-positive organisms, similar to benzylpenicillin (see Fig. 12.3).

Route of administration: Erythromycin is administered orally or intravenously.

Adverse effects: Side effects of erythromycin include gastrointestinal disturbance, which is common after oral administration. Liver damage and jaundice can occur after chronic administration.

Therapeutic notes: Resistance to erythromycin results from a mutation of the binding site on the 50S subunit.

Fusidic acid

Mechanism of action: Fusidic acid is a steroid that prevents binding of tRNA to the ribosome (Fig. 12.4).

Spectrum of activity: Fusidic acid has a narrow spectrum of activity, particularly against *Staphylococcus aureus* (see Fig. 12.3).

Route of administration: Fusidic acid is administered orally and intravenously.

Adverse effects: Common side effects of fusidic acid include gastro-intestinal disturbance. Skin eruptions and jaundice may occur.

Therapeutic notes: Resistance to fusidic acid can occur via mutation or by plasmid-borne mechanisms.

Miscellaneous antibacterials

Miscellaneous antibacterials include:

- Polymyixins.
- Bacitracin.
- Metronidazole.
- Nitrofurantoin.

Polymyixins

Examples of polymyixins include polymyixin B and polymyixin E.

Mechanism of action: Polymixins are bactericidal. They are peptides that interact with phospholipids on the outer plasma cell membranes of Gram-negative bacteria, disrupting their structure. This disruption destroys the

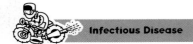

bacteria's osmotic barrier, leading to lysis (Fig. 12.2).

Spectrum of activity: Polymixins are active only against Gram-negative bacteria (see Fig. 12.3).

Route of administration: Polymyixins are seriously toxic systemically, and are currently used only topically on the ear, eye, and skin.

Adverse effects: Side effects of polymyixins are few when used topically. Serious neuro- and nephrotoxicity occurs if they are used systemically.

Therapeutic notes: Resistance to polymyixins is rare.

Bacitracin

Mechanism of action: Bacitracin is a natural antibiotic, isolated from *Bacillus subtilis*, that inhibits bacterial cell wall formation.

Spectrum of activity: Bacitracin is similar in its spectrum of activity to penicillin (see Fig. 12.3).

Route of administration: Bacitracin is applied topically only, for infections of the mouth, nose, eyes, and skin, as it is seriously toxic when given systemically.

Adverse effects: Side effects of bacitracin are few when it is used topically. Serious nephrotoxicity can occur if it is used systemically.

Therapeutic notes: Bacitracin is much less likely to cause hypersensitivity reactions than penicillin. Acquired resistance is rare.

Metronidazole

Mechanism of action: Metronidazole is bactericidal. It is metabolized to an intermediate that inhibits bacterial DNA synthesis and degrades existing DNA. Its selectivity is due to the fact that the intermediate toxic metabolite is not produced in mammalian cells.

Spectrum of activity: Metronidazole is antiprotozoal (p. 209). It has antibacterial activity against anaerobic bacteria (see Fig. 12.3).

Route of administration: Metronidazole is administered orally, rectally, and vaginally.

Contraindications: Metronidazole should not be given to pregnant women.

Adverse effects: Side effects of metronidazole commonly include mild headache and gastrointestinal disturbance. Adverse drug reactions occur with alcohol.

Therapeutic notes: Acquired resistance to metronidazole is rare.

Nitrofurantoin

Mechanism of action: The mechanism of action of nitrofurantoin is uncertain but possibly involves bacterial

DNA disruption by metabolites.

Spectrum of activity: Nitrofurantoin is active against Gram-positive and *Escherichia coli* infections of the UTI (see Fig. 12.3).

Route of administration: Nitrofurantoin is administered orally; it reaches high therapeutic concentrations in the urine.

Adverse effects: Common side effects of nitrofurantoin include gastrointestinal disturbance. Pulmonary complications can occur with chronic therapy.

Therapeutic notes: Rarely, chromosomal resistance to nitrofurantoin can occur.

Antimycobacterial drugs

The mycobacteria are slow-growing intracellular bacilli that cause turberculosis (*Mycobacterium tuberculosis*) and leprosy (*M. leprae*) in humans.

Mycobacteria differ in their structure and lifestyle from Gram-positive and Gram-negative bacteria and are treated with different drugs.

Antituberculosis therapy

The first-line drugs used in the treatment of tuberculosis are:

- Isoniazid, which inhibits the production of mycolic acid, a component of the cell wall unique to mycobacteria, and is bactericidal against growing organisms. Taken orally it penetrates tuberculous lesions well. Adverse effects occur in about 5% of patients and include peripheral neuropathy, hepatotoxicity, and autoimmune phenomena. Resistance is rare in developed countries, but not in less-developed areas.
- Rifampicin, which inhibits DNA-dependent RNA polymerase, causing a bactericidal effect. It is a potent drug, active orally. Adverse effects are infrequent but can be serious, e.g. hepatotoxicity and 'toxic syndromes'. There are many drug interactions, and resistance can develop rapidly.
- Ethambutol, which is bacteriostatic. The mechanism of action is uncertain, involving impaired synthesis of the mycobacterial cell wall. Ethambutol is administered orally. Adverse effects are uncommon but reversible optic neuritis may occur. Resistance often develops.
- Pyrazinamide, the mechanism of action of which is uncertain but may involve metabolism of drug within *M. tuberculosis* to produce a toxic product, pyrazinoic acid, which works as a bacteriostatic agent in the low pH environment of the phagolysosome. It is active

orally. Adverse effects are hepatotoxicity and raised plasma urate levels that can lead to gout. Resistance can develop rapidly.

- Streptomycin, which is now rarely used in the UK for tuberculosis (p. 194).

The second-line drugs used for tuberculosis infections when first-line drugs have been discontinued owing to resistance or adverse effects are:

- Capreomycin, which is a peptide drug given intramuscularly. It can cause ototoxicity and kidney damage.
- Cycloserine, which is a broad-spectrum drug that inhibits peptidoglycan synthesis. This drug is admininstered orally, and can cause CNS toxicity.
- New macrolides, e.g. azithromycin and clarithromycin.
- Quinolones, e.g. ciprofloxacin.

To reduce the emergence of resistant organisms, a compound drug therapy is used to treat tuberculosis, involving:

- An initial phase of 2 months when at least three drugs are used, until the bacterial sensitivities are known.

- A continuation phase of up to ten months when the most effective two drugs are continued to achieve a cure.

Antileprosy therapy

Tuberculoid leprosy is treated with dapsone and rifampicin for 6 months.

Lepromatous leprosy is treated with dapsone, rifampicin, and clofazimine for up to 2 years.

Dapsone resembles sulphonamides chemically and may inhibit folate synthesis in a similar way. It is active orally. Adverse effects are numerous and some are serious.

Clofazimine is a chemically complex dye that accumulates in macrophages, possibly acting on mycobacterial DNA. It literally acts as a dye, turning skin and bodily wastes red. Other adverse effects are numerous and some are serious. It is active orally.

Grouping of antibacterial drugs by their mechanism of action rather than chemical structure is easier, more important, and more relevant to your understanding.

- What are the differences between bacterial (prokaryotic) cells and mammalian (eukaryotic) cells, and how are these differences exploited by selective antibacterial agents?
- Define the terms bacteristatic, bactericidal, and spectrum of activity with reference to antibiotics.
- Describe the difference between innate and acquired antibiotic resistance, the biochemical mechanisms of resistance, and the genetic mechanisms by which it is acquired.
- For each of the following antibacterial drug categories, give examples of drugs in that class, their mechanism of action, approximate spectrum of activity, route of administration, adverse effects, and state whether antibiotic resistance is a problem:
  −Antibacterial drugs that inhibit cell wall synthesis.
  −Antibacterial drugs that inhibit nucleic acid synthesis.
  −Antibacterial drugs that inhibit protein synthesis,
  −Other antibacterial drugs.
- Outline the classification of mycobacterial diseases and the drugs used in their treatment.

ANTIVIRAL DRUGS

Concepts of viral infection

Viruses are obligate intracellular parasites that lack independent metabolism and can only replicate within the host cells they enter and infect. A virus particle, or virion, consists essentially of DNA or RNA enclosed in a protein coat (capsid). In addition, certain viruses may possess a lipoprotein envelope and replicative enzymes (see Fig. 12.5).

Viruses are classified largely according to the architecture of the virion and the nature of the genetic material. In different viruses the nucleic acid may be single stranded (ss) or double stranded (ds) (Fig. 12.6).

Antiviral agents

Because viruses have an intracellular replication cycle and share many of the metabolic processes of the host cell, it has proved extremely difficult to find drugs that are selectively toxic to them. Additionally, by the time a viral infection becomes detectable clinically, the viral replication process tends to be very far advanced, making chemotherapeutic intervention difficult. All current antiviral agents are virustatic rather than virucidal and thus rely upon host immunocompetence for a complete clinical cure.

Nevertheless, antiviral chemotherapy is clinically effective against some viral diseases (identified with an

asterisk in Fig. 12.6). The viruses include:
- Herpesviruses [herpes simplex virus (HSV), varicella zoster virus (VZV), and cytomegalovirus (CMV)].
- Influenza virus A.
- Respiratory syncytial virus, arenaviruses.
- HIV-1.

The selective inhibition of these viruses by drugs depends on either:
- Inhibition of unique steps in the viral replication pathways, such as adsorption of the virion to a cell receptor, penetration, uncoating, assembly, and release.
- Preferential inhibition of steps shared with the host cell, which include transcription and translation.

In addition to chemotherapy, immune based therapies, such as the use of immunoglobulins and cytokines in viral infection, are also mentioned below.

Inhibition of attachment to or penetration of host cells
Amantadine

Mechanism of action: Amantadine, and its analogue rimantadine, inhibit penetration into the host cell by preventing uncoating of the influenza virion. Uncoating is the process by which the virus genome is released inside

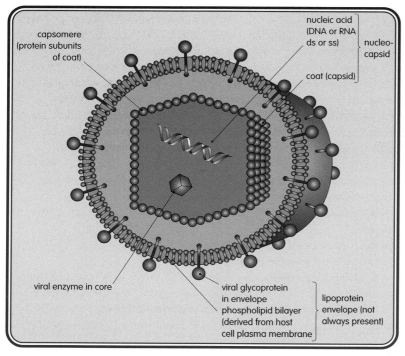

Fig. 12.5 Diagrammatic representation of the components of a virion.

nucleic acid (DNA or RNA ds or ss)
nucleo-capsid
coat (capsid)
capsomere (protein subunits of coat)
viral enzyme in core
viral glycoprotein in envelope
phospholipid bilayer (derived from host cell plasma membrane)
lipoprotein envelope (not always present)

Classification of medically important viruses and the diseases they cause

Family	ss/ds	Viruses	Diseases
DNA viruses			
herpes viruses	ds	herpes simplex (HSV)*	cold sores, genital herpes
		varicella-zoster (VZV)*	chickenpox, shingles
		cytomegalovirus (CMV)*	cytomegalic disease
		Epstein Barr virus (EBV)*	infectious mononucleosis
poxviruses	ds	variola	smallpox
adenoviruses	ds	adenoviruses	acute respiratory disease
hepadnaviruses	ds	hepatitis B	hepatitis
papovaviruses	ds	papilloma	warts
parvoviruses	ss	B19	erythema infectiosum
RNA viruses			
orthomyxoviruses	ss	influenza A* and B	influenza
paramyxoviruses	ss	measles virus	measles
		mumps virus	mumps
		parainfluenza	respiratory infection
		respiratory syncytal*	respiratory infection
coronaviruses	ss	coronavirus	respiratory infection
rhabdoviruses	ss	rabies virus	rabies
picornoviruses	ss	enteroviruses	meningitis
		rhinoviruses	colds
		hepatitis A	hepatitis
calciviruses	ss	Norwalk virus	gastroenteritis
togaviruses	ss	alphaviruses	encephalitis, haemorrhagic fevers
		rubivirus	rubella
reoviruses	ds	rotavirus	gastroenteritis
arenavirus	ss	lymphocytic choriomeningitis	meningitis
		lassa virus*	lassa fever
retroviruses	ss	HIV I, II*	AIDS

Fig. 12.6 Classification of selected medically important viruses and the diseases they cause (*, viruses for which effective chemotherapy exists; ds, double stranded; ss, single stranded.)

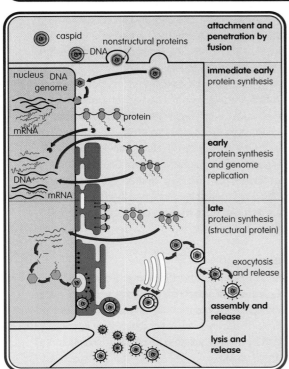

Fig. 12.7 Schematic diagram of the life cycle of a DNA virus (e.g. *Herpes simplex*) showing the various stages that may be inhibited by antiviral agents. (Reproduced with permission from *Medical Microbiology, 3rd Edition,* by PR Murray, Mosby-Yearbook, 1998.)

the host cell prior to replication. Amantadine binds to the M2 viral protein to prevent this process (Fig. 12.7).

Route of administration: Amantadine is administered orally.

Indications: Amantadine is used for the prophylaxis and treatment of acute influenza A in groups at risk. It is not effective against influenza B.

Adverse effects: Amantadine is well tolerated, with no serious renal, hepatic, or haematological adverse effects. Some patients (5–10%) report non-serious dizziness, slurred speech, and insomnia. Neurological side effects and renal failure can occur at high concentrations.

Therapeutic notes: Emergence of resistance to amantidine associated with clinical failure has been reported in 25–50% of patients. Amantadine is not used widely because of problems with resistance, its narrow spectrum of activity, and because influenza vaccines are often preferred.

Immunoglobulins

Examples of immunoglobulins include human normal immunoglobulin (HNIG/gamma globulin) and specific immunoglobulins, e.g. hepatitis B (HBIG), rabies (RIG), varicella zoster (VZIG), and cytomegalovirus (CMVIG) immunoglobulins.

Mechanism of action: Immunoglobulins or antibodies bind specifically to antigenic determinants on the outside of virions. By specifically binding to a virus, the immunoglobulins may neutralize it by coating the virus and preventing its attachment and entry into host cells.

HNIG is prepared from pooled plasma of ~1000 donors and contains antibodies to measles, mumps, varicella, and hepatitis A.

Specific immunoglobulins are prepared by pooling the plasma of selected donors with high levels of the antibody required.

Route of administration: Immunoglobulins are administered by intramuscular injection.

Indications: HNIG is administered for the protection of susceptible contacts against hepatitis A, measles, mumps, and rubella. Specific immunoglobulins may attenuate or prevent hepatitis and rabies following a known exposure, and before the onset of signs and symptoms, e.g. following exposure to a rabid animal. VZIG and CMVG are indicated for prophylactic use to prevent chickenpox, and cytomegalic disease in immunosuppressed patients at risk.

Contraindications: Immunoglobulins should not be given to people with known antibody against IgA.

Adverse effects: Side effects of immunoglobulins include malaise, chills, fever, and (rarely) anaphylaxis.

Therapeutic notes: Protection with immunoglobulins is immediate and lasts several weeks. HNIG may interfere with vaccinations for 3 months.

Inhibition of nucleic acid synthesis

The advent of nucleotide analogue drugs that selectively interfere with viral nucleic acid synthesis has opened up a new era of effective selective antiviral therapies.

Acyclovir and related drugs

Mechanism of action: Acyclovir and related drugs are characterized by their selective phosphorylation in herpes-infected cells. This takes place by a viral thymidine kinase rather than host kinase, as a first step.

Phosphorylation yields a triphosphate nucleotide that inhibits viral DNA polymerase and viral DNA synthesis.

These drugs are selectively toxic to infected cells because, in the absence of viral thymidine kinase, the host kinase activates only a small amount of the drug. Also, the DNA polymerase of herpes virus has a much

higher affinity for the activated drug than has cellular DNA polymerase (Fig. 12.7).

Route of administration: Acyclovir and related drugs are administered topically, orally, and parentally; the choice depends on the site and severity of infection.

Indications: Acyclovir and related drugs are used for the prophylaxis and treatment of herpes simplex and varicella zoster superficial and systemic infections, particularly in immunocompromised people.

Adverse effects: Side effects of acyclovir and related drugs are minimal. Rarely, renal impairment and encephalopathy occur.

Therapeutic notes: The herpes genome in latent (non-replicating) cells is not affected by acyclovir therapy and so recurrence of infection after cessation of treatment is to be expected.

CMV is resistant to acyclovir because its genome does not encode thymidine kinase.

Ganciclovir

Mechanism of action: Ganciclovir is an acyclic analogue structurally related to acyclovir. It also requires conversion to the triphosphate nucleotide form, though by a different kinase. Ganciclovir acts as a substrate for viral DNA polymerase and as a chain terminator aborting virus replication.

Route of administration: Ganciclovir is administered orally and intravenously.

Indications: Though as active as acyclovir against HSV and VZV, ganciclovir is reserved for the treatment of severe CMV infections in immunocompromised people, owing to its toxicity (neutropenia).

Adverse effects: Side effects of ganciclovir include reversible neutropenia in 40% of patients. There is occasional rash, nausea, and encephalopathy.

Therapeutic notes: Maintenance therapy with ganciclovir at a reduced dose may be necessary to prevent recurrence of CMV.

Ribavirin

Mechanism of action: Ribavirin is a nucleoside analogue that selectively interferes with viral nucleic acid synthesis in a manner similar to acyclovir.

Route of administration: For respiratory syncytial virus (RSV) by aerosol within a hood; for Lassa virus intravenously.

Indications: Severe respiratory syncytial virus bronchiolitis in infants. Lassa fever.

Adverse effects: Reticulocytosis; respiratory depression.

Therapeutic notes: The necessity of aerosol administration for RSV limits the usefulness of this effective drug.

Immunomodulators

Interferons

Mechanism of action: Interferons (IFNs) are endogenous cytokines with antiviral activity, that are normally produced by leucocytes and other cells in response to viral infection. Three major classes have been identified (α, β, and γ) and have been shown to have immunoregulatory and antiproliferative effects.

The mechanism of the antiviral effect of IFN varies for different viruses and cells. IFNs have been shown to bind to cell-surface receptors and signal a cascade of events that interfere with viral penetration, uncoating, synthesis, or methylation of mRNA, translation of viral protein, viral assembly, and viral release (Fig. 12.7).

Probably the most important effect of IFNs is the induction of enzymes in the host cell that inhibit the translation of viral mRNA.

The relatively recent production of IFNs in large quantities by cell culture and recombinant DNA technology has allowed their evaluation and prescription as antiviral agents.

Route of administration: IFNs are administered intravenously only.

Indications: The exact role of interferons (IFNs) in the treatment of viral infections remains to be elucidated. They have a wide spectrum of activity and have been shown to be effective in the treatment of chronic hepatitis (B and C), among others.

Adverse effects: Common side effects of IFNs include an influenza-like syndrome with fatigue, fever, myalgia, nausea, and diarrhoea. Chronic administration can cause bone-marrow depression and neurological effects.

Therapeutic notes: The role of IFNs remains to be established. Their usefulness has been limited by the need for repeated injections, dose-limiting adverse effects, and a relative lack of efficacy. They may find a use in conjunction with other chemotherapeutic agents.

Drugs used in HIV infection

The pandemic of HIV-1 infection has resulted in an intensive search for new antiretroviral agents. There are a variety of potential sites for antiviral drug action in the HIV-1 replicative cycle (Fig. 12.8).

Two different classes of drug have been shown to be effective. These are:

- Nucleoside reverse transcriptase inhibitors (see Fig. 12.8, site 3).
- Protease inhibitors (see Fig. 12.8, site 5).

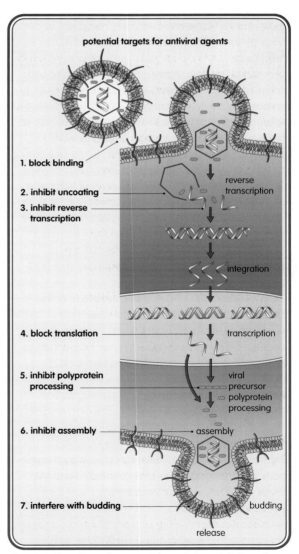

Fig. 12.8 The HIV replicative cycle and potential sites of antiviral drug action.

Nucleoside reverse transcriptase inhibitors

Examples of nucleoside reverse transcriptase inhibitors include zidovudine (azidothymidine, AZT)—this is the prototype of this class of drugs—and the newer drugs, didanosine (dideoxyadenosine, DDI) and zalcitabine (dideoxycytidine, DDC).

Mechanism of action: These nucleotide analogues all require intracellular conversion to the corresponding triphosphate nucleotide for activation. The active triphosphates competitively inhibit reverse transcriptase, and cause termination of DNA chain elongation once incorporated. Affinity for viral reverse transcriptase is 100 times that for host DNA polymerase (Fig. 12.8, site 3).

Route of administration: Nucleoside reverse transcriptase inhibitors are administered orally.

Indications: Nucleoside reverse transcriptase inhibitors are used for the management of asymptomatic and symptomatic HIV infections, and the prevention of maternal–fetal HIV transmission.

Adverse effects: Side effects of AZT are uncommon at the recommended low dosage in patients with asymptomatic or mild HIV infections, but more common in AIDS patients on higher dosage regimes.

Toxicity to human myeloid and erythroid progenitor cells commonly causes anaemia and neutropenia, i.e. bone-marrow suppression. Other side effects include nausea, insomnia, headaches, and myalgia.

The major dose-limiting effects of DDI are pancreatitis and peripheral neuropathy, and of DDC, peripheral neuropathy.

Therapeutic notes: Drug resistance evolves to all the current nucleoside reverse transcriptase inhibitors by the development of mutations in reverse transcriptase, although the kinetics of resistance development varies for the different drugs (e.g. ~6–18 months for AZT). Combined therapies may have a place in increasing efficacy synergistically and reducing emergence of resistant strains.

Protease inhibitors

Examples of protease inhibitors include sanquinavir—this is the prototype of this class of drugs—and the newer drugs, ritonavir and indinavir.

Mechanism of action: Protease inhibitors interfere with HIV replication by inhibiting post-translational processing of viral precursor polypeptides (see Fig. 12.8, site 5).

Route of administration: Protease inhibitors are administered orally.

Indications: Protease inhibitors are used for the management of asymptomatic and symptomatic HIV infections, in combination with nucleoside reverse transcriptase inhibitors. This is under evaluation.

Adverse effects: Protease inhibitors are well tolerated. However, nausea, vomiting diarrhoea are common. In addition, indinavir and ritonavir may cause taste disturbances, and saquinavir may cause buccal and mucosal ulceration.

Therapeutic notes: Combination treatment between protease inhibitors and nucleoside reverse transcriptase inhibitors produces additive antiviral effects and reduces the incidence of resistance.

Future anti-HIV drug therapy

A number of strategies are being pursued in research laboratories across the world in the quest for effective drugs to treat HIV infection. These strategies include:

- Recombinant, truncated, or synthetic CD4 receptor-specific peptides that would compete with HIV for attachment to CD4 T-cell lymphocytes, inhibiting viral binding (see Fig 12.8, site 1).
- Synthetic peptide inhibitors of the HIV-encoded protease that is responsible for cleavage, and release of mature reverse transcriptase from its precursor polypeptide (see Fig 12.8, site 5).
- Antisense oligonucleotides, which are synthetic stretches of single-stranded nucleic acid that can be designed to bind to viral genome by complementary base pairing, thus inhibiting viral replication *in vivo* (see Fig. 12.8, site 4).
- Avarol and avarone, which are two drugs that are thought to interfere with cytoskeletal processes

The development of antiviral drugs is a rapidly-moving field and, with HIV especially, one that is currently topical. Keep up to date, as knowledge of recent developments in this area should impress examiners.

involved in the assembly (see Fig. 12.8, site 6) and budding (see Fig. 12.8, site 7) of HIV virus particles.
- Non-nucleotide reverse transcriptase inhibitors (Fig. 12.8, site 3)

- What are the peculiar features of viruses as infective pathogens and how does their life cycle make selective chemotherapy difficult?
- What is the broad classification of viruses and what are the major human diseases caused by viruses.
- Which viral diseases can be pharmacologically treated?
- Describe the mechanism of action of the different classes of antiviral drug and the point in the viral replicative cycle that they act.
- Name an example from each of the major antiviral drug classes, when they are used, and the major adverse effects associated with their use.
- Name the drugs currently used in the treatment of infections with HIV.

ANTIFUNGAL DRUGS

Concepts of fungal infection

Fungi are members of a kingdom of eukaryotic organisms that live as saprophytes or parasites. A few species of fungi are pathogenic to humans.

Fungal infections are termed mycoses and may be superficial, affecting the skin, nails, hair, mucous membranes, etc., or systemic, affecting deep tissues and organs.

Three main groups of fungi cause disease in humans (Fig. 12.9).

Fungal pathogenicity results from mycotoxin production, allergenicity/inflammatory reactions, and tissue invasion. Opportunistic fungal infections are important causes of disease in immunosuppressed people.

Antifungal drugs

There are three main classes of antifungal drugs (Fig. 12.10). These are the:
- Polyene macrolides.
- Antifungal azoles.
- Allylamines.

The routes of administration and the sites of action of the antifungal drugs are summarized in Fig. 12.10 and 12.11, respectively.

Polyene macrolides

Examples of polyene macrolides include amphotericin B and nystatin.

Fungi causing disease in humans			
Fungal class	**Form**	**Example**	**Disease caused**
moulds	filamentous branching mycelia	dermatophytes e.g. *Tinea* spp. *Aspergillus fumigatus*	athlete's foot, ringworm and other superficial mycoses pulmonary or disseminated aspergillosis
true yeasts	unicellular (round or oval)	*Cryptococcus neoformans*	cryptococcal meningitis and lung infections in the immunocompromised
yeast-like fungi	similar to yeasts but can also form long (non branching) filaments	*Candida albicans*	oral and vaginal thrush, endocarditis and septicaemias

Fig. 12.9 Main groups of fungi causing disease in humans.

Mechanism of action: Polyene macrolides bind to ergosterol in the fungal cell membrane, forming pores through which cell constituents are lost. This results in fatal damage (Fig. 12.12). These drugs are selectively toxic because in human cells the major sterol is cholesterol, not ergosterol.

Route of administration: Amphotericin B is administered topically and intravenously. Nystatin is too toxic for intravenous use. It is not absorbed orally at all and so is applied topically as a cream or vaginal pessaries, or tablets sucked so as to deliver the drug via the oral membranes.

Indications: Amphotericin is a broad-spectrum antifungal used in potentially fatal systemic infections. Nystatin is used to suppress candidiasis (thrush) on the skin and mucous membranes (oral and vaginal).

Adverse effects: Side effects of amphotericin given parenterally include fever, chills, and nausea. Long-term therapy invariably causes renal damage. Nystatin may cause oral sensitization.

Therapeutic notes: Creatinine clearance must be monitored during amphotericin therapy to observe renal damage. Resistance can develop *in vivo* to amphotericin, but not to nystatin.

Antifungal drugs and their routes of administration		
Drug class	**Drug name**	**Route of administration**
polyene macrolides	amphotericin B nystatin	topical, intravenous topical (oral for gastrointestinal tract only)

azoles
    imidazoles
 	
    triazoles
	clotrimazole
	miconazole
	ketoconazole
	fluconazole
	itraconazole
		topical
		topical, intravenous
		topical, oral
		oral
		oral

allylamines	terbinafine	topical, oral
other	flucytosine griseofulvin	oral oral

Fig. 12.10 Antifungal drugs and their routes of administration.

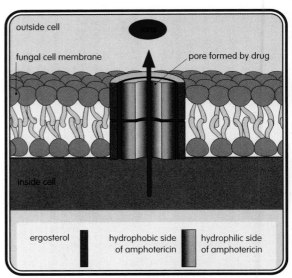

Fig. 12.12 Mechanism of action of polyene antifungal agents.

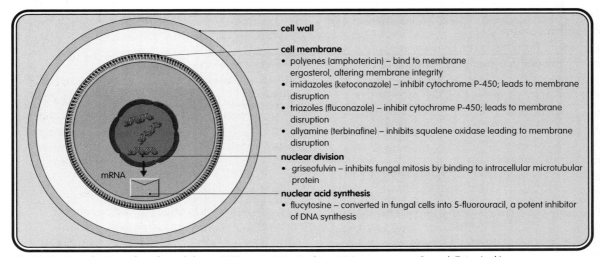

Fig. 12.11 Sites of action of antifungal drugs. (GIT, gastrointestinal tract; I, intraveneous; O, oral; T, topical.)

Imidazoles

Examples of imidazoles include clotrimazole, miconazole, and ketoconazole.

Mechanism of action: Imidazoles have a broad spectrum of activity. They inhibit fungal lipid (especially ergosterol) synthesis in cell membranes. Interference with fungal oxidative enzymes results in the accumulation of 14α-methyl sterols, which may disrupt the packing of acyl chains of phospholipids, inhibiting growth and interfering with membrane-bound enzyme systems.

Route of administration: The imidazoles are administered intraveneously or topically. Ketoconazole is given orally as, unlike the other imidazoles, it is well absorbed by this route.

Indications: Imidazoles are used for candidiasis and dermatophyte mycoses. Miconazole can also be used intravenously as an alternative to amphotericin in disseminated mycoses. Because ketonazole is active orally, it can be used for systemic mycoses.

Adverse effects: Topical use of imidazoles tends to be unproblematic. Intravenous miconazole is often limited by side effects of nausea, faintness, and haematological disorders. Oral ketonazole can cause serious hepatotoxicity and adrenosuppression.

Therapeutic notes: Resistance rarely develops to imidazoles.

Triazoles

Examples of triazoles include fluconazole and itraconazole.

Mechanism of action: Triazoles are similar to imidazoles (see above), although they have greater selectivity against fungi and cause less endocrinological problems.

Route of administration: Fluconazole and itraconazole are administered orally.

Indications: Fluconazole can be used for a wide range of systemic and superficial infections, including cryptococcal meningitis, as it reaches the CSF in high concentrations. Itraconazole is similarly indicated, although unlike fluconazole, it can be used against *Aspergillus*.

Adverse effects: Side effects of fluconazole include nausea, diarrhoea, and rashes, although, unlike itraconazole, it does not severely affect the liver or endocrine systems. Itraconazole is well tolerated though nausea, headaches and abdominal pain can occur.

Therapeutic notes: Resistance rarely develops to the triazoles.

Allylamines

Terbinafine is an example of an allylamine.

Mechanism of action: Terbinafine prevents ergosterol synthesis by inhibiting the enzyme squalene oxidase, resulting in squalene accumulation, which leads to membrane disruption and cell death. It is lipophilic and penetrates superficial tissues well, including the nails.

Route of administration: Terbinafine is administered orally or applied topically.

Indications: Terbinafine has been recently introduced against dermatophyte infections including ringworm, where oral therapy is appropriate because of the site and severity of extent of infection.

Adverse effects: Side effects to terbinafine are few, but include mild nausea, abdominal pain, and skin reactions. Loss of taste has been reported.

Therapeutic notes: Resistance rarely develops. Initial trials with terbinafine show impressive clinical and mycological cure rates.

Flucytosine

Mechanism of action: Flucytosine is imported into fungal, but not human, cells, where it is converted into 5-fluorouracil, a potent inhibitor of DNA synthesis.

Route of administration: Flucytosine is administered orally.

Indications: Flucytosine is most active against yeasts, and is indicated for use in systemic candidiasis and as an adjunct to amphotericin in cryptococcal meningitis.

Adverse effects: Side effects from flucytosine are uncommon but include hepatotoxicity, hair loss, and bone-marrow suppression.

Therapeutic notes: Weekly blood counts of patients on flucytosine are necessary to monitor bone marrow suppression.

Griseofulvin

Mechanism of action: The action of griseofulvin is not fully established, but it probably interferes with microtubule formation or nucleic acid synthesis and polymerization. It is selectively concentrated in keratin and therefore is suitable for treating dermatophyte mycoses.

Route of administration: Griseofulvin is administered orally.

Indications: Griseofulvin is the drug of choice for widespread or intractable dermatophyte infections, where topical therapy has failed.

Adverse effects: Side effects from griseofulvin are uncommon, but include hypersensitivity, headaches,

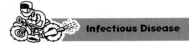
rashes, and photosensitivity.

Therapeutic notes: Because griseofulvin is fungistatic rather than fungicidal, treatment regimes are long amounting to several weeks or months.

Griseofulvin is more effective for skin than nail infections.

Superficial mycoses (e.g. 'athletes foot'/'thrush') are common and usually easily treated with topical drugs that have few adverse effects. Deep mycoses are rare (except in the immunocompromised), serious, and may be fatal despite therapy with systemic drugs, which often have adverse effects.

○ **Describe the classification of fungi and the types of infection (mycoses) that fungi can cause.**
○ **What are the main classes of antifungal drugs? Describe their mechanism and site of action.**
○ **For each class of antifungal name examples of the drugs, their route of administration, indications, and major adverse effects.**

ANTIPROTOZOAL DRUGS

Concepts of protozoal infection

Protozoa are members of a phylum of unicellular organisms, some of which are parasitic pathogens in humans, causing several diseases of medical and global importance. Parasitic protozoa replicate within the host's body and are usually divided into four subphyla according to their type of locomotion (Fig. 12.13).

Malaria

Malaria is the most important protozoan disease in tropical medicine. It is responsible for two million deaths per year and much morbidity in the 200 million people worldwide who are infected.

Malaria is caused by four species of plasmodial parasites that are transmitted by female anopheline mosquitoes.

Antimalarial drugs target different phases of the malarial life cycle (Fig. 12.14). This life cycle proceeds as follows:

- When an infected mosquito feeds on a human it injects sporozoites into the bloodstream from its salivary glands.
- The sporozoites rapidly penetrate the liver where they transform and grow into tissue schizonts containing large numbers of merozoites. In the case of *Plasmodium vivax* and *P. ovale*, some schizonts remain dormant in the liver for years (hypnozoites), before rupturing to cause a relapse.
- The large tissue schizonts rupture after 5–20 days, releasing thousands of merozoites that invade circulating red blood cells (RBCs), and multiply inside the cell.
- The host's RBCs rupture, leading to the release of more merozoites. These then invade and destroy more RBCs. This cycle of invasion/destruction causes the episodic chills and fever that characterize malaria.
- Some merozoites develop into gametocytes. If these are taken up by a feeding mosquito, the insect becomes infected, thus completing the cycle.

The clinical features and severity of malaria depend on the species of parasite and the immunological status of the person infected. Clinically significant malaria is rarer in adults who have always lived in endemic areas, as partial immunity develops.

The four types of plasmodium causing malaria are:

- *P. falciparum,* which is widespread and causes malignant tertian (fever every third day) malaria. There is no exo-erythrocytic stage, so that, if the erythrocytic forms are eradicated, relapses do not occur.
- *P. vivax,* which is widespread and causes benign, tertian relapsing malaria. Exo-erythrocytic forms may persist in the liver for years and cause relapses.
- *P. malariae,* which is rare and causes benign quartan (fever every fourth day) malaria. There is no exo-erythrocytic stage, so that, if the erythrocytic

Classification of medically important protozoan species causing disease in humans			
Sub-phyla	**Defining characteristics**	**Medically important species**	**Disease**
amoebae (sarcodina)	ameoboid movement with pseudopods	*Entameoba histolytica*	amoebiasis (ameobic dysentery)
flagellates (mastigophora)	flagella that produces a whip-like movement	*Giarda lamlia* *Trichonomas vaginalis* *Leishmania* spp. *Trypanosoma* spp.	giardiasis trichomonal vaginitis leishmaniasis trypanosomiasis (sleeping sickness and Chaga's disease)
ciliates (ciliophora)	cilia beat to produce movement	—	—
sporozoans (sporozoa)	no locomotor organs in adult stage	*Plasmodium* spp.	malaria

Fig. 12.13 Classification of medically-important protozoan species causing disease in humans.

forms are eradicated, relapses do not occur.

- *P. ovale*, which is mainly African and causes a rare form of benign relapsing malaria. Exo-erythrocytic forms may persist in the liver for years and cause relapses.

Approaches to antimalarial chemotherapy

Antimalarial drugs are usually classified in terms of their action against different stages of the parasite (Fig.

12.14). They are used to protect against or cure malaria or to prevent transmission.

Prophylactic use

The aim of prophylactic use is to prevent the occurrence of infection in a previously healthy individual who is at potential exposure risk.

Suppressive prophylaxis involves the use of blood schizontocides to prevent acute attacks; causal

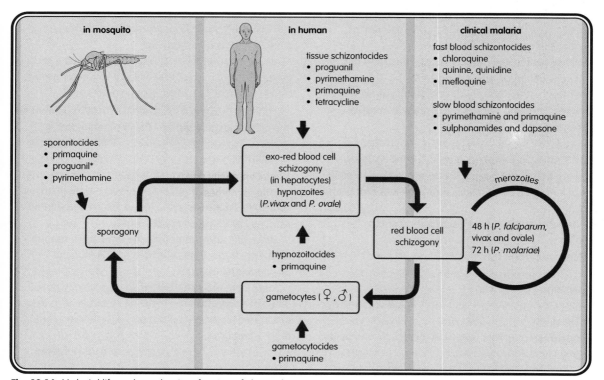

Fig. 12.14 Malarial life cycle and point of action of chemotherapeutic agents.

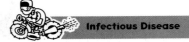

prophylaxis involves the use of tissue schizontocides or drugs against the sporozoite to prevent the parasite becoming established in the liver.

Curative (therapeutic use)

Antimalarial drugs can be used curatively (therapeutically) against an established infection.

Suppressive treatment aims to control acute attacks, usually with blood schizontocides; radical treatment aims to kill dormant liver forms, usually with a hypnozoitocide, to prevent relapsing malaria.

Antimalarial drugs

4-Aminoquinolines

Chloroquine is an example of a 4-aminoquinoline.

Mechanism of action: Chloroquine is a rapidly acting blood schizontocide (Fig. 12.14). It is concentrated 100-fold in erythrocytes that contain plasmodial parasites; this occurs because ferriprotoporphyrin IX, a degradation product of haemoglobin digestion by the parasites, acts as a chloroquine receptor. It is unclear how the high chloroquine concentrations kill the parasites; possibly, the digestion of haemoglobin is inhibited.

Route of administration: Orally; however, in severe falcipanum malaria, injections or infusions can be used.

Indications: Chloroquine is the drug of choice for suppressive chemoprophylaxis and treatment of susceptible strains of plasmodium.

Adverse effects: Side effects from chloroquine are unusual with the low doses taken for chemoprophylaxis. Higher treatment doses may cause nausea, vomiting, headache, rashes, and, rarely, neurological effects.

Therapeutic notes: Chloroquine is considered safe for use in pregnant women. It rapidly controls fever (24–48 hours) but cannot produce a lasting radical cure in *P.vivax* and *P.ovale* strains as it does not affect hypnozoites.

In most areas, *P.falciparum* is resistant to chloroquinine, necessitating combination chemoprophylaxis with antifolates (see later).

Quinoline–methanols

Examples of quinoline–methanols include quinine and mefloquine.

Mechanism of action: Quinoline-methanols are rapidly acting blood schizontocides (Fig. 12.14). It is not precisely known how the quinoline–methanols work but, like chloroquine, they are known to bind to a product of haemoglobin digestion.

Route of administration: Quinine is administered orally or by rate-controlled infusion in severe cases. Mefloquine is given orally only.

Indications: Quinine is the drug of choice for treating the acute clinical attack of falciparum malaria resistant to chloroquine. Mefloquine is effective against all malarial species including multidrug-resistant *P. falciparum,* and can also be used for chemoprophylaxis.

Adverse effects: Common side effects of quinine include tinnitus, headache, nausea, blurring of vision, hypoglycaemia, and, rarely, blood disorders. Overdose results in profound hypotension due to peripheral vasodilatation and myocardial depression (see Chapter 4). Quinine is safe in pregnancy.

Mefloquine can cause nausea, vomiting, gastro-intestinal disturbance, and postural hypotension. Rarely, acute neuropathic conditions may occur. Mefloquine may cause fetal abnormalities.

Therapeutic notes: The quinoline–methanols are used in combination therapy with other agents such as the sulphonamides or tetracyclines.

Antifolates

Examples of antifolates include type 1 drugs, e.g. sulphonamides and dapsone, and type 2 drugs, e.g. pyrimethamine and proguanil.

Mechanism of action: Antifolates are slow-acting (in comparison with chloroquine, quinine, and mefloquine) blood schizontocides, tissue schizontocides, and sporontocides. These drugs inhibit the formation of folate compounds and thus inhibit DNA synthesis and cell division. Hence, all growing stages of the malarial parasite are affected.

The sulphonamides and dapsone are known as type 1 antifolate drugs. They compete with P-aminobenzoic acid (PABA) for the enzyme dihydropteroate synthetase, which is found only in the parasites.

Proguanil and pyrimethamine are known as type 2 antifolate drugs. They selectively inhibit malarial dihydrofolate reductase.

Hence the drugs act on the same pathway but at different points; they are used in combination as their synergistic blockade is more powerful than any one drug acting alone.

Route of administration: Antifolates are administered orally.

Indications: Antifolates are used in combination for the causal chemoprophylaxis of malaria, or in combination with quinine for the treatment of acute chloroquine-resistant malaria.

Adverse effects: Antifolates have almost no side effects if used in therapeutic doses. In toxic doses, type 2 antifolates can inhibit mammalian dihydrofolate reductase and cause a megoblastic anaemia. Skin rashes occasionally occur.

Therapeutic notes: Common chemoprophylactic combinations include chloroquine plus pyrimethamine with a sulphonamide or dapsone.

8-Aminoquinolines

Primaquine is an example of an 8-aminoquinoline.

Mechanism of action: Primaquine is an hypnozoitocide and gametocytocide. It is unclear how the drug works, but it may cause oxidative damage to the parasite. It is effective against the non-growing stages of malaria, i.e. hypnozoites and gametocytes (Fig. 12.14).

Route of administration: oral.

Indications: Primaquine is used for the radical cure of relapsing malarias (*P. ovale* and *P. vivax*) and prevention of transmission of *P. falciparum*.

Contraindications: Primaquine should not be given to pregnant women.

Adverse effects: Side effects of primaquine include nausea, vomiting, and bone- marrow depression. Intravenous haemolysis can occur in people with glucose-6-phosphate deficiency.

Therapeutic notes: Primaquine is usually used in combination with chloroquine. Resistance is rare.

Treatment of other protozoal infections
Amoebiasis

Amoebic dysentery is caused by infection with *Entamoeba histolytica,* which is ingested in a cystic form. Dysentery results from invasion of the intestinal wall by the parasite. Occasionally, the organism encysts in the liver, forming abscesses.

Metronidazole (an imidazole) (p. 196) is the drug of choice for acute invasive amoebic dysentery, it kills the trophozoites but has no activity against the cyst forms. Diloxanide furoate (a dichloracetamide) is active against the cysts.

Giardiasis

Giardiasis is a bowel infection caused by the flagellate *Giardia lamblia.* Infection follows ingestion of contaminated water or food and involves flatulence and diarrhoea.

Metronidazole (p. 196) is the drug of choice for giardiasis.

Trichomonas vaginitis

Trichomonas vaginitis is caused by the flagellate *Trichomonas vaginalis.* It is a sexually transmitted inflammatory condition of the female vagina and, occasionally, male urethra.

Metronidazole (p. 196) is the drug of choice for trichomonas vaginitis.

Trypanosomiasis and leishmaniasis
Trypanosomiasis

African sleeping sickness and South American Chagas' disease are caused by species of flagellate trypanosome.

Insect vectors introduce the parasites into the human host, where they reproduce, causing bouts of parasitaemia and fever. Toxins released cause damage to organs—the CNS in the case of sleeping sickness, and the heart, liver, spleen, bone, and intestine in Chagas' disease.

Leishmaniasis

Leishmania species are flagellated parasites that are transmitted by a sandfly vector, assuming a non-flagellated intracellular form that resides within macrophages on infecting humans.

Clinical infections range from simple, resolving cutaneous infections to systemic 'visceral' forms with hepatomegaly, splenomegaly, anaemia, and fever.

The prophylaxis and treatment of trypanosomiasis and leishmaniasis are difficult and of variable efficacy. The drugs used are generally toxic and dangerous, making specialized knowledge essential.

A decent knowledge of the plasmodial life cycle is a prerequisite to understanding the mechanism and site of action of antimalarial drugs.

ANTHELMINTIC DRUGS

Concepts of helminthic infection

Helminth is derived from the Greek *helmins*, meaning worm. Anthelmintic drugs are therefore medicines acting against parasitic worms.

The three groups of helminths that parasitize humans are:

- Cestoda (tapeworms).
- Nematoda (roundworms).
- Trematoda (flukes).

Fig. 12.15 lists medically important helminth infections and the main drugs used in their treatment.

Anthelmintic drugs

To be effective, an anthelmintic drug must be able to penetrate the cuticle of the worm, or gain access to its alimentary tract, so that it may exert its pharmacological effect on the physiology of the worm.

Anthelmintic drugs act on parasitic worms by a number of mechanisms. These include:

- Damaging or killing the worm directly.
- Paralysing the worm.
- Damaging the cuticle of the worm so that host defences, such as digestion and immune rejection, can affect the worm.
- Interfering with worm metabolism.

Because there is great diversity across the different helminth classes, drugs highly effective against one species of worm are often ineffectual against another species.

Niclosamide

Mechanism of action: Niclosamide, a salicylamide derivative, is the most used drug for tapeworm infestations. It blocks glucose uptake at high concentrations, irreversibly damaging the scolex (attachment end) of the tapeworm, leading to the release and expulsion of the tapeworm. It is a safe, selective drug since very little is absorbed from the gastrointestinal tract.

Route of administration: Niclosamide is administered orally.

Indications: Niclosamide is used for tapeworm infestation (see Fig. 12.15).

Adverse effects: Side effects of niclosamide include mild gastrointestinal disturbance.

Therapeutic notes: Patients are fasted before treatment with niclosamide. Purgatives to expel the dead worm segments (proglottides) can be used, but are probably unnecessary, since the worm may be digested after the effects of the drug.

Praziquantel

Mechanism of action: Praziquantel increases the permeability of the helminth plasma membrane to calcium. At low concentrations this causes contraction and spastic paralysis and, at higher concentrations, vesiculation and vacuolization damage is caused to the tegument of the worm.

Route of administration: Praziquantel is administered orally.

Indications: Praziquantel is the drug of choice for all schistosome infections (see Fig. 12.15), and for cysticercosis (a rare cestode condition caused by encystation of larvae of the tapeworm *Taenia solium,* in human organs).

Classification of medically important helminth infection and the main drugs in their treatment		
	Helminth species	**Drugs used in treatment**
• **cestodes**		
beef tapeworm	*Taenia saginata*	niclosamide, praziquantel
pork tapeworm	*Taenia solium*	niclosamide, praziquantel
fish tapeworm	*Diphyllobothrium latum*	niclosamide, praziquantel
hyatid tapeworm	*Echinococcus granulosus*	albendazole
• **nematodes**		
intestinal species		
common round worms	*Ascaris lumbricoides*	mebendazole, piperazine
threadworm/pin worm	*Enterobius vermicularis*	mebendazole, piperazine
threadworm (USA)	*Strongyloides stecoralis*	thiabendazole, albendazole
whipworm	*Trichuris trichuria*	mebendazole
hookworms	*Necator americanus*	mebendazole
	Ankylostoma duodenale	mebendazole
tissue species		
trichella	*Tricheinella spiralis*	thiabendazole
guinea worm	*Dracunulus medinesis*	metronidazole*
filariaroidea	*Wucheria bancrofti*	diethylcarbamazine
	Loa loa	diethylcarbamazine
	Brugia malayi	diethylcarbamazine
	Onchocera volvulus	ivermectin
• **trematodes**		
blood flukes/	*Schistosoma japoniicum*	praziquantel
schistosomes	*Schistosoma mansoni*	praziquantel
	Schistosoma haematobium	praziquantel

Fig. 12.15 Classification of medically important helminth infections and the main drugs used in their treatment. (* see p. 196.)

Adverse effects: Side effects of praziquantel include mild gastrointestinal disturbance, and headache and dizziness may occur shortly after administration.
Therapeutic notes: Praziquantel should be taken after meals three times a day for 2 days only.

Piperazine

Mechanism of action: Piperazine is a reversible neuromuscular blocker that causes a flaccid paralysis in worms, leading to their expulsion by gastrointestinal peristalsis. It has very little effect on the host.
Route of administration: Piperazine is administered orally.
Indications: Piperazine is used for roundworm and threadworm gastrointestinal infestation.
Adverse effects: Side effects of piperazine include occasional gastrointestinal disturbance, and neurotoxic effects (dizziness) may occur.
Therapeutic notes: A single dose of piperazine is usually effective for treating roundworm infection; threadworm iinfestation may require a longer course (7 days).

Benzimidazoles
Examples of benzimidazoles include mebendazole, thiabendazole, and albendazole.

Mechanism of action: Benzimidazoles bind with high affinity to a site on tubulin dimers, thus preventing the polymerization of microtubules. Subsequent depolymerization leads to complete breakdown of the microtubule.

The selectivity of benzimidazoles arises because they are 250–400 times more potent in helminth than in mammalian tissue. The process takes time to have effect, and the worm may not be expelled for days.
Route of administration: Benzimidazoles are administered orally.
Indications: Benzimidazoles are used in the treatment of hydatid disease, and many nematode infestations (Fig. 12.15).
Contraindications: Benzimidazoles should not be given to pregnant women as they are teratogenic and embryotoxic.
Adverse effects: Side effects of mebendazole and albendazole include occasional gastrointestinal disturbance. Thiabendazole causes more frequent gastrointestinal disturbance, headache, and dizziness. Serious hepatotoxicity rarely occurs.
Therapeutic notes: Dosage regimes of benzimidazoles range from a single dose for pinworm infestation to multiple doses for up to 5 days for trichinosis.

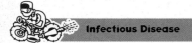
Diethylcarbamazine

Mechanism of action: It is not clear exactly how diethylcarbamazine exerts its filaricidal effect. It has been suggested that it damages or modifies the parasites in such a way as to make them more susceptible to host immune defences.

Diethylcarbamazine kills both microfilariae in the peripheral circulation and adult worms in the lymphatics.

Route of administration: Diethylcarbamazine is administered orally.

Indications: Diethylcarbamazine is the drug of choice for lymphatic filiariasis caused by *Wucheria bancrofti, Loa loa,* and *Brugia malayi* (see Fig. 12.15).

Adverse effects: Common side effects of diethylcarbamazine include transient gastrointestinal disturbance, headache, and lassitude.

Material from the damaged and dead worms causes allergic side effects, including skin reactions, lymph gland enlargement, dizziness, and tachycardia, lasting from 3 to 7 days.

Therapeutic notes: To minimize the dangerous sudden release of dead worm material, the initial dose of diethylcarbamazine is started low and then increased and maintained for 21 days.

Ivermectin

Mechanism of action: Ivermectin immobilizes the tapeworm *Onchocerca volvulus* by causing tonic paralysis of the peripheral muscle system. It does this by potentiating the effect of GABA at the worm's neuromuscular junction.

Route of administration: Ivermectin is administered orally.

Indications: Ivermectin is the drug of choice for *Onchocerca volvulus,* which causes river blindness (Fig. 12.15).

Adverse effects: Side effects from ivermectin are uncommon and include ocular irritation, transient electrocardiographic changes, and somnolence. An immediate immune reaction to dead microfilariae (Mazzotti reaction) can be severe.

All the anthelmintic drugs described in this chapter are administered orally.

- Describe the classification of the helminths that parasitize humans.
- Name the medically important helminths in each group, the diseases they cause, and the drugs used in their treatment.
- Discuss the mechanisms of action of the drugs used in the treatment of helminth infections.

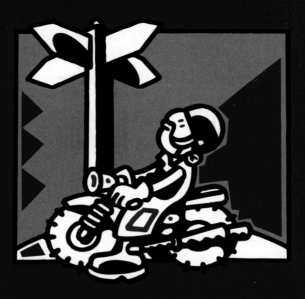

SELF-ASSESSMENT

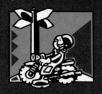

Multiple-choice Questions

Indicate whether each answer is true or false.

1. L-Dopa reduces the symptoms of Parkinson's disease because:

(a) There is a deficiency of dopamine in some areas of the brain in patients with this condition.
(b) It is converted to serotonin in serotonergic neurons.
(c) It is converted to dopamine in the central nervous system.
(d) It is an inhibitory transmitter.
(e) It antagonizes cholinergic receptors in the corpus striatum.

2. γ-aminobutyric acid (GABA):

(a) Is an inhibitory transmitter.
(b) Reduces chloride permeability in central neurons.
(c) Acts on receptors that are potentiated by some hypnotics.
(d) Has its actions blocked selectively by fluoxetine.
(e) Acts on receptors that are antagonized by barbiturates.

3. Benzodiazepines:

(a) Are safer if taken in overdose than are other hypnotics.
(b) Are potent inducers of hepatic enzyme systems.
(c) Do not produce tolerance and physical dependence, unlike barbiturates.
(d) Are sometimes used intravenously in status epilepticus.
(e) Are GABA-receptor antagonists with neuroexcitatory effects.

4. Treatments for depression may include:

(a) Muscarinic receptor antagonists.
(b) Monoamine oxidase inhibitors.
(c) Neuroleptics.
(d) Dopamine-receptor antagonists.
(e) Serotonin reuptake inhibitors.

5. Side effects of chlorpromazine administration may include:

(a) Hallucinations.
(b) Movement disorders.
(c) Hyperactivity and insomnia.
(d) Endocrine irregularities.
(e) Dry mouth, blurred vision, and constipation.

6. The following drugs are effective in treating grand mal epilepsy:

(a) Ethosuximide.
(b) Carbamazepine.
(c) Haloperidol.
(d) Choral hydrate.
(e) Phenytoin.

7. Drugs used in premedication and induction prior to inhalation anaesthesia include:

(a) Opioids.
(b) Benzodiazepines.
(c) Barbiturates.
(d) Muscarinic agonists.
(e) Halothane.

8. Side effects of morphine used as an analgesic include:

(a) Pupillary constriction.
(b) Nausea and vomiting.
(c) Respiratory depression.
(d) Diarrhoea.
(e) Euphoria in most patients.

9. Alcohol withdrawal syndrome can involve:

(a) Piloerection.
(b) Hallucinations.
(c) Epileptic-type fits.
(d) Death.
(e) Treatment with chlormethiazole.

10. Salbutamol:

(a) Must be given prior to an asthma attack.
(b) Is most commonly administered via a metered-dose inhaler, but can be taken orally and intravenously.
(c) Is a β_2-antagonist of use in the treatment of mild to moderate asthma.
(d) Is longer-acting than salmeterol.
(e) Causes bronchodilatation and may decrease the release of inflammatory mediators from mast cells.

11. Drugs used in the treatment of asthma include:

(a) Theophylline by aerosol.
(b) β_2-adrenoceptor agonists given by aerosol, orally, or intravenously.
(c) Mineralocorticoids by aerosol, orally, or intravenously.
(d) Ipratopium aerosol.
(e) H_1 histamine receptor antagonists.

12. The following drugs are useful for treating peptic ulcers:

(a) Cimetidine.
b) Histamine H_1 receptor antagonists.
(c) Bismuth chelate.
(d) Prostaglandin antagonists.
(e) Sodium chloride.

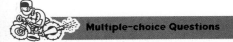

13. The following statements are true:

(a) Loperamide inhibits gastrointestinal motility by reducing acetylcholine secretion from nerve endings.
(b) Smooth muscle spasm in irritable bowel syndrome can be treated with atropine.
(c) Postoperative atony of the gut (paralytic ileus) can be treated with neostigmine.
(d) Metoclopramide is useful in reducing nausea, vomiting, and diarrhoea.
(e) Corticosteroid foams are used to treat serious infective diarrhoeas.

14. The following features about drug dependence and tolerance are correct:

(a) Dependence is confined to drugs that alter state of consciousness.
(b) Psychological dependence leads to emotional distress if the drug is withheld.
(c) Physical dependence is a major factor with cocaine.
(d) Physical dependence is a major factor with heroin.
(e) Physical and psychological withdrawal are moderate with legal drugs like alcohol and tobacco.

15. Side effects of systemic glucocorticoid use can include:

(a) Loss of bone and muscle tissue.
(b) Renal failure.
(c) Hyperglycaemia and sometimes diabetes.
(d) Increased susceptibility to infections.
(e) Hallucinations.

16. Drugs that have their major effect on immune function include:

(a) Cyclosporine.
(b) Histamine H_2 antagonists.
(c) Sulphonamides.
(d) Ibuprofen.
(e) Methotrexate.

17. The following adverse effects can result from treatment with cytotoxic chemotherapeutic agents:

(a) Nausea and vomiting.
(b) Immunosuppression due to reduced numbers of circulating leucocytes.
(c) Renal failure.
(d) Amenorrhoea and infertility.
(e) Cancers

18. The drugs below are matched correctly with their mechanism of action:

(a) 5-Fluorouracil: antimetabolite.
(b) Mustine: alkylating agent.
(c) Actinomycin: antimetabolite.
(d) Vincristine: cytotoxic antibiotic.
(e) Mercaptopurine: alkylating agent.

19. The drugs below are correctly matched with their mechanism of action:

(a) Erythromycin: binds to bacterial ribosome inhibiting DNA replication.
(b) Benzylpenicillin: destroys the integrity of the bacterial plasma membrane.
(c) Trimethoprim: inhibits the metabolism of DNA precursors.
(d) Vancomycin: inhibits the synthesis of peptidoglycan.
(e) Rifampicin: binds to RNA polymerase preventing DNA transcription.

20. Penicillins:

(a) As a group all share the same range of antibacterial activity.
(b) Are all resistant to gastric acid degradation allowing oral administration.
(c) Are only active against multiplying organisms.
(d) Are bacteriostatic.
(e) Are no longer of clinical use due to bacterial resistance.

21. The drugs below are correctly matched with their mechanism of action:

(a) Interferon-α: binds to virus particles to inhibit attachment.
(b) Amantadine: prophylactic against influenza A by inhibiting attachment and penetration.
(c) Acyclovir: metabolized in viral-infected cells to a false nucleotide.
(d) Zidovudine: a false nucleotide chain that terminates viral DNA replication.
(e) Amphotericin: binds to viral DNA polymerase inhibiting DNA replication.

22. Properties of acyclovir include the following:

(a) Has excellent oral absorption.
(b) Inhibits herpes simplex and varicella–zoster virus.
(c) Has limiting side effects at therapeutic concentrations.
(d) Has topical activity.
(e) May cause renal tubular obstruction.

23. The following mechanisms of action are correct:

(a) Micronidazole inhibits the synthesis of fungal lipids, especially ergosterol.
(b) Terbinafine prevents the synthesis of ergosterol by inhibiting the enzyme squalene oxidase.
(c) Nystatin interferes with fungal oxidative enzymes.
(d) Amphotericin B is thought to act by interfering with microtubule function.
(e) Flucytosine is converted in fungal cells to metabolites that inhibit DNA synthesis.

24. Metronidazole:

(a) Disrupts DNA in susceptible organisms, resulting in strand breakage and loss of helical structure.
(b) Is a first-line drug in the treatment of falciparum malaria.
(c) Has to be given parenterally as it is destroyed by gastric acidity.
(d) Has antibacterial, antiprotozoal, and anthelmintic actions.
(e) Is a first-line drug in the treatment of amoebic dysentery.

25. The drugs below are correctly matched with their mechanism of action:

(a) Praziquantel: increases permeability of worm membrane to calcium.
(b) Diethylcarbamazine: unknown mechanism of activity against tapeworms.
(c) Benzimidazoles: bind tubulin in helminth tissue leading to microtubule depolymerization.
(d) Niclosamide: damages tapeworm scolexes.
(e) Piperazine: exposes worm to host immune system.

26. The following are muscarinic antagonistsl:

(a) Suxamethonium.
(b) Tropicamide.
(c) Hyoscine.
(d) Neostigmine.
(e) Pilocarpine.

27. Suxamethonium:

(a) Its action is reversed by anticholinesterases.
(b) Is a competitive blocker of the neuromuscular junction.
(c) Is used clinically as a skeletal muscle relaxant.
(d) Shows tetanic fade.
(e) Binds to voltage-operated sodium channels causing block of muscle action potential.

28. The following are used as abortifacients:

(a) Nifedipine.
(b) Prostaglandin E_2.
(c) Ergometrine.
(d) Oxytocin.
(e) Mifepristone.

29. In renal pharmacology:

(a) Thiazides block the Na^+/Cl^- co-transporter in the luminal membrane of the renal tubular cells.
(b) Carbonic anhydrase inhibitors produce a highly acidic urine and loss of water.
(c) Loop diuretics provide rapid relief of acute pulmonary oedema.
(d) Frusemide and polythiazide are equipotent diuretics.
(e) The diuretic effect of the diuretics correlates with their antihypertensive effect.

30. Cardiac β-adrenoceptors:

(a) Are linked by G-proteins to cause the stimulation of phospholipase C.
(b) Are of the β_1 subtype.
(c) Are present only in the sinoatrial node.
(d) Are activated by cardiac glycosides.
(e) Can be activated by adrenaline released from sympathetic nerve terminals in the heart.

31. Regarding drugs acting at α-adrenoceptors:

(a) Prazocin is a selective α_1-adrenoceptor agonist.
(b) Oxymetazoline is an agonist used as a nasal decongestant.
(c) Yohimbine is is a selective α_2-adrenoceptor antagonist used in the treatment of hypotension.
(d) Phenylephrine is a selective α_1-adrenoceptor agonist used in the treatment of hypotension.
(e) Clonidine is a selective α_1-adrenoceptor agonist used in the treatment of hypertension.

32. Heparin is:

(a) Administered orally.
(b) Contraindicated in haemophilia.
(c) Counteracted by the administration of protamine sulphate.
(d) Contraindicated in deep vein thrombosis.
(e) Rapid in onset of action.

33. Which of the following statements are true?

(a) Thyroid peroxidase catalyses the conversion of iodide to iodine and the formation of thyroxine.
(b) The thionamides stimulate thyroid peroxidase.
(c) High doses of iodine paradoxically inhibit thyroid function and are used in thyrotoxic crisis.
(d) Propranolol is used in the treatment of hypothyroidism.
(e) Liothyronine has an onset of action that is faster than thyroxine.

34. The combined oral contraceptive pill:

(a) Commonly increases menstrual blood loss.
(b) Is taken for 21 days with a 7-day break to induce a withdrawal bleed.
(c) Is the most reliable reversible method of contraception.
(d) May protect against thrombosis.
(e) May protect against ovarian and uterine cancer.

35. Vasoconstrictor drugs can act by:

(a) Activating α-adrenoceptors on the plasma membrane of vascular smooth muscle cells.
(b) Mimicking the effect of endogenous bradykinin.
(c) Mimicking the vasoconstrictor effect of vasopressin.
(d) Activating phospholipase C.
(e) Inhibiting the release of acetylcholine from perivascular parasympathetic nerve terminals.

217

36. In relation to competitive antagonists:

(a) They shift the agonist dose–response curve in a parallel manner to the right.
(b) The pA_2 is defined as the dose of antagonist required to halve the agonist response.
(c) The maximum response of the agonist dose–response curve is depressed.
(d) The affinity of yohimbine differs between α-receptor subtypes.
(e) Antagonist affinity can be quantified in terms of the dose ratio.

37. Local anaesthetics act by:

(a) Selectively blocking nociceptive fibres.
(b) Blocking calcium channels.
(c) Blocking potassium channels.
(d) Blocking sodium channels.
(e) Interfering with synaptic transmission.

38. In the treatment of classical angina:

(a) It is essential to increase coronary blood flow.
(b) Organic nitrates provide rapid relief.
(c) Glyceryl trinitrate works by elevating myocardial inositol triphosphate levels.
(d) Isoprenaline is beneficial because of its myocardial stimulant properties.
(e) Rapidly acting analgesics are the mainstay of therapy.

39. Ganglionic transmission:

(a) Is blocked by pancuronium.
(b) Is potentiated by pyridostigmine.
(c) Is blocked by α-bungarotoxin.
(d) Requires extracellular calcium.
(e) Is potentiated by hexamethonium.

40. The following are intracellular messengers:

(a) Cyclic adenosine monophosphate.
(b) Inositol tetraphosphate.
(c) Cyclic guanosine monophosphate.
(d) Cyclic uridine monophosphate.
(e) Diacylglycerol.

41. Acetylcholinesterase inhibitors:

(a) Can be used to assist the reversal of suxamethonium-induced neuromuscular block.
(b) Can be used as pesticides.
(c) Are used to reduce intraocular pressure in the treatment of glaucoma.
(d) Can be used as nerve gases.
(e) Are sometimes used in conjunction with muscarinic antagonists.

42. Vitamin K antagonists are useful anticoagulants:

(a) Because they can be given orally.
(b) Because they have a rapid onset of action.
(c) In the treatment of cerebral thrombosis.
(d) In the treatment of deep vein thrombosis.
(e) As emergency treatment.

43. Phase I drug oxidation:

(a) Is mediated by the hepatic mitochondrial electron transport system.
(b) Is the most common phase I reaction.
(c) Is restricted to the liver.
(d) Terminates all drug action.
(e) Prepares drugs for phase II conjugation.

44. The following drugs are used in the treatment of hypertension:

(a) Captopril.
(b) Hydralazine.
(c) Prazocin.
(d) Milrinone.
(e) Propranolol.

45. The following are true statements:

(a) The neurotransmitter at autonomic ganglia is noradrenaline.
(b) The receptors in parasympathetic ganglia are of the nicotinic type.
(c) The neurotransmitter released from postganglionic parasympathetic nerves is acetylcholine.
(d) The postganglionic receptors of the parasympathetic nerves are of the nicotinic type.
(e) The adrenal medulla releases adrenaline, noradrenaline, and dopamine in response to stress.

46. In ocular pharmacology:

(a) Muscarinic antagonists cause mydriasis.
(b) Acetazolamide is indicated in the treatment of closed-angle glaucoma.
(c) Muscarinic agonists increase intraocular pressure.
(d) Timolol reduces intraocular pressure by blocking β_1-adrenoceptors.
(e) Edrophonium is an anticholinesterase used in the treatment of open-angle glaucoma.

47. Class Ia antiarrhythmics:

(a) Depress the fast sodium current by blocking inactivated voltage-dependent sodium channels.
(b) Depress conduction in the atrioventricular node.
(c) Prolong the refractory period.
(d) Prolong action potential duration.
(e) Are indicated in ventricular and supraventricular arrhythmias.

48. The following are associated with ganglion block:

(a) Paralysis of accommodation of the eye.
(b) Diarrhoea.
(c) Postural hypotension.
(d) Increased skin temperature.
(e) Sweating.

49. The following are correct combinations:

(a) Agonist/high efficacy/conformational change.
(b) pA_2/measure of agonist affinity/related to the dose ratio.
(c) Partial agonist/low efficacy/affinity.
(d) Competitive antagonist/parallel shift to the left of agonist dose–response curve/no efficacy.
(e) Antagonist/high efficacy/zero affinity.

50. Cardiac inotropic agents:

(a) Of the cardiac glycoside class act by enzyme inhibition.
(b) Of the β-adrenoceptor agonist class increase intracellular calcium.
(c) Of the cardiac glycoside class have a narrow therapeutic window.
(d) Of the cardiac glycoside class act by increasing activating adenylyl cyclase.
(e) Of the cardiac glycoside class increase intracellular calcium.

Short-answer Questions

1. Discuss the use of premedication in anaesthesia.

2. Discuss the therapy of hay fever.

3. Describe the classes of drugs used in the treatment of peptic ulcers.

4. What are the main classes of drug used to treat fungal diseases and what are their mechanisms of action?

5. Which drugs exert their action by modifying γ-amino-butyric acid (GABA) synaptic transmission, and when are they used clinically?

6. Explain the analgesic effect of opioids.

7. How are intestinal worm infestations treated?

8. Explain the concept of selective toxicity with reference to cytotoxic drugs used in the treatment of cancer.

9. Discuss the different classes of drug used as laxatives.

10. Describe the neurochemical imbalance found in the brains of people suffering from Parkinson's disease, and list the classes of drug used to correct this imbalance.

11. Compare and contrast suxamethonium and atracurium.

12. Explain first-pass metabolism.

13. Desribe the therapeutic uses of vasoconstrictors.

14. Explain the differences between lignocaine and amiodarone in their use as antiarrhythmics.

15. Compare and contrast competitive and non-competitive antagonists.

16. Explain the effects and clinical use of warfarin.

17. Explain how local anaesthetics inhibit nerve conduction.

18. Give an outline of the drug treatment of diabetes mellitus.

19. Explain the clinical use of anticholinesterases and how this is influenced by their duration of action.

20. Explain the role of cAMP as an intracellular messenger in the cardiovascular system.

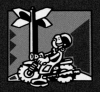

Essay Questions

1. Describe, using examples, how drugs can act presynaptically and postsynaptically to alter transmission at the sympathetic neuroeffector junction.

2. Describe the drugs used in the treatment of congestive heart failure, outlining their mechanism of action, route of administration, and the reasons for their use.

3. Explain how a drug molecule or transmitter can interact with a receptor to induce intracellular events involving second messengers.

4. Describe the site and mechanism of action and the pharmacological properties of the loop diuretics and the thiazides. How are these used clinically?

5. Give an account of the drugs used in the prevention and treatment of thrombosis, indicating their mechanism of action and the clinical circumstances of their use.

6. What are the main classes of drugs used to treat reversible airways obstruction in the respiratory system? Outline their overall pharmacology, their uses, and side effects?

7. Do the drugs used in the treatment of Parkinson's disease reflect the underlying defects in the brain? What side effects may be encountered in the use of these drugs?

8. What is the mechanism of action of antipsychotic drugs, and what are the side effects associated with their use?

9. Discuss the classification and possible mechanisms of action of the antidepressant drugs. Does this information reveal anything about the primary neurochemical defect, in the brain, of endogenous depression?

10. Outline the special features of the viral life cycle and how drugs have been developed to target viral diseases by acting at different points of this cycle.

Remember, the use of diagrams is strongly encouraged!

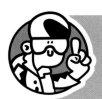

You should spend an hour on each question.

221

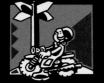

MCQ Answers

1. (a) T, (b) F, (c) T, (d) F, (e) F
2. (a) T, (b) F, (c) T, (d) F, (e) F
3. (a) T, (b) F, (c) F, (d) T, (e) F
4. (a) F, (b) T, (c) F, (d) F, (e) T
5. (a) F, (b) T, (c) F, (d) T, (e) T
6. (a) F, (b) T, (c) F, (d) F, (e) T
7. (a) T, (b) T, (c) T, (d) F, (e) F
8. (a) T, (b) T, (c) T, (d) T, (e) T
9. (a) F, (b) T, (c) T, (d) F, (e) T
10. (a) F, (b) T, (c) F, (d) F, (e) T
11. (a) F, (b) T, (c) F, (d) T, (e) F
12. (a) T, (b) F, (c) T, (d) F, (e) F
13. (a) T, (b) T, (c) T, (d) F, (e) F
14. (a) F, (b) T, (c) F, (d) T, (e) F
15. (a) T, (b) F, (c) T, (d) T, (e) T
16. (a) T, (b) F, (c) F, (d) T, (e) T
17. (a) T, (b) T, (c) F, (d) T, (e) T
18. (a) T, (b) T, (c) F, (d) F, (e) F
19. (a) F, (b) F, (c) T, (d) T, (e) T
20. (a) F, (b) F, (c) T, (d) F, (e) F
21. (a) F, (b) T, (c) T, (d) F, (e) F
22. (a) T, (b) T, (c) F, (d) T, (e) T
23. (a) T, (b) T, (c) F, (d) F, (e) T
24. (a) T, (b) F, (c) F, (d) F, (e) T
25. (a) T, (b) F, (c) T, (d) T, (e) F

26. (a) F, (b) T, (c) T, (d) F, (e) F
27. (a) F, (b) F, (c) T, (d) F, (e) F
28. (a) F, (b) T, (c) F, (d) F, (e) T
29. (a) T, (b) F, (c) T, (d) F, (e) F
30. (a) F, (b) T, (c) F, (d) F, (e) T
31. (a) F, (b) T, (c) F, (d) T, (e) F
32. (a) F, (b) T, (c) T, (d) F, (e) T
33. (a) T, (b) F, (c) T, (d) F, (e) T
34. (a) F, (b) T, (c) T, (d) F, (e) T
35. (a) T, (b) F, (c) T, (d) T, (e) F
36. (a) T, (b) T, (c) F, (d) T, (e) F
37. (a) T, (b) F, (c) F, (d) T, (e) F
38. (a) T, (b) T, (c) F, (d) F, (e) F
39. (a) F, (b) F, (c) F, (d) T, (e) F
40. (a) T, (b) F, (c) T, (d) F, (e) T
41. (a) F, (b) T, (c) T, (d) T, (e) T
42. (a) T, (b) F, (c) F, (d) T, (e) F
43. (a) T, (b) T, (c) T, (d) F, (e) F
44. (a) T, (b) T, (c) T, (d) F, (e) F
45. (a) F, (b) T, (c) T, (d) F, (e) T
46. (a) T, (b) F, (c) F, (d) F, (e) F
47. (a) F, (b) T, (c) T, (d) T, (e) T
48. (a) F, (b) F, (c) T, (d) T, (e) F
49. (a) T, (b) F, (c) T, (d) F, (e) F
50. (a) F, (b) T, (c) T, (d) F, (e) T

1. Premedication is given before the patient is taken to the operating theatre, and has four component aims. A selection of drugs are used as no one compound has all the desired effects:
   (a) Benzodiazepines (give two examples) are used to relieve apprehension and anxiety before anaesthesia, to reduce the amount of anaesthetic required to induce unconsciousness, and, possibly, to sedate postoperatively.
   (b) Muscarinic antagonists (give two examples) are used to prevent salivation and bronchial secretions, and more importantly to protect the heart from arrhythmias, particularly bradycardia caused by some inhalation agents and neuromuscular blockers.
   (c) Opioid analgesics (give an example) are often given before an operation as, although the patient is unconscious during surgery, adequate analgesia is important to stop physiological stress reactions to pain.
   (d) Antiemetic drugs (give an example) can be given to inhibit postoperative emesis. Nausea and vomiting are common after general anaesthesia, often owing to the administration of opioid drugs.

2. Hay fever (seasonal allergic rhinitis) is caused by a type I hypersensivity reaction to pollen and is characterized by features such as a streaming nose, inflamed eyes, etc.

   Precipitating factors (allergens) should be avoided, but symptomatic relief is often necessary. Antihistamines (H_1 histamine receptor antagonists) are the mainstay of treatment, the initial choice being governed by the degree of sedation required. Older drugs (e.g. chlopheniramine, trimeprazine) that cross the blood–brain barrier are much more sedative than the newer drugs that don't (e.g. astemizole, terfenadine).

   Other drugs that can be of use are topical nasal formulations of corticosteroids (beclamethasone) and nasal or eye drop preparations of sodium cromoglycate, but these must be used prophylactically. An anticholinergic spray (e.g. ipratopium) can be used for persistent rhinorrhoea.

3. Drugs that are effective in the treatment of peptic ulcers can be classified as follows:
   - Acid secretion inhibitors such as Proton pump inhibitors (e.g. omeprazole) irreversibly inhibit the H^+/K^+ ATPase that is responsible for H^+ secretion from parietal cells. Histamine H_2-receptor antagonists (e.g. cimetidine) competitively block the action of histamine on parietal cell H_2-receptors. Muscarinic antagonists (e.g. pirenzipine) reduce gastric acid and pepsin secretion by blocking muscarinic M_1-receptors in the enteric nervous system and M_3-receptors on the parietal cell.
   - Mucosal strengtheners such as sucralfate and bismuth chelate polymerize below pH 4 to a gel substance that adheres to and protects ulcer craters. Bismuth chelate has an additional weak antibacterial effect on *Helicobacter pylori*. Misoprostol is a synthetic analogue of prostaglandin E that imitates the action of endogenous prostaglandins (PGE_2 and PGI_2) in maintaining the integrity of the gastroduodenal mucosal barrier.
   - Antacids such as aluminium hydroxide and sodium bicarbonate are alkaline salts that are used to raise the luminal pH of the stomach.
   - *H. pylori* eradication regimes under evaluation include: 'classic' triple therapy (bismuth, metronidazole, and tetracycline) and dual therapy (omeprazole and amoxycillin or clarithromycin).

4. The main classes of drug used to treat fungal infections (mycoses) are the polyene macroglides, the imidazoles, and the triadazoles.
   - Polyene macroglides (amphotericin B, nystatin) bind to ergosterol in the fungal cell membrane, forming pores through which the cell constituents are lost. This causes fatal damage.
   - Imidazoles and triadazoles (clotrimazole, fluconazole) inhibit fungal lipid (especially ergosterol) synthesis in cell membranes and also interfere with fungal oxidative enzymes.

   Additionally, three other drugs are increasingly being used:
   - Allylamines (terbinafine) prevents ergosterol synthesis by inhibiting the enzyme squalene oxidase, resulting in squalene accumulation, which leads to membrane disruption and cell death.
   - Flucytosine, which is imported into fungal (but not human) cells, where it is converted into 5-fluorouracil, a potent inhibitor of DNA synthesis.
   - Griseofulvin, the mechanism of action of which is not fully established, but it probably interferes with microtubule formation or nucleic acid synthesis and polymerization.

5. Refer to Fig. 1

6. Opioid analgesic drugs, whether naturally occurring like morphine or chemically synthesized, possess agonist action at opioid receptors. μ-Receptors are thought to be responsible for most of the analgesic effects of opioids, though δ-receptors and κ-receptors are probably important in the periphery and at the spinal level, respectively, and may also contribute to analgesia.

   Opioids act on these opioid receptors and affect the transmission of pain information from the periphery via the dorsal horn of the spinal cord to higher brain centres.

   Opioid drugs affect the activity of the dorsal horn relay neurons by several inhibitory inputs. This constitutes the 'gate-control mechanism':
   • Opioid receptor agonism (inhibitory) on the dorsal horn relay neurons themselves.
   • Activation of descending inhibitory noradrenergic fibres from the locus ceruleus area of the brainstem.
   • Activation of descending inhibitory serotonergic fibres from the nucleus raphe magnus and periaqueductal grey areas of the brainstem.
   The combined effect of this is to reduce the activity of the dorsal horn relay neurons, 'shutting the gate', and causing analgesia. Note that the sense of euphoria produced by strong opioids undoubtedly contributes to their analgesic activity by helping to reduce the anxiety and emotive components associated with pain.

7. To be effective, an anthelmintic drug must be able to penetrate the cuticle of the worm, or gain access to its alimentary tract, so that it may exert its pharmacological effect on the physiology of the worm.

   Anthelmintic drugs act on intestinal parasitic worms by a number of mechanisms:
   • Damaging or killing the worm directly.
   • Paralysing the worm, leading to its expulsion by gastrointestinal peristalsis.
   • Damaging the cuticle of the worm so that host defences such as digestion and immune rejection can affect the worm.
   • Interfering with worm metabolism.
   Refer to Fig. 2.

8. Selectively toxic cytotoxic cancer chemotherapy is the use of chemicals or drugs (both natural and synthetic) in an attempt to kill malignant cancer cells preferentially while aiming to cause the minimum of damage to normal host cells. The problem that exists with selective toxicity in the chemotherapy of cancers is that whereas in, e.g., antibacterial chemotherapy, where the target (prokaryote) is of a very different cell type to host (eukaryote), cancer cells are very similar in most ways to normal host cells. This makes identification of targets for selective chemotherapy very difficult.

   Cytotoxic drugs are therefore not specifically toxic to cancer cells; the selectivity they show is marginal at best, and they affect all rapidly dividing tissues (both normal and malignant) and thus have a number of general toxic effects: myelosuppression, inhibition of mucosal cell division, alopecia, sterility, etc. Relative selectivity (a higher proportional kill of cancer cells) can be achieved with some cancers because:
   • In the malignant tumours, more cells are undergoing proliferation than in normal proliferating tissues.
   • Normal cells seem to recover from chemotherapeutic inhibition faster than some cancer cells.
   • Synchronized cell cycling may leave discrete periods of vulnerability to cytotoxic drugs.

9. Laxatives are drugs used to increase the motility of the gut and encourage defecation. They are used to relieve constipation (an infrequent or difficult passage of stool) and to clear the gastrointestinal tract before medical or

Classes of drug that act by modifying γ- aminobutyric acid (GABA) synaptic transmission		
Drug class & examples	**Mechanism of action**	**Clinical uses**
Benzodiazepines *e.g. clonazepam temazepam lorazepan*	occupation of the benzodiazepine site on the GABA/Cl⁻ channel complex by benzodiazepine receptor agonists enhances the actions of GABA on the Cl⁻ conductance of the neuronal membrane (increase frequency of opening)	sleep disorders anxiety disorders premedication status epilepticus alcohol withdrawal
Barbiturates *e.g. thiopentone phenobarbitone*	occupation of the barbiturate site on the GABA/Cl⁻ channel complex enhances the actions of GABA on the Cl⁻ conductance of the neuronal membrane (increase duration of opening)	anaesthetic induction epilepsy
Anticonvulsants *e.g. vigabatrin valproate?*	irreversible inhibition of GABAγ, increasing brain GABA levels and central GABA release	epilepsy

Fig. 1 Classes of drug that act by modifying γ-aminobutyric acid (GABA) synaptic transmission.

surgical procedures.

Four main classes of laxative are used:

(a) Bulk laxatives (bran, methylcellulose), which increase the volume of non-absorbable solid residue, distending the colon and stimulating peristaltic activity.

(b) Osmotic laxatives (lactulose, saline purgatives—magnesium sulphate, sodium acid phosphate), which are poorly absorbed compounds that increase the water content of the bowel by osmosis.

(c) Stimulant laxatives (castor oil, senna, cascara, bisacodyl, sodium picosulphate), which increase gastro-intestinal peristalsis by stimulating the mucosa of the gut (probably by irritating local reflexes), the signal arising in the mucosa and being transmitted through the intramural plexi to the smooth muscle of the intestine.

(d) Faecal softeners (liquid paraffin, dioctyl sodium sulphosuccinate), which promote defecation by softening (e.g. dioctyl sodium sulphosuccinate) and/or lubricating (e.g. liquid paraffin) the faeces to aid their passage through the gastrointestinal tract.

10. The main pathology in Parkinson's disease is a progressive degeneration of the dopaminergic neurons of the substantia nigra, which project in the nigrostriatal pathway to the corpus striatum (analysis of post-mortem brains of parkinsonian patients shows a substantially reduced concentration of dopamine (less than 10% of normal) in the basal ganglia).

In Parkinson's disease, the inhibitory dopaminergic activity of the nigrostriatal pathway is therefore considerably reduced (20–40%). This results in cholinergic neuron hyperactivity from the corpus striatum, which contributes to the pathological features of parkinsonism. Usually, the activity of this cholinergic neuronal pathway is restrained by inhibition from the dopaminergic pathway that projects from the substantia nigra.

The treatment of parkinsonism is based on correcting the imbalance at the basal ganglia between the dopaminergic and cholinergic systems. Two major groups of drugs are used:

1. Drugs that increase dopaminergic activity between the substantia nigra and the corpus striatum. These are:
   - Dopamine precursors.
   - Dopamine agonists.
   - Drugs stimulating the release of dopamine.
   - Monoamine oxidase B (MAO_B) inhibitors.
2. Drugs that inhibit striatal cholinergic activity. These are:
   - Anticholinergic drugs.

11. Refer to Fig. 3.

12. Orally administered drugs, which are usually absorbed in the small intestine, reach the liver via the portal circulation. At this stage, or within the small intestine, they may be extensively metabolized, which is known as first-pass metabolism, and means that considerably less drug reaches the systemic circulation than enters the portal vein. This causes problems because it means that higher doses of drug must be given and, owing to individual variation in the degree of first-pass metabolism, the effects of the drug can be unpredictable. Drugs that are subject to a high degree of first-pass metabolism, such as the local anaesthetic lignocaine, cannot be given orally and must be administered by some other route.

13. Vasoconstrictors are used in the treatment of shock (a state of circulatory collapse, characterized by an arterial blood pressure unable to maintain adequate tissue perfusion) and hypotension.
   - Sympathomimetic amines, including adrenaline, noradrenaline, phenylephrine, and ephedrine, can be administered intravenously. These activate α-receptors, stimulating phospholipase C and causing vasoconstriction and a consequent increase in arterial blood pressure. However, these raise blood pressure at the expense of vital organs such as the kidneys,

Main drugs used in treatment of intestinal helminth infestations		
Drug	**Use**	**Mechanism of action**
Niclosamide	tapeworm infestations	blocks glucose uptake, irreversibly damaging the scolex, leading to release and expulsion of the tapeworm
Nyrantel	intestinal nematode infestations	a depolarising neuromuscularblocker that causes a spastic paralysis allowing worm expulsion from the gastrointestinal tract
Piperazine	roundworm and pinworm infestations	a reversible neuromuscular blocker that causes a flaccid paralysis in the worm leading to its expulsion by gastrointestinal peristalsis
Benzimadaz-oles	many nematode infestations	bind with high affinity to a site on tubulin dimers thus preventing the polymerisation of microtubules leading to depolymerisation of microtubules

Fig. 2 Main drugs used in the treatment of intestinal helminth infestations.

Fig. 3 A comparison of atracurium and suxamethonium.

	Atracurium	Suxamethonium
Block	non-depolarising/ competitive	depolarising/ non-competive
Tetanic fade	present	absent unless repeatedly or continuously administered
Initial spasms	absent	present
Effect of anticholinesterase	block reversed	block enhanced unless repeatedly or continuously administered
Effect of competive antagonist	block enhanced	block reduced
Effect of depolarising agents	block reversed	block enhanced
Route of administration	quaternary ammonium compounds are poorly absorbed orally and must be admisistered by intravenous injection	quaternary ammonium compounds are poorly absorbed orally and must be administered by intravenous injection
Rate of onset	fast	very fast
Duration	40 minutes	4 minutes
Myasthenia gravis patients	block enhanced	block reduced
Side effects	minimal histamine release tachycardia	postopertive muscle pain bradycardia K+ release
Clinical use	neuromuscular blockers for surgery	neuromuscular blockers for surgery

and raise peripheral resistance, which is already high in patients with shock.

- Dobutamine and dopamine given by intravenous infusion are a more appropriate form of treating shock than α-adrenoceptor agonists, as renal perfusion is not impaired. Dopamine is a precursor of noradrenaline and activates dopamine receptors and α- and β-adrenoceptors.

- Vasopressin, desmopressin, and felypressin are antidiuretic peptides. They activate V_1 receptors on smooth muscle cells, stimulating phospholipase C and causing vasoconstriction.

14. Refer to Fig. 4.

15. Refer to Fig. 5.

16. Warfarin is the most commonly used oral anticoagulant. It is a vitamin K antagonist. Vitamin K is needed for the post-transcriptional γ-carboxylation of glutamic acid residues of prothrombin and clotting factors VII, IX, and X by the liver. Warfarin works by blocking the reduction of vitamin K epoxide, a step necessary for its action as a co-factor. It is indicated in the prophylaxis and treatment of deep vein thrombosis and pulmonary embolism, in the prophylaxis of embolization in atrial fibrillation, in patients with prosthetic heart valves, and in rheumatic heart disease.

Warfarin is well absorbed and can therefore be given orally. The onset of action of these drugs takes several hours, owing to the time needed for the degradation of factors that have already been carboxylated. ($t_{1/2}$: VII = 6 hours, IX = 24 hours, X = 40 hours, II = 60 hours).

Haemorrhage is the main adverse effect and can be treated by administering vitamin K.

17. Local anaesthetics are drugs used to inhibit pain by reversibly blocking nerve conduction.

Small nerve fibres are preferentially blocked, owing to the high surface-area to volume ratio. This results in a differential block whereby the small nocioceptive (pain) and autonomic fibres are blocked but not the larger fibres responsible for the mediation of movement and touch.

	Lignocaine	Amiodarone
Class	1b	111
Mechanism of action	blocks voltage-dependent Na+ channels in their refractory (inactivated) state	K+ channel blocker which also blocks Na+ and Ca2+ channels, i.e. slows phase 0 and 3, and blocks α and β adrenoceptors
Effect on action potential duration	decreased	increased
Effect on effective refractory period	increased	increased
Effect on atrioventricular conduction	no effect	decreased
Route of administration	intravenously	oral and intravenous
Indications	ventricular arrhythmias following myocardial infarction	ventricular and supraventricular arrhythmias in patients resistant to other drugs
Adverse effects	hypotension bradycardia respiratory depression	thyroid dysfunction liver damage pulmonary disorders photosensitivity neuropathy

Fig. 4 A comparison of lignocaine and amiodarone.

	Competitive antagonists	Non-competitive antagonists
Example	isoprenaline	nifedipine
Binding to receptor	reversible	irreversible
Effect on receptors	dilution	effectively remove receptors from the system
Effect on dose-response curve	parallel shift to the right	parallel shift to the right
Effect on maximum response of the agonist dose-response curve	not depressed - reflects the fact that the block is surmountable by the addition of greater doses of agonist	depressed, reflecting the fact that the antagonist's effect cannot be overcome by the addition of greater doses of agonist
Other notes	making the assumption that the competive antagonist is acting in a totally reversible manner, then the pA_2 is equal to the negative logarithm of the Kd for the antagonist	at low concentrations, a parallel shift may occur without a reduced maximum response; since irreversible antagonists effectively remove receptors from the system, this reflects the fact that there must be a number of spare receptors

Fig. 5 A comparison of competitive and non-competitive antagonists.

Local anaesthetics are weak bases (pK_a = 8–9). Only the uncharged form can penetrate lipid membranes; thus, quaternary ammonium compounds, which are fully protonated, must be injected into the nerve axon if they are to work.

The majority of local anaesthetics block by two routes—hydrophobic and hydrophilic. The hydrophobic route involves the uncharged form entering the membrane and blocking the channel from a site in the protein membrane interface. The hydrophilic route involves the uncharged form crossing the membrane to the inside where the charged form blocks the channel. This latter pathway depends on the channel being open and therefore this type of block is use dependent. Use dependency is especially important in the antiarrhythmic action of local anaesthetics.

Nerve block occurs when the number of non-inactivated channels is insufficient in order to bring about depolarization to threshold.

Examples of local anaesthetics include cocaine, procaine, lignocaine, and prilocaine, which vary in their rate of onset, duration, tissue penetration, chemistry, and clinical use.

18. Insulin preparations aim to mimic basal levels of insulin, and meal-induced increases in insulin. They are indicated in insulin-dependent diabetes mellitus. The insulin may be from human, porcine, or bovine sources. The preparations are available as short-, medium- and long-acting agents. The short-acting preparations consist of soluble insulin with zinc to maintain solubility, and most resemble endogenous insulin. The intermediate-acting preparations are not as soluble, owing to the presence of a buffer such as large insulin crystals or the addition of protamine; examples include semilente, lente, isophane insulin, and biphasic fixed mixtures. The long-acting preparations such as ultralente consist of insulin zinc crystals. Insulin must always be given parenterally, as it is a peptide and thus destroyed in the gastrointestinal tract. Short-acting insulin is given intravenously in emergencies, but administration of the insulin preparations in maintenance treatment is usually subcutaneous.

The sulphonylureas are given orally and include tolbutamide, chlorpropamide, and glibenclamide. They block the ATP-dependent potassium channels in the membrane of the pancreatic β-cells, causing depolarization, calcium influx, and insulin release. They are indicated in non-insulin dependent diabetes mellitus, in patients with some β-cell activity

The biguanides include metformin. They are administered orally and are indicated in non-insulin dependent diabetes mellitus. They increase the peripheral utilization of glucose and decrease gluconeogenesis, but require the presence of endogenous insulin; thus, patients must have some functioning β-cells.

19. Anticholinesterases inhibit acetylcholinesterase and thus increase the amount of acetylcholine in the synaptic cleft, and enhance cholinergic transmission.

Short-acting anticholinesterases include edrophonium, which is selective for the neuromuscular junction (NMJ) and clinically relevant in the diagnosis of myasthenia gravis. Its duration of action is only 2–10 minutes; it is therefore not used therapeutically.

Intermediate-acting anticholinesterases include neostigmine, which is used intravenously to reverse the effects of non-depolarizing blockers. It has a duration of 2–4 h and is used orally in the treatment of myasthenia gravis. Although neostigmine shows some selectivity for the NMJ, atropine is sometimes co-administered to block the muscarinic effects of the drug. Pyridostigmine has few parasympathetic actions, lasts for 3–6 h, and is also used orally in myasthenia gravis. Physostigmine shows selectivity for the postganglionic parasympathetic junction. It is a tertiary amine and its use is therefore associated with central effects such as initial excitation followed by depression and possible respiratory depression and unconsciousness. The central effects can be antagonized by atropine. It is used in the form of eye drops to constrict the pupil and contract the ciliary muscle in the treatment of glaucoma.

Most long-lasting or irreversible anticholinesterases are organophosphorous compounds. Sarin and tabun were developed as nerve gases, and parathion was developed as an insecticide as well as for clinical use. These have many adverse effects, such as bradycardia, hypotension, respiratory problems, depolarizing neuromuscular block, central effects, and possible death from peripheral nerve demyelination. Ecothiopate shows selectivity for the postganglionic parasympathetic junction and is used in the treatment of glaucoma.

20. The sympathetic system mediates its effects on the cardiovascular system through activation of β_1-receptors. These are linked to adenylyl cyclase, an enzyme that catalyses the conversion of ATP to cAMP within the myocardial cells. The cAMP produced causes activation of cAMP-dependent protein kinase A, which phosphorylates serine and threonine residues of voltage-operated calcium channels resulting in their opening. There is a subsequent elevation in intracellular calcium levels, resulting in an increased rate and force of contraction of the heart.

β_1-Adrenoceptor antagonists prevent the activation of adenylyl cyclase and the subsequent rise in cAMP and thus calcium. These are used in the treatment of heart failure and arrhythmias.

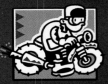

Index

Readers are advised to refer to both the individual drugs and their respective drug groups. Cross-references have not been inserted. Drug names are in **bold**.

DNA-linked receptors, 7
DNA synthesis, cytotoxic drug action, 181
dobutamine, 35, 97
domperidone, 40, 128–9
[SC]L[sc]-dopa (levodopa), 17, 32, 40
dopa decarboxylase, 32, 40
dopamine/5-HT blockers, 54
dopamine
  agonists, 40–1
  antagonists, motility stimulant, 128–9
  degradation reduction, 42
  drugs stimulating release, 41
  precursors, 40
  reduced in Parkinson's disease, 39
  shock management, 97
  vasodilatation/vasoconstriction, 97
dopamine receptors, 40, 41, 97
  antipsychotic drugs blocking, 52, 53
  classes (location/function), 53
  D_2, 52, 53
  D_2 agonists, 41
  D_2 blockade, 53, 54, 55
dopaminergic pathways, 54, 55
  adverse effects of neuroleptics, 54–6
  drugs increasing activity, 40
  overactivity in schizophrenia, 40, 52
  reduced activity in Parkinson's disease, 39
dorsal horn, pain transmission, 68
dorzolamide, 158
dose ratio, 9
dose–response curves, 9
dosing schedule, 11
doxapram, 113
doxazocin, 94–5
doxorubicin, 184
doxycycline, 194–5
dracontiasis, 212
dromotropic, definition, 91
droperidol, 53
drug abuse, 72
  see also drug misuse
drug dependence, 72, 74
  benzodiazepines, 44
  opioid analgesics, 70, 71, 76
drug misuse, 72–8
  concepts, 72
  drugs associated, 74–7
  legal aspects, 72–4
drug resistance
  antibiotics, 190, 191, 193, 195
  antifungal drugs, 204, 205
  antimalarial drugs, 208
  chemotherapy, 181–3
drugs, 3
  absorption, 11–12, 13, 163
  adverse effects, 17–18
  affinity for receptors, 8
  competition between, 14
  compliance, 10–11
  controlled, 72, 73
  distribution, 12–13
  dosage forms, 11
  excretion, 14–15

half-life ($t_{1/2}$), 12, 15
  interactions, 12, 17, 177
  mechanisms of action, 3
  medicinal and non-medicinal (social), 3
  metabolism *see* metabolism of drugs
  names and classification, 3
  receptor interactions, 8–10
  route of administration, 11
  size of molecules, 12
drug tolerance, 72, 73, 74
  opioids, 70, 71, 76
duodenal ulcers, 123
dynorphins, 69
dysentery, amoebic, 209
dyskinesias, levodopa causing, 40
dysrhythmia, 87

E
EC_{50}, 10
ecothiopate, 30
Ecstasy, 75
eczema (dermatitis), 148, 160
edrophonium, 29
effective dose, 10
efficacy, 9
eicosanoids, 165–6
elderly, adverse effects of drugs, 18
electrolyte balance, in rehydration, 131
elimination rate constant (K_{el}), 15
emollients, 163
enalapril, 94
encainide, 89
'end of dose deterioration', 40, 41
endocrine systems, 135–48
endocrine therapy, 186
endometrial cancer, 152, 186
endorphins, 69
endothelium-derived relaxing factor (EDRF), 92
end-plate potential (EPP), 26
energy-dependent carriers (pumps), 3, 21
energy-independent carriers, 3
enflurane, 66
enkephalins, 69
enteral administration, drugs, 11
enteric nervous system, 128
enterohepatic circulation, 15, 98
enzymes, 3–4
  drug metabolism, 13, 14
  induction, 14, 17
ephedrine, 17, 33
  nasal decongestion, 174
  shock management, 97
epidural anaesthesia, 24
epigenetic carcinogens, 18
epilepsy, 57–61
epileptic syndromes, 57
ergometrine, 154
erythromycin, 190, 195
ethacrynic acid, 118
ethambutol, 196
ethamsylate, 107

ethanol (alcohol), 75–6
  benzodiazepine action increased, 44
  withdrawal syndrome, 76
ethinyloestradiol, 150, 151, 152
ethisterone, 152
ethmivan, 113
ethosuximide, 59
ethyloestrenol, 153
etomidate, 64
etoposide, 184–5
eukaryotic cells, 189
euphoria, 69, 70, 75, 76
excitatory amino acids, drugs inhibiting, 59
excretion, drugs, 14–15
EXP3174, 94
eyes, 155–9
  anatomy and physiology, 155–6

F
factor VII, 103
factor VIII, 104
factor IX, 104
faecal softeners, 131
f current, 81
felypressin, 97–8
female reproductive system, 148–50
fenemates, 168
fenoprofen, 167
fibrates, 100
fibrin, 103
fibrinogen, 103
fibrinolysis, 104
fibrinolytic drugs, 103, 106
fight-or-flight response, 37
filariasis, lymphatic, 212
filgrastim, 186
first-pass metabolism, 11, 13
flagellates, 207
flecainide, 89
flucloxacillin, 191
fluconazole, 205
flucytosine, 204, 205
fludrocortisone, 148
fluid, maintenance/replacement, 131
flumazenil, 44
5-fluorouracil, 183, 185, 205
fluoxetine, 49
fluoxymesterone, 153
flupenthixol, 53
fluphenazine, 53
flutamide, 186
fluticasone propionate, 174
folates, 192
folic acid antagonists, 185
follicle-stimulating hormone (FSH), 148, 149, 150
food allergies, 172
Frank–Starling curves, 85, 86
free fatty acids (FFAs), 98
frusemide, 118
fungal infections, 203
fungi, groups, 203
fusidic acid, 195

G

GABA, 43, 44
   agonists, 51, 59, 61
   antiepileptic mechanism of action, 59, 60
   benzodiazepine mechanism of action, 43, 44, 59
   degradation, drugs inhibiting, 59, 60
   in depression, 48
   drugs enhancing inhibitory action, 44, 59, 61, 63
   GABA$_A$ receptors, 4, 43, 44
   receptor structure, 43
GABA$_A$/Cl$^-$ channels, 43
   chloride current potentiation, 43, 44, 59, 61, 63
gabapentin, 59, 61
GABA transaminase, inhibition, 59, 60
gallamine, 28
gall stones, 133
gamma globulin (human normal immunoglobulin), 199–200
ganciclovir, 200
ganglia, autonomic, 30–1
ganglion-blocking drugs, 31
ganglion-stimulating drugs, 30–1
gastric acid, secretion, 124, 125
   drugs reducing, 124–6
gastric stasis, 128
gastric ulcers, 123
gastrin receptors, 124
gastrointestinal excretion, drugs, 15
gastrointestinal haemorrhage, 106
gastrointestinal tract, drugs in, 123–34
gastro-oesophageal reflux disease (GERD), 128, 129
'gate-control mechanism', pain, 68
'gating', ion channels, 3
gemeprost, 154
gemfibrozil, 100, 101
general anaesthesia, 62
   balanced technique, 62
   induction, 62, 64–5
   maintenance, 62
   neuromuscular blockers in, 67
general anaesthetics, 62–6
   inhalational, 63, 64–5, 64–6
   intravenous, 62–4
   mechanisms of action/theories, 64–5
   pharmacokinetics, 65
generic names, 3
gentamycin, 192, 194
giardiasis, 209
glaucoma, 118, 156–8, 159
   closed-angle, 156, 158
   open-angle, 156, 157, 158
   treatment, 29, 121, 156–8
glibenclamide, 141–2
glomerular capillaries, 14
glomerular filtration, 14, 116
glomerulus, 115
glucagon, 139
glucocorticoids, 142, 143, 144, 145

allergic disorders, 174
   anti-inflammatory actions, 112, 132–3, 145–6, 165, 168–9, 174
   asthma, 112
   as immunosuppressants, 177
   inflammatory bowel disease, 132–3
   specific drugs, 145, 147–8
   see also corticosteroids
glucose
   plasma, control, 139
   receptors, 139
glucose-6-phosphate dehydrogenase deficiency, 18
glutathione, 14
glycerol, in closed-angle glaucoma, 158
glyceryltrinitrate (GTN), 89–90
glycogen, 7
glycopeptides, 191–2
glycosuria, 140
goitre, 137
gold salts, 169
gonadotrophin-releasing hormone (GnRH), 148
   agonists/antagonists, 153–4, 186
gonadotrophin-surge-attenuating factor, 149
gossypol, 152
gout, drug therapy, 170–1
G-protein-linked receptors, 4, 5
   mechanism of action, 4–6
G-proteins, 4, 4–6
   adrenoceptor action via, 32
   a-subunits, 6, 7
   muscarinic receptor transduction via, 34
   subunits, 4–5
   targets, 6–7
graft rejection, prevention, 175, 176
graft-versus-host disease, 175, 176
granulocyte colony-stimulating factor (G-CSF), 186
granulocyte-macrophage colony-stimulating factor (GM-CSF), 187
Graves' disease (diffuse toxic goitre), 137
'grey baby syndrome', 195
griseofulvin, 204, 205–6
GTP, 5
guanethidine, 32, 157
guanylyl cyclase, 7, 89, 92, 95
guinea-worm infection, 212

H

H$^+$/K$^+$ ATPase, inhibition, 124
H$_2$ receptors see histamine H$_2$ receptors
haemophilia, 104
haemorrhage, 105
haemostasis, 102–7
   management of disorders, 104–7
   principles, 102–4
half-life (t$_{1/2}$), drugs, 12, 15
hallucinogens, 77
haloperidol, 53
halothane, 66
'hangover', 76
Hashimoto's thyroiditis, 136

hashish, 77
hay fever, 172, 173, 174
heart, 79–91
   abnormal impulse conduction, 84, 85
   action potential, 79, 80, 81
   anatomy and physiology, 79–85
   autonomic control, 81
   block, 84
   conducting system, 79, 80
   contractility, 82
   nodal/non-nodal cells, action potential, 80–1
   rate and rhythm, 79
   see also entries beginning cardiac
heart failure, 83
   drug treatment, 85–7, 91
   types/characteristics, 83
Helicobacter pylori, 123
   eradication, 126, 127
helminthic infections, 210, 211
hemicholinium, 27
Henderson–Hasselbalch equation, 12, 23
Henle, loop, 116, 117
heparin, 103, 105
hepatic necrosis, halothane causing, 66
hepatitis, viral, 199, 200, 201
hepatotoxicity, paracetamol, 168
heroin (diamorphine), 70, 76–7
herpes simplex virus, 200, 201
herpesviruses, 198
hexamethonium, 31
high density lipoprotein (HDL), 98, 100, 101
histamine, 27, 70, 124, 173
histamine H$_1$ receptors, 173
   antagonists (antihistamines), 46, 173
   blockade by neuroleptics, 56
histamine H$_2$ receptors, 124, 173
   antagonists, 124–5, 133
histamine H$_3$ receptors, 173
HIV infections, drug therapy, 201–2
HMG CoA reductase inhibitors, 98–100
Hodgkin's lymphoma, 185
hookworms, 211
hormone replacement therapy (HRT), 152
hormones, 4, 8
   adrenal, 142–3
   endocrine therapy, 186
   intestinal motility control, 128
   sex, 148
hydatid disease, 212
hydralazine, 18, 95
hydrate theory, anaesthesia, 64–5
hydrochloric acid, secretion see gastric acid
hydrochlorothiazide, 120
hydrocortisone (cortisol), 132–3, 143, 144, 147
   intravenous, 174
   skin disorders, 161
hydrogen ion

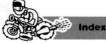

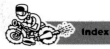

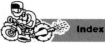